T0293725

Handbook of Clinical Medicine

Handbook of Clinical Medicine

Editor: Maxim Clement

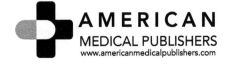

AMERICAN
MEDICAL PUBLISHERS
www.americanmedicalpublishers.com

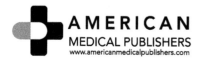

AMERICAN
MEDICAL PUBLISHERS
www.americanmedicalpublishers.com

Cataloging-in-Publication Data

Handbook of clinical medicine / edited by Maxim Clement.
    p. cm.
Includes bibliographical references and index.
ISBN 978-1-63927-679-0
1. Clinical medicine. 2. Medical care. 3. Medicine. I. Clement, Maxim.
RC48 .H36 2023
616--dc23

American Medical Publishers,
41 Flatbush Avenue,
1st Floor, New York,
NY 11217, USA

ISBN 978-1-63927-679-0 (Hardback)

Contents

Preface...VII

Chapter 1   **Specialized Staff for the Care of People with Parkinson's Disease in Germany**..1
Tino Prell, Frank Siebecker, Michael Lorrain, Lars Tönges, Tobias Warnecke, Jochen Klucken, Ingmar Wellach, Carsten Buhmann, Martin Wolz, Stefan Lorenzl, Heinz Herbst, Carsten Eggers and Tobias Mai

Chapter 2   **The Complex Balance between Analgesic Efficacy, Change of Dose and Safety Profile Over Time, in Cancer Patients Treated with Opioids: Providing the Clinicians with an Evaluation Tool**..13
Oscar Corli, Luca Porcu, Claudia Santucci and Cristina Bosetti

Chapter 3   **Efficacy and Safety of Ceftaroline for the Treatment of Community-Acquired Pneumonia**...23
Shao-Huan Lan, Shen-Peng Chang, Chih-Cheng Lai, Li-Chin Lu and Chien-Ming Chao

Chapter 4   **Patient Experience in Home Respiratory Therapies: Where we are and Where to Go**..34
Cátia Caneiras, Cristina Jácome, Sagrario Mayoralas-Alises, José Ramon Calvo, João Almeida Fonseca, Joan Escarrabill and João Carlos Winck

Chapter 5   **Comparison of Oncologic Outcomes in Laparoscopic versus Open Surgery for Non-Metastatic Colorectal Cancer: Personal Experience in a Single Institution**.............58
Chong-Chi Chiu, Wen-Li Lin, Hon-Yi Shi, Chien-Cheng Huang, Jyh-Jou Chen, Shih-Bin Su, Chih-Cheng Lai, Chien-Ming Chao, Chao-Jung Tsao, Shang-Hung Chen and Jhi-Joung Wang

Chapter 6   **Relationship between Morbidity and Health Behavior in Chronic Diseases**........................76
Munjae Lee, Sewon Park and Kyu-Sung Lee

Chapter 7   **Factors Associated with Health-Related Quality of Life in Community-Dwelling Older Adults: A Multinomial Logistic Analysis**...87
Encarnación Blanco-Reina, Jenifer Valdellós, Ricardo Ocaña-Riola, María Rosa García-Merino, Lorena Aguilar-Cano, Gabriel Ariza-Zafra and Inmaculada Bellido-Estévez

Chapter 8   **Epidemiology and Burden of Diabetic Foot Ulcer and Peripheral Arterial Disease in Korea**...99
Dong-il Chun, Sangyoung Kim, Jahyung Kim, Hyeon-Jong Yang, Jae Heon Kim, Jae-ho Cho, Young Yi, Woo Jong Kim and Sung Hun Won

Chapter 9   **The Optimal Range of Serum Uric Acid for Cardiometabolic Diseases: A 5-Year Japanese Cohort Study**............107
Masanari Kuwabara, Ichiro Hisatome, Koichiro Niwa, Petter Bjornstad,
Carlos A. Roncal-Jimenez, Ana Andres-Hernando, Mehmet Kanbay,
Richard J. Johnson and Miguel A. Lanaspa

Chapter 10   **Re-Evaluating the Protective Effect of Hemodialysis Catheter Locking Solutions in Hemodialysis Patients**............121
Chang-Hua Chen, Yu-Min Chen, Yu Yang, Yu-Jun Chang, Li-Jhen Lin and
Hua-Cheng Yen

Chapter 11   **The Efficacy and Safety of Eravacycline in the Treatment of Complicated Intra-Abdominal Infections**............139
Shao-Huan Lan, Shen-Peng Chang, Chih-Cheng Lai, Li-Chin Lu and
Chien-Ming Chao

Chapter 12   **Predictors of Discordance in the Assessment of Skeletal Muscle Mass between Computed Tomography and Bioimpedance Analysis**............148
Min Ho Jo, Tae Seop Lim, Mi Young Jeon, Hye Won Lee, Beom Kyung Kim,
Jun Yong Park, Do Young Kim, Sang Hoon Ahn, Kwang-Hyub Han and
Seung Up Kim

Chapter 13   **Evaluation of Transfer Learning with Deep Convolutional Neural Networks for Screening Osteoporosis in Dental Panoramic Radiographs**............162
Ki-Sun Lee, Seok-Ki Jung, Jae-Jun Ryu, Sang-Wan Shin and Jinwook Choi

Chapter 14   **A Scoping Review of the Efficacy of Virtual Reality and Exergaming on Patients of Musculoskeletal System Disorder**............175
Hui-Ting Lin, Yen-I Li, Wen-Pin Hu, Chun-Cheng Huang and Yi-Chun Du

Chapter 15   **Use of Secukinumab in a Cohort of Erythrodermic Psoriatic Patients**............192
Giovanni Damiani, Alessia Pacifico, Filomena Russo, Paolo Daniele Maria Pigatto,
Nicola Luigi Bragazzi, Claudio Bonifati, Aldo Morrone, Abdulla Watad and
Mohammad Adawi

Chapter 16   **The Efficacy and Safety of Doripenem in the Treatment of Acute Bacterial Infections**............201
Chih-Cheng Lai, I-Ling Cheng, Yu-Hung Chen and Hung-Jen Tang

Chapter 17   **Prospective Evaluation of Intensity of Symptoms, Therapeutic Procedures and Treatment in Palliative Care Patients in Nursing Homes**............211
Daniel Puente-Fernández, Concepción B. Roldán-López,
Concepción P. Campos-Calderón, Cesar Hueso-Montoro,
María P. García-Caro and Rafael Montoya-Juarez

Chapter 18   **Multidiscipline Stroke Post-Acute Care Transfer System: Propensity-Score-Based Comparison of Functional Status**............222
Chung-Yuan Wang, Hong-Hsi Hsien, Kuo-Wei Hung, Hsiu-Fen Lin,
Hung-Yi Chiou, Shu-Chuan Jennifer Yeh, Yu-Jo Yeh and Hon-Yi Shi

Permissions

List of Contributors

Index

Preface

Clinical medicine is a medical field that involves the study of technical medical subjects and a practical experience of medicine. It covers a comprehensive understanding of a patient's medical status through observations, diagnosis, as well as treatment and management of real-life patients. In the field of clinical medicine, a patient's clinical history is documented through a series of different examinations and investigations. It also involves gaining knowledge from different sources such as a theoretical study of books and taught-courses. This knowledge is then applied to gain a comprehensive understanding of the medical condition of a patient. The physical diagnosis of a patient makes use of diagnostic devices such as tongue depressor, thermometer and stethoscope. This book contains some path-breaking studies in the field of clinical medicine. It provides significant information of this discipline to help develop a good understanding of clinical medicine and related fields. With state-of-the-art inputs by acclaimed experts of this field, this book targets medical science students and professionals.

The information shared in this book is based on empirical researches made by veterans in this field of study. The elaborative information provided in this book will help the readers further their scope of knowledge leading to advancements in this field.

Finally, I would like to thank my fellow researchers who gave constructive feedback and my family members who supported me at every step of my research.

Editor

Specialized Staff for the Care of People with Parkinson's Disease in Germany

Tino Prell [1,2,*]🄳, Frank Siebecker [3], Michael Lorrain [4], Lars Tönges [5]🄳, Tobias Warnecke [6]🄳, Jochen Klucken [7,8,9], Ingmar Wellach [10,11], Carsten Buhmann [12]🄳, Martin Wolz [13], Stefan Lorenzl [14,15,16], Heinz Herbst [17]🄳, Carsten Eggers [18] and Tobias Mai [19]🄳

1   Department of Neurology, Jena University Hospital, 07740 Jena, Germany
2   Center for Healthy Ageing, Jena University Hospital, 07740 Jena, Germany
3   Praxis Neurologie, 48291 Telgte, Germany; fs@neurologie-telgte.de
4   Neuroärzte Gerresheim-Pempelfort, 40625 Düsseldorf, Germany; dr.lorrain@volggerconsult.de
5   Department of Neurology, St. Josef-Hospital, Ruhr-University Bochum, 44801 Bochum, Germany; lars.toenges@rub.de
6   Department of Neurology, University of Muenster, 48149 Münster, Germany; Tobias.Warnecke@ukmuenster.de
7   Department of Molecular Neurology, Universitätsklinikum Erlangen, Schwabachanlage 6, 91054 Erlangen Neurology, Ev. Amalie Sieveking Hospital, 22359 Hamburg, Germany; Jochen.Klucken@uk-erlangen.de
8   AG Digital Health Pathways, Fraunhofer Institute for Integrated Circuits, Am Wolfsmantel 33, 91058 Erlangen, Germany
9   Münster Medical Center Hamburg-Eppendorf, 20246 Hamburg, Germany
10 Department of Neurology, Ev. Amalie Sieveking Hospital, 22359 Hamburg, Germany; ingmar.wellach@immanuelalbertinen.de
11 Office for Neurology and Psychiatry Hamburg Walddörfer, 22359 Hamburg, Germany
12 Department of Neurology, University Medical Center Hamburg-Eppendorf, 20246 Hamburg, Germany; buhmann@uke.uni-hamburg.de
13 Department of Neurology, Elblandklinikum Meißen, 01662 Meißen, Germany; Martin.Wolz@elblandkliniken.de
14 Professorship for Palliative Care, Paracelsus Medical University, 5020 Salzburg, Austria; stefan.lorenzl@pmu.ac.at
15 Department of Palliative Medicine, Ludwig-Maximilians-University Munich, 81377 Munich, Germany
16 Department of Neurology, Klinikum Agatharied, 83734 Hausham, Germany
17 Neurozentrum Sophienstrasse, 70178 Stuttgart, Germany; heinz.herbst@t-online.de
18 Department of Neurology, University Hospital Marburg, 35037 Marburg, Germany; Carsten.Eggers@uk-gm.de
19 Department of Nursing, University Hospital Frankfurt, Goethe University, 60590 Frankfurt, Germany; tobias.mai@kgu.de
*   Correspondence: Tino.prell@med.uni-jena.de

Abstract: Access to specialized care is essential for people with Parkinson´s disease (PD). Given the growing number of people with PD and the lack of general practitioners and neurologists, particularly in rural areas in Germany, specialized PD staff (PDS), such as PD nurse specialists and Parkinson Assistants (PASS), will play an increasingly important role in the care of people with PD over the coming years. PDS have several tasks, such as having a role as an educator or adviser for other health professionals or an advocate for people with PD to represent and justify their needs. PD nurse specialists have been established for a long time in the Netherlands, England, the USA, and Scandinavia. In contrast, in Germany, distinct PDS models and projects have been established. However, these projects and models show substantial heterogeneity in terms of access requirements, education, theoretical and practical skills, principal workplace (inpatient vs. outpatient), and reimbursement. This review provides an overview of the existing forms and regional models for PDS in Germany. PDS reimbursement concepts must be established that will foster an implementation throughout Germany. Additionally, development of professional roles in nursing and more specialized care in Germany is needed.

Keywords: networks; multimodal complex treatment; day clinic; advanced care planning

1. Background

Parkinson's disease (PD) is a common neurodegenerative disorder characterized by motor symptoms such as tremor, rigidity, bradykinesia, and a plethora of nonmotor symptoms (NMS). The appearance and severity of motor symptoms and NMS vary throughout the disease course and contribute to different degrees of functional impairment and reduced quality of life [1]. Therefore, access to different levels of care is essential for the increasing number of people with PD [2]. An important factor here is specialized outpatient and inpatient medical care as well as the well-coordinated trans-sectoral transition from hospitalized inpatient to outpatient to homecare, and vice versa [3]. Patients with PD need continuous specialized outpatient care, which can be supplemented by more intensive inpatient treatment (such as PD multimodal complex treatment (PD-MCT), PD day clinic, telemedicine) if necessary [4–6]. Frequently, PD patients also must consult emergency care at local hospitals [7,8]. Reasons for hospital admission are PD-related symptoms [9] as well as infections, gastrointestinal disorders, falls, neuropsychiatric, and other health problems. In hospitals and wards without specialized neurological knowledge, there is an increased risk of discontinuation, inappropriate change of medication, or use of inappropriate or contraindicated drugs. Such can lead to the worsening of motor function, falls, and delirium or comorbidity with all its known secondary complications, especially in the elderly with PD. Such complications are often associated with a higher risk of long term care in nursing homes [10].

People with PD need specially structured and cooperative therapy, education, and care concepts both in the short and long run. Qualified PD-specific nonphysician staff (PDS), such as PD nurse specialists (PD nurse) and Parkinson Assistants (PASS), can play an important role. Among others, PDS can fulfill a role as an educator or adviser for other health professionals in hospitals and be an advocate for the people with PD to represent and justify their needs. Such is also relevant given the lack of general practitioners (GP) and neurologists in rural areas [11]. Experiences in other countries (e.g., the Netherlands, England) show that PD nurses can provide a large part of care and treatment [12–15]. Given the growing number of PD patients, it is difficult to provide comprehensive care solely through physicians and nurses alone. PD nurses and other PDS could engage in routine support and could spend more time on more complex cases [16]. Moreover, in Germany, the majority of PD nurses work in hospitals, so there is a lack of qualified specialists, especially in outpatient care and in nursing homes. However, the German S3 PD guideline recommends that every PD patient should have access to PD nurses [17]. Over the disease course, the caregiver burden is often high, and specialized staff in outpatient care should play a key role in addressing potential problems. This article provides an overview of the existing forms and regional models of PDS in Germany.

2. Field of Activities and Responsibilities

The expenditure of time needed to care for people with PD has increased enormously recently. Such is based on a higher complexity of revised clinical diagnostic criteria, new technical diagnostic methods, and individualized therapeutic care considering the growing known spectrum of PD symptoms defining different motor and nonmotor subtypes of PD [18]. Specialized, holistic, lifelong care of people with PD requires practices that focus on the disease-specific needs of the individual, their family members, and caregivers. However, the treatment should not only account for the individual course of the disease with its plethora of motor symptoms and NMS. The often far-reaching psychosocial problems must also be taken into consideration (e.g., coping with the diagnosis, fear of uncertainty about the individual course of the disease, changes in family structures, job and pension problems, need for care). Given the high prevalence of cognitive impairment and dementia in PD, these symptoms also need special attention. Patients, relatives and caregivers need advice how to cope with cognitive decline and what kind of therapies and strategies are available. The PDS can provide assistance and support for many aspects and challenges during the PD course. Such assistance can maintain and improve the quality of life for people with PD, provide support and education to patients and healthcare professionals, and support and provide a seamless service throughout the disease trajectory [19]. Especially the complex aspects of palliative care at the late stage of PD require a well-positioned interdisciplinary team of PD specialists.

Discontinued care and lack of self-management are frequently associated with improper handling of PD medication. Nonadherence to medication is a significant issue in PD. It results in frequent hospitalizations, reduced quality of life, and causes a financial burden for the health system [20–26]. There are various reasons why people do not or cannot follow the given recommendations and instructions for the prescribed treatment. PDS can improve knowledge about medication or identify reasons for nonadherence. In summary, PDS can [12–14,27–31]:

- Help to cope with PD, answer frequent and everyday questions and give advice where doctors lack the necessary time: Typical questions are for example "What do I have to pay attention to with the medication?", "Can I go on holiday?", or "Can I do sports?"
- Use assessments to identify and monitor symptoms, side effects, and family problems
- Advise on the motor and NMS and complications.
- Counsel relatives and monitor their burden
- Teach other health and social care professionals (e.g., for handling pumps or deep brain stimulation (DBS))
- Inform comprehensively about therapy options, self-help groups or socio-medical aspects, such as applying for care levels or certificates for severely disabled persons
- Help to improve adherence to medication
- Assist in the initiation and adjustment of continuous therapies or take over most of them independently
- Support in making the PD diagnosis (e.g., performing an L-dopa or apomorphine challenge test)
- Make referrals to other professionals such as speech and language therapists, occupational therapists, physiotherapists or social workers and support networking between different therapeutic players
- Assist in advanced care planning (ACP)

In the UK, distinct competency levels for PD nurses were defined, ranging from a registered competent nurse (Level 5 of the Career Framework for Health), experienced specialist nurse (Level 6), expert specialist nurse (Level 7) to consultant nurse (Level 8) [19]. In contrast, in Germany officially certified and reimbursed models for PD do not exist. Distinct models and projects show a relevant heterogeneity in terms of access requirements, education, theoretical and practical skills, and principal workplace (inpatient vs. outpatient). In the following, we present established PDS in the German healthcare system.

3. Parkinson's Disease Nurse Specialist (PD Nurse)

Specialized nurses for patients with PD (hereinafter, PD nurse) have been available for over 40 years in several countries, including England, the USA, and the Scandinavian countries. PD nurses are acknowledged and valued as part of the multi-professional PD team [30]. The work tasks for PD nurses as mentioned above vary between different workplaces. However, they can include case management tasks, care of patients with complex therapies such as pen/pump therapies and DBS, scoring and assessments, and clinical research tasks. The experience with this specialized nurse function has been consistently positive. It shows improved care for patients with PD, improved productivity and quality of clinical research, as well as improved job satisfaction of the participating employees [12,13,27,29]. For many patients, the PD nurse is the primary link to medical care as most PD specialist nurses have an open phone line [14].

The German Parkinson Society (DPG), the German Parkinson Association (dPV), the Competence Network Parkinson (KNP) and the Association of Parkinson Nurses and Assistants (VPNA e.V.) have developed an education curriculum representing the standard for PD nurses in Germany. The first training course started in 2007. Applicants should be qualified health and nursing professionals and have a minimum of two years of professional experience in acute neurological departments or PD hospitals (Table 1). Training comprises four days of theoretical training and two weeks of work shadowing, spread over a year. Knowledge of the disease and the treatment are crucial for the work of a PD nurse [28,31]. The duties of the PD nurse also includes practical tasks (e.g., examine and evaluate the patient's health and motor functions, collect blood samples, adjust the settings in DBS and pumps) [12]. They play a vital role in the new concept of Parkinson Day Clinics in Germany [32].

The most reported tasks of PD nurses in Germany are giving information and advice to people with PD and their next of kin in the context of medication and side effects, education and counseling to PD symptoms and specialized therapies (and education of other nursing staff) [13,29]. Additionally, nursing functions include screening and offering prevention, supporting patients and caregivers in psychosocial well-being, care coordination and case management, and palliative care and multidisciplinary collaboration. According to the European Qualification Framework, the more expanded international role of a PD nurse is on level 6 or 7 [13,19]. Most PD nurses have completed specialized modules as part of a master course. In Germany, the PD nurse course is based on level 5 of the German Qualification Framework. It is similar to the registered competent nurse at level 5 of the Career Framework for Health [19]. For example, a qualified training course for PD nurse comprises 30 to 40 credit points. The German qualification course is shorter, and there is no state certificate. Recognition as specialized training in Germany usually requires 720 h or more (e.g., a professional training in critical care). Such may explain the different PD nurse role expansion in Germany and international comparison. As in other countries, counseling and education, information on medication management, educational advertising on PD and training of other professionals are at the center of German PD nurses [29]. German PD nurses also stated that they have not enough time for appropriate care and nursing, just like PD nurses have mentioned in the UK (16). PD nurses have a more extensive caseload than the suggested manageable number of 300 patients [15] and therefore need to be substantially supported.

As a future goal, PD nurses can support palliative outpatient teams when caring for the patient and the relative in the last phase since PD patients often suffer from symptoms unknown to palliative care teams. They might visit the patient together with the team or could be the specialist visiting the patient while a telemedical approach discusses symptom control [33].

Table 1. An overview of the existing forms and regional models of Parkinson's disease (PD)-specific nonphysician staff.

	Target Group and Prerequisite	Education Curriculum	State Certificate	Setting	Organization
Parkinson's disease specialist nurse	health and nursing professionals minimum of 2 years of professional experience in acute neurological departments or PD hospitals	4 × 2 days of theoretical training +2 weeks of hospital observation, spread over one year	none	inpatient outpatient	Deutsche Parkinson-Gesellschaft, DPG, Deutsche Parkinsonvereinigung, dPV, Kompetenznetz Parkinson, KNP, Verein der Parkinsonnurses u.–assistenten, VPNA
Parkinson assistant	mainly medical assistants with formerly three-year training	basic course (24 teaching hours) advanced course (1-day workshop)	none	inpatient outpatient	QUANUP e. V.
Parkinson care specialist	nurse	two days training in PD center	none	inpatient outpatient	Verein der Parkinsonnurses u.–assistenten, VPNA
VERAH (Versorgungsassistentin in der Hausarztpraxis)	medical assistant	200 teaching units + internship of 40 units	yes	outpatient (GP)	Deutscher Hausärzteverband
AGnESzwei (Arztentlastende, Gemeindenahe, E-health-gestützte systemische intervention)	nurse or medical assistant	129 theoretical teaching units	yes	outpatient (GP)	Arbeitsgemeinschaft "Innovative Gesundheitsversorgung in Brandenburg" (IGiB)–der KVBB
EVA (Entlastende Versorgungsassistentin)	nurse or medical assistant	at least 300 teaching h	yes	outpatient (GP)	Nordrheinische Akademie

4. Parkinson Assistant (PASS Concept)

At the end of 2000, the Association for Quality Development in Neurology and Psychiatry (QUANUP e.V) was founded as a joint initiative of the Professional Association of German Neurologists (BVDN) and the Professional Association of German Neurologists (BDN). QUANUP has developed a training program for nonmedical staff in neurological doctor´s practices and neurological units in hospitals to qualify them as PASS. Participants were mainly medical assistants with formerly three-year training (Table 1). Since 2009, QUANUP has regularly conducted these structured advanced training events at several locations throughout Germany. The PASS basic course-advanced training is conducted on two weekends on Friday afternoons and Saturday full-time with a total of 14-course hours per weekend. Between the two weekends, homework with self-study should be completed. The participants of the further training courses will receive a certificate after passing the final examination. The first course discusses essential topics (e.g., occurrence and frequency of the disease, possible causes, and mechanisms of PD). The teaching of the PASS includes knowledge about symptoms and complications of the disease, diagnostic procedures, medication and non drug-related treatment options. Case presentations, role playing, and video demonstrations improve practical skills in addition to theoretical knowledge. Neurologists from PD specialist practices and registered PASS lead the PASS courses. An advance course supplements this basic course after 6–12 months. This course includes the teaching of specialized treatment methods such as handling pumps, pens or DBS, provides knowledge about atypical Parkinson's syndrome in more detail and allows the discussion of problems that have arisen in daily practice. Furthermore, in all courses, advice on efficient, practical organization is given.

The PASS should be a competent contact person for patients with PD and their relatives in outpatient settings, Parkinson day clinics, and the wards in the hospitals. Through the joint, coordinated deployment of qualified physicians and qualified PASS, work processes in the practices should be made more efficient. PASS cares for people with PD and relatives through short distances and low-threshold contact offers. They provide necessary information for patients and their families and are the hub between patients, neurologists, therapists, and care institutions. Among others, PASS can also be involved in: (1) visits of neurological practice unspecialized in PD, (2) PD-specialized practices (Parkinson's Practice) [34], and (3) video-supported homecare of patients in a telemedical approach.

For the certificate "Parkinson's Practice" awarded by the German Parkinson Association (Deutsche Parkinsonvereinigung, dPV), a list of criteria has been compiled [34]. The certificate is issued for three years upon application and after an appropriate review. These criteria include, among others, the continuous care of a minimum number of 120 patients with PD and regular training and counseling offers for patients. Additionally, treating physicians must provide proof of regular training in the field of PD, and at least one practice employee must have completed training as a PASS. Further criteria are the standardized collection and documentation of findings in a PD database and guideline-based treatment concepts.

For PD care in rural areas, telemedicine supplied as outpatient video-supported therapy is a suitable option to provide many PD patients access to specific PD care. Homecare via telemedicine may improve patient satisfaction, increase participation, and adherence to therapy substantially. A low-threshold connection between patients and relatives through PASS in neurological practices is another critical issue. This, for example, can significantly reduce complications due to incorrectly taken medication. A structured approach must be developed for Germany on how televisits should be carried out by PDS. Moreover, a reimbursement of this service by the health insurance companies is required.

5. Parkinson Care Specialist (Parkinson Pflegespezialist/In)

The target group for the Parkinson care specialist includes nursing staff from wards and outpatient clinics from nursing homes and outpatient nursing and care services as well as staff from nursing support and advice centers (Table 1). To become a Parkinson care specialist, training for two days in a PD center must be completed. The aim of the training is to provide participants with better knowledge regarding PD and allow participants to correctly and professionally implement medical prescriptions and recommendations from PD nurses, PASS or therapists. Parkinson care specialists support their colleagues and organize the appropriate implementation of prescriptions for therapies and therapeutical settings as well as the appropriate care planning and documentation in their department. Moreover, they are familiar with the unique features and effects of PD drugs, the variety of NMS, nutritional aspects, DBS, and pumps. Advanced courses are offered once a year and should be part of this qualification. VPNA e.V organizes the courses.

6. Support of Health Care Assistants in General Practice and Outpatient Clinics

Due to the increasing number of chronically ill people and the increasing shortage of GPs but also of hospital-based care, especially in rural areas [4,35], there are many courses to provide healthcare assistants to support medical doctors. There is a high diversity in these training courses [36] (Table 1). Furthermore, Advanced Nurse Practitioners (ANP) are implemented in hospitals to support PD patients. In the outpatient setting, healthcare assistants are trained to support medical doctors. In the review by Günther and colleagues, many projects are mentioned for primary care (e.g., VERAH, AGnES, EVA, MoNi, and MoPra). These training courses for healthcare assistants should comprise at least 150 h. VERAH relates to care assistants in general practice (Versorgungsassistentin in der Hausarztpraxis) and who can do home visits. They also take over delegated tasks from the physicians and advise patients regarding prevention and other health-related questions. They are working as case managers and wound managers as well. AGnES is an acronym for physician-relieving, community-oriented intervention with E-health support (Arztentlastende, gemeindenahe, E-health-gestützte systemische intervention). This approach focuses on older and chronically ill patients who are living at home. In addition to VERAH, the healthcare assistants assess diagnostic parameters and do standardized health monitoring. The tasks are much broader than in the VERAH project, but they also do no nursing tasks. The nursing process is a statutory duty of qualified nurses; it is a certified and reimbursed service (Education Act, Pflegeberufereformgesetz–PflBRefGe §4). However, it is not easy to maintain this distinction because in real work life, the borders are blurring.

MoNi stands for Model of Lower Saxony (Modell Niedersachsen). It is a similar project to AGnES and VERAH in cooperation with the Ministry for Social Affairs, Women, Family, Health Care and Integration of Lower Saxony and the physician Association of Lower Saxony. MoPra means mobile practice assistant (Mobile Praxisassistentin) and meets the criteria and tasks of AGnES. MoPra is well established in Saxony-Anhalt.

In cooperation with the Association of Statutory Health Insurance Physicians North Rhine-Westphalia, the North Rhine-Westphalian Academy offers in-service training to become a "relieving care assistant" (EVA–Entlastende Versorgungsassistentin). The prerequisite for participation is a qualified professional qualification as a Medical Specialist Assistant or nurse. Moreover, at least three years of professional activity in a family doctor's practice must be proven. Depending on the professional experience, the total EVA training comprises 170–221 h of theoretical instruction and 20–50 h of practical training. In this course, approximately 30% self-study is integrated on a learning platform. The specialization qualification EVA concludes with a certificate from the Association of Statutory Health Insurance Physicians of North Rhine-Westphalia. The further training aims to give the medical assistant the skills to take over delegable services in outpatient practice. The EVA acquires the competence to take over services in the outpatient practice eligible for delegation. In this way, EVA relieves the physician of the burden of accompanying and supporting patients and their relatives in various tasks relating to the treatment process. The training includes different aspects, such as geriatric syndromes, care and support of oncology and palliative patients, pharmaceutical supply, wound care and wound management, coordination and organization of therapy and social measures, telemedical basics, communication management, medical documentation, and practical training (home visits). Details are given on the homepage of the North Rhine-Westphalian Academy: http://www.akademienordrhein.info/eva-entlastende-versorgungsassistentin.

In terms of PD, the North Rhine-Westphalian Academy offers advanced training to become a "Support Care Assistant in Neurology/Psychiatry (EVA-NP)." This training includes skills required to take over delegated services in specialist neurological and psychiatric practice. EVA-NPs are familiar with many neurological and psychiatric clinical syndromes and disorders and are a qualified contact person for patients. Depending on the professional experience, the complete training for the EVA-NP comprises 197–247 h of theoretical instruction and 20 h of practical training (home visits). Various modules are offered within the theoretical instruction. A PD module (24 lessons) can be taken as part of the optional part.

The tasks in every project/position are quite similar. There is an increasing effort to relieve medical doctors and to support the patients. Many healthcare services delegated to healthcare assistants are appreciated and accepted by patients [37]. The increasing shortage of medical doctors in rural areas is the base of increasing demand for qualified healthcare assistants. Nevertheless, doctors are right in their critical view of whether this need for medical delegation of tasks can be taken on by medical assistants with 200 h training [36]. Such is a crucial aspect, especially in distinction of these qualifications from Physician Assistants courses at Bachelor Level or ANP at master level.

7. Community Matrons

Because of the high workload of PD nurses in the UK, they usually work in collaboration with community matrons as generic practitioners [15]. Community Matrons are experienced registered nurses with academic training. They have advanced competencies (e.g., in case management or assessments) [38,39] and perform advanced nursing practice, especially for patients with high risk of hospital admission such as people with complex and chronic conditions. Community Matrons can be seen as the extension role of healthcare assistants—but they operate more autonomously. Their qualification is nursing education and an academic training (e.g., a course of community health nursing). In Germany, the German Nurses Association developed a concept for community health nursing (Deutscher Berufsverband für Pflegeberufe) [38]. In a project funded by the Robert Bosch Foundation and the Agnes-Karll-Corporation in the German Nurses Association, three German universities developed a community health nursing course in 2020. Community Health Nurses in Germany should have their tasks in routine activities. These include health and chronic disease related assessments, ensuring adherence to medication, monitoring of symptoms of chronically ill patients, support on self-management, health promotion and prevention, patient and caregiver education, and counseling. They should manage and coordinate health care services as case managers. The authors focus on the care of patients (e.g., with diabetes or PD).

8. Proposal of Core Elements for Future PDS Education in Germany

Today, PDS training in Germany is very heterogeneous and differs in terms of duration, content, and target group. There are courses for health care assistants in general or neurological practices. Within these courses are differences in the specialized view on PD (e.g., PASS with a broader view than AGnES). Additionally, there are existing trainings for nurses. While PD nurses mainly work in specialized hospitals and outpatient clinics, the community health nursing will be operating more in an outpatient setting. In the future, it should be discussed how to integrate more specific PD knowledge in community health nursing qualification, especially for supporting long term care settings and in the community. Moreover, it is essential to develop approaches how these different qualifications could create a functional network for supporting people with PD and their next of kin [40]. In particular, the role of PDS in PD telemedicine needs special attention and standardized procedures. This review was not intended to propose a comprehensive model for future PDS education. However, we propose the core elements given in Figure 1 which is from analysis of the Career Framework for Health [19]. We want to point out that PDS education in Germany needs harmonization, standardization, and reimbursement to improve PD care for all PD patients. In particular, the missing certification and reimbursement are main barriers for the implementation of PDS in outpatient and inpatient structures today.

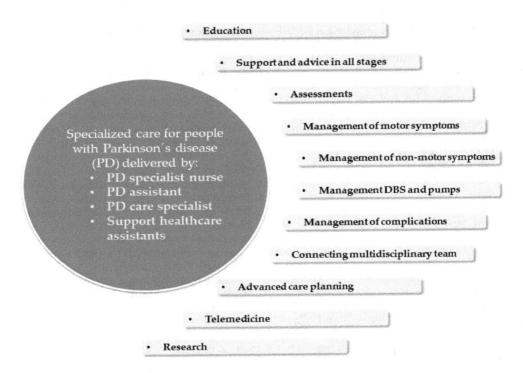

Figure 1. Proposed core elements for future PD staff (PDS) education in Germany.

9. Concluding Remarks

Due to the increasing complexity of PD therapy and the availability of specialized therapies for different stages of the disease, an optimized PD treatment requires expert and multi-professional care. However, for many PD patients in Germany, care is provided only by non-specialized neurological practices or GPs without close exchange with neurologists or specialized university outpatient clinics for movement disorders [34]. PDS are important links between outpatient and inpatient care, physicians and therapists, and PDS transfer specialized PD care into so far nonspecialized neurological practices and hospitals. Unfortunately, there is no institutionalized financial support for PDS training. Moreover, the Association of Statutory Health Insurance Physicians does not support or finance independent activity of PDS in outpatients or inpatient setting, which is already possible in other countries such as Great Britain or the Netherlands.

We also need more research on how PDS can improve patient reported outcome and aspects like management/medication adherence, quality of life, palliative care, and functional status/improving function [41]. PDS still require a delegation by responsible physician. To counteract against the current and increasing shortage of physicians, the professional profile and self-image of the physician will have to change, which does not only apply to the PD care setting [36]. It is expected that the physician will have a leading role in an inter-professional team. To establish these teams and include a high standard of continuous education for PDS, reimbursement concepts must be established that will foster an implementation throughout Germany. Furthermore, the development of professional roles in nursing and specialized care in Germany is needed.

Author Contributions: Conceptualization: T.P., F.S., M.L. and M.W. Writing—Original Draft Preparation: T.P. Writing—Review and Editing: F.S., M.L., M.W., T.M., L.T., S.L., I.W., J.K., H.H., C.E. T.W. and C.B. All authors have read and agreed to the published version of the manuscript.

Acknowledgments: Some of the authors met in Cologne in 2019 for a roundtable discussion and to organize the foundation of the working group PD Networks and Integrated Care, part of the Deutsche Gesellschaft für Parkinson und Bewegungsstörungen (DPG). We would like to thank DPG for covering the travel costs for the experts' meeting for T.P., F.S., M.L., L.T., T.W., J.K. and M.W.

Conflicts of Interest: Tino Prell has received a BMBF research grant, and honoraria for presentations/lectures AbbVie GmbH, UCB Pharma GmbH, Desitin GmbH, Licher MT GmbH, and Bayer AG Deutschland. Frank Siebecker reports no conflict of interest. Michael Lorrain has received honoraria and compensation for consultancy and lecturing from Abbvie, Afi, Bayer, Bial, Biogen, Desitin, Merck, Nordrheinische Akademie, Teva, Ucb, and Zambon. Lars Tönges received travel funding and/or speaker honoraria from Abbvie, Bayer, Bial, Desitin, GE, UCB, Zambon and consulted for Abbvie, Bayer, Bial, Desitin, UCB, Zambon in the last 3 years. Tobias Warnecke has received honoraria from AbbVie (lecture fees, consultant). AbbVie acts as coinitiator of the Parkinsonnetwork Muensterland+ (PNM+) and is cocontractor of the University Hospital of Muenster. Jochen Klucken reports institutional research grants from Bavarian Research Foundation; Emerging Field Initiative, FAU, EIT-Health, EIT-Digital, EU (H2020), German Research Foundation (DFG), and BMBF, and industry-sponsored institutional IITs and grants from Teva GmbH, Licher MT GmbH, Astrum IT GmbH, and Alpha-Telemed AG. He is coemployed by the University Hospital Erlangen, Germany, Fraunhofer Institute for Integrated Circuits e.V., Germany, and the Medical Valley Digital Health Application Center GmbH, Bamberg, Germany. He works on advisory boards in the field of healthcare technologies and digital health of different associations of medical professionals, industries, and political authorities. He holds shares of Portabiles HealthCare Technologies GmbH, Portabiles GmbH, Alpha-Telemed AG, and received compensation and honoraria from serving on scientific advisory boards for LicherMT GmbH, Abbvie GmbH, UCB Pharma GmbH; he has lectured at UCB Pharma GmbH, TEVA Pharma GmbH, Licher MT GmbH, Desitin GmbH, Abbvie GmbH, Solvay Pharmaceuticals, Bial Deutschland GmbH; Celgene GmbH, Lundbeck-Foundation. Dr. Klucken has a patent related to gait assessments pending. Ingmar Wellach has received honoraria as compensation for consultancy and lecturing from AbbVie GmbH, UCB Pharma GmbH, Desitin GmbH, Bial Deutschland GmbH, Zambon Deutschland GmbH, Fagron GmbH & Co. KG, Grünenthal GmbH, and Bayer AG Deutschland. Carsten Buhmann received fees as speaker and/or advisor from Abbvie, Bial, Desitin, Grünenthal, Licher, Novartis, TAD Pharma, UCB, and Zambon in the last 3 years. Martin Wolz has received honoraria for presentations/lectures from Zambon, Valeant, Desitin, TEVA, UCB Pharma, Abbvie, Bial, Licher, and Daiichi Sankyo. Stefan Lorenzl reports no conflict of interest. Heinz Herbst received honoraria and compensation for consultancy and lecturing from AbbVie GmbH, UCB Pharma GmbH, Desitin GmbH, Bial Deutschland GmbH, Zambon Deutschland GmbH, Grünenthal GmbH, and Bayer AG Deutschland. Carsten Eggers CE received payments as a consultant for Abbvie Inc. CE received honoraria as a speaker from Abbvie Inc., Daiichi Sankyo Inc., Bayer Vital Inc. CE received payments as a consultant for Abbvie Inc. and Philyra Inc. Tobias Mai reports no conflict of interests.

References

1. Pfeiffer, R.F. Non-motor symptoms in Parkinson's disease. *Parkinsonism Relat. Disord.* **2016**, *22*, S119–S122. [CrossRef] [PubMed]

2. Ascherio, A.; Schwarzschild, M.A. The epidemiology of Parkinson's disease: Risk factors and prevention. *Lancet Neurol.* **2016**, *15*, 1257–1272. [CrossRef]

3. Feldmann, F.; Zipprich, H.M.; Witte, O.W.; Prell, T. Self-Reported Nonadherence Predicts Changes of Medication after Discharge from Hospital in People with Parkinson's Disease. *Parkinsons Dis.* **2020**, *2020*, 4315489. [CrossRef] [PubMed]

4. Richter, D.; Bartig, D.; Muhlack, S.; Hartelt, E.; Scherbaum, R.; Katsanos, A.H.; Muller, T.; Jost, W.; Ebersbach, G.; Gold, R.; et al. Dynamics of Parkinson's Disease Multimodal Complex Treatment in Germany from 2010–2016, Patient Characteristics, Access to Treatment, and Formation of Regional Centers. *Cells* **2019**, *8*, 151. [CrossRef]

5. Müller, T.; Öhm, G.; Eilert, K.; Möhr, K.; Rotter, S.; Haas, T.; Küchler, M.; Lütge, S.; Marg, M.; Rothe, H. Benefit on motor and non-motor behavior in a specialized unit for Parkinson's disease. *J. Neural Transm.* **2017**, *124*, 715–720. [CrossRef]

6. Scherbaum, R.; Hartelt, E.; Kinkel, M.; Gold, R.; Muhlack, S.; Tonges, L. Parkinson's Disease Multimodal Complex Treatment improves motor symptoms, depression and quality of life. *J. Neurol.* **2019**, *267*. [CrossRef]

7. Gerlach, O.H.; Winogrodzka, A.; Weber, W.E. Clinical problems in the hospitalized Parkinson's disease patient: Systematic review. *Mov. Disord.* **2011**, *26*, 197–208. [CrossRef]

8. Harris, M.; Fry, M. The utilisation of one district hospital emergency department by people with Parkinson's disease. *Australas. Emerg. Nurs. J.* **2017**, *20*, 1–5. [CrossRef]

9. Okunoye, O.; Kojima, G.; Marston, L.; Walters, K.; Schrag, A. Factors associated with hospitalisation among people with Parkinson's disease-A systematic review and meta-analysis. *Parkinsonism Relat. Disord.* **2020**, *71*, 66–72. [CrossRef]

10. Vossius, C.; Nilsen, O.B.; Larsen, J.P. Parkinson's disease and nursing home placement: The economic impact of the need for care. *Eur. J. Neurol.* **2009**, *16*, 194–200. [CrossRef]

11. Binder, S.; Groppa, S.; Woitalla, D.; Müller, T.; Wellach, I.; Klucken, J.; Eggers, C.; Liersch, S.; Amelung, V.E. Patients' Perspective on Provided Health Services in Parkinson's Disease in Germany—A Cross-Sectional Survey. *Akt Neurol.* **2018**, *45*, 703–710.

12. Hellqvist, C.; Bertero, C. Support supplied by Parkinson's disease specialist nurses to Parkinson's disease patients and their spouses. *Appl. Nurs. Res.* **2015**, *28*, 86–91. [CrossRef] [PubMed]

13. Lennaerts, H.; Groot, M.; Rood, B.; Gilissen, K.; Tulp, H.; van Wensen, E.; Munneke, M.; van Laar, T.; Bloem, B.R. A Guideline for Parkinson's Disease Nurse Specialists, with Recommendations for Clinical Practice. *J. Parkinsons Dis.* **2017**, *7*, 749–754. [CrossRef] [PubMed]

14. MacMahon, D.G. Parkinson's disease nurse specialists: An important role in disease management. *Neurology* **1999**, *52*, S21–S25. [PubMed]

15. Osborne, L. Marking 20 years of Parkinson's disease nurse specialists: Looking to the future. *Br. J. Neurosci. Nurs.* **2013**, *5*, 450–455. [CrossRef]

16. Axelrod, L.; Gage, H.; Kaye, J.; Bryan, K.; Trend, P.; Wade, D. Workloads of Parkinson's specialist nurses: Implications for implementing national service guidelines in England. *J. Clin. Nurs.* **2010**, *19*, 3575–3580. [CrossRef]

17. German Society of Neurology (DGN). S3 Leitlinie Idiopathisches Parkinson Syndrom. Available online: https://www.deutsche-apotheker-zeitung.de/daz-az/2016/daz-17-2016/leitlinien-update-morbus-parkinson (accessed on 29 June 2020).

18. Titova, N.; Chaudhuri, K.R. Personalized Medicine and Nonmotor Symptoms in Parkinson's Disease. *Int. Rev. Neurobiol.* **2017**, *134*, 1257–1281.

19. A competency Framework for Nurses Working in Parkinson's Disease Management. Available online: https://www.parkinsons.org.uk/sites/default/files/2017-12/competency_framework_for_parkinsons_nurses_2016.pdf (accessed on 29 June 2020).

20. Brown, M.T.; Bussell, J.K. Medication adherence: WHO cares? *Mayo Clin. Proc.* **2011**, *86*, 304–314. [CrossRef]

21. Grosset, D.; Antonini, A.; Canesi, M.; Pezzoli, G.; Lees, A.; Shaw, K.; Cubo, E.; Martinez-Martin, P.; Rascol, O.; Negre-Pages, L.; et al. Adherence to antiparkinson medication in a multicenter European study. *Mov. Disord.* **2009**, *24*, 826–832. [CrossRef]

22. Sabaté, E. *Adherence to Long-Term Therapies: Evidence for Action*; World Health Organization: Geneva, Switzerland, 2003.

23. Straka, I.; Minar, M.; Skorvanek, M.; Grofik, M.; Danterova, K.; Benetin, J.; Kurca, E.; Gazova, A.; Bolekova, V.; Wyman-Chick, K.A.; et al. Adherence to Pharmacotherapy in Patients With Parkinson's Disease Taking Three and More Daily Doses of Medication. *Front. Neurol.* **2019**, *10*, 799. [CrossRef]

24. Valldeoriola, F.; Coronell, C.; Pont, C.; Buongiorno, M.T.; Camara, A.; Gaig, C.; Compta, Y.; ADHESON Study Group. Socio-demographic and clinical factors influencing the adherence to treatment in Parkinson's disease: The ADHESON study. *Eur. J. Neurol.* **2011**, *18*, 980–987. [CrossRef] [PubMed]

25. Yap, A.F.; Thirumoorthy, T.; Kwan, Y.H. Systematic review of the barriers affecting medication adherence in older adults. *Geriatr. Gerontol. Int.* **2016**, *16*, 1093–1101. [CrossRef] [PubMed]

26. Mendorf, S.; Witte, O.W.; Grosskreutz, J.; Zipprich, H.M.; Prell, T. What Predicts Different Kinds of Nonadherent Behavior in Elderly People With Parkinson's Disease? *Front. Med.* **2020**, *7*, 103. [CrossRef] [PubMed]

27. Bhidayasiri, R.; Boonpang, K.; Jitkritsadakul, O.; Calne, S.M.; Henriksen, T.; Trump, S.; Chaiwong, S.; Chaiwong, S.; Boonrod, N.; Sringean, J.; et al. Understanding the role of the Parkinson's disease nurse specialist in the delivery of apomorphine therpy. *Parkinsonism Relat. Disord.* **2016**, *33*, S49–S55. [CrossRef]

28. Hagell, P. Nursing and multidisciplinary interventions for Parkinson's disease: What is the evidence? *Parkinsonism Relat. Disord.* **2007**, *13*, S501–S508. [CrossRef]

29. Mai, T. Status and development of the role as Parkinson Nurse in Germany—An online survey. *Pflege* **2018**, *31*, 181–189. [CrossRef]

30. Reynolds, H.; Wilson-Barnett, J.; Richardson, G. Evaluation of the role of the Parkinson's disease nurse specialist. *Int. J. Nurs. Stud.* **2000**, *37*, 337–349. [CrossRef]

31. Shin, J.Y.; Hendrix, C.C. Management of patients with Parkinson disease. *Nurse Pract.* **2013**, *38*, 34–43. [CrossRef]

32. Frundt, O.; Mainka, T.; Schonwald, B.; Muller, B.; Dicusar, P.; Gerloff, C.; Buhmann, C. The Hamburg Parkinson day-clinic: A new treatment concept at the border of in- and outpatient care. *J. Neural Transm.* **2018**, *125*, 1461–1472. [CrossRef]

33. Weck, C.E.; Lex, K.M.; Lorenzl, S. Telemedicine in Palliative Care: Implementation of New Technologies to Overcome Structural Challenges in the Care of Neurological Patients. *Front. Neurol.* **2019**, *10*, 510. [CrossRef]

34. Tonges, L.; Ehret, R.; Lorrain, M.; Riederer, P.; Mungersdorf, M. Epidemiology of Parkinson's Disease and Current Concepts of Outpatient Care in Germany. *Fortschr. Neurol. Psychiatr.* **2017**, *85*, 329–335.

35. Tonges, L.; Bartig, D.; Muhlack, S.; Jost, W.; Gold, R.; Krogias, C. Characteristics and dynamics of inpatient treatment of patients with Parkinson's disease in Germany: Analysis of 1.5 million patient cases from 2010 to 2015. *Der Nervenarzt* **2019**, *90*, 167–174.

36. Gunther, H.J.; Bader, C.; Erlenberg, R.M.; Hagl, C.; Schirrmacher, B.; Schuster, A. From AGnES to PA-medical assistant professions in Germany: Who still keeps the track? *MMW Fortschr. Med.* **2019**, *161*, 21–30. [PubMed]

37. Mergenthal, K.G.C.; Beyer, M.; Gerlach, F.M.; Siebenhofer, A. Wie bewerten und akzeptieren Patienten die Betreuung durch Medizinische Fachangestellte in der Hausarztpraxis? Ergebnisse einer Patienten-Befragung in der HzV in Baden-Württemberg [How Patients View and Accept Health Care Services Provided by Health Care Assistants in the General Practice: Survey of Participants of the GP-centered Health Care Program in Baden-Wuerttemberg]. *Das Gesundh.* **2018**, *80*, 1077–1083.

38. DBfP (DBfK). *Community Health Nursing in Deutschland. Konzeptionelle Ansatzpunkte Für Berufsbild und Curriculum.* 2019. Available online: https://www.dbfk.de/media/docs/Bundesverband/CHN-Veroeffentlichung/Broschuere-Community-Health-Nursing-09-2019.pdf (accessed on 29 June 2020).

39. Geithner, L.; Doris, A.; Alexandra, F.; Anna, H.; Maike, S.; Tatjana, S. Advanced Nursing Practice: Rahmenbedingungen in Deutschland und Literaturübersicht zu Nationalen und Internationalen Modellen Erweiterter Pflegepraxis. Available online: https://www.e-hoch-b.de/fileadmin/user_upload/Dokumente/Geithner_et_al-2016-ANP.pdf (accessed on 29 June 2020).

40. Prell, T.; Siebecker, F.; Lorrain, M.; Eggers, C.; Lorenzl, S.; Klucken, J.; Warnecke, T.; Buhmann, C.; Tonges, L.; Ehret, R.; et al. Recommendations for Standards of Network Care for Patients with Parkinson's Disease in Germany. *J. Clin. Med.* **2020**, *9*, 1455. [CrossRef] [PubMed]

41. Shin, J.Y.; Habermann, B. Nursing Research in Parkinson's Disease From 2006 to 2015. *Clin. Nurs. Res.* **2017**, *26*, 142–156. [CrossRef]

The Complex Balance between Analgesic Efficacy, Change of Dose and Safety Profile Over Time, in Cancer Patients Treated with Opioids: Providing the Clinicians with an Evaluation Tool

Oscar Corli [1],*, Luca Porcu [2], Claudia Santucci [3] and Cristina Bosetti [3]

[1]   Department of Oncology, Laboratory of Methodology for Clinical Research, Unit of Pain and Palliative Care Research, Istituto di Ricerche Farmacologiche Mario Negri IRCCS, 20156 Milan, Italy
[2]   Department of Oncology, Laboratory of Methodology for Clinical Research, Unit of Methodological Research, Istituto di Ricerche Farmacologiche Mario Negri IRCCS, 20156 Milan, Italy; luca.porcu@marionegri.it
[3]   Department of Oncology, Laboratory of Methodology for Clinical Research, Unit of Cancer Epidemiology, Istituto di Ricerche Farmacologiche Mario Negri IRCCS, 20156 Milan, Italy; claudia.santucci@marionegri.it (C.S.); cristina.bosetti@marionegri.it (C.B.)
*   Correspondence: oscar.corli@marionegri.it

Abstract: Background: Scanty data exist on the integration between the analgesic effect of opioids, dose changes, and adverse events in cancer patients. Methods: To provide further information on this issue, we analysed data on 498 advanced-stage cancer patients treated with strong opioids. At baseline and three visits (at days 7, 14, and 21), pain intensity, oral morphine-equivalent daily dose, and the prevalence of major adverse events were measured. The proportion of responders (pain intensity decrease ≥30% from baseline) and non-responders, as well as of patients with low or high dose escalation, was calculated. Results: Pain intensity strongly decreased from baseline (pain intensity difference −4.0 at day 7 and −4.2 at day 21) in responders, while it was quite stable in non-responders (pain intensity difference −0.8 at day 7 and −0.9 at day 21). In low dose escalation patients (82.4% at final visit), daily dose changed from 52.3 to 65.3 mg; in high dose escalation patients (17.6%), it varied from 94.1 to 146.7 mg. Among responders, high dose escalation patients experienced significantly more frequent adverse events compared to low or high dose escalation patients, while no differences were observed in non-responders. Conclusions: The response to opioids results from the combination of three clinical aspects, which are strongly interrelated. These results provide some thoughts to help clinical evaluations and therapeutic decisions regarding opioid use.

Keywords: analgesic response; cancer; dose escalation; opioids; safety

1. Introduction

Opioids are considered the most effective drugs to relieve severe cancer pain, as indicated by several guidelines and recommendations [1–3]. The opioid treatment over time, however, cannot only be evaluated on the basis of the analgesic effect but should also consider the dose necessary to obtain and maintain pain reduction and a safety profile.

In general, analgesia is not a constant outcome but tends to vary among patients and time [4,5]. Given a pain reduction by at least 30% as a cut-off for satisfactory clinical results [6], good pain control has been reported in 50%–90% of cancer patients [7,8]. Non-responsiveness is not a rare condition and, up to now, it has only been partially investigated in the literature. Cancer pain is a singular clinical entity, defined by multimorphic characteristics, that can be modified during cancer progression by various factors. These include both cancer etiology, physiopathology, and clinical presentation, as well as disruptive elements, as concomitant treatments, pain from associated diseases, comorbidities and complications, and modifications in the environment [9]. Furthermore, the presence of neuropathic and breakthrough pain worsens pain intensity and induces a poorer response to analgesics [10,11].

Personalised, interventional, and multimodal management, aiming to give an exhaustive approach to all factors influencing pain, must be carefully considered. Moreover, facing poor analgesia, the clinician tends to apply a compensatory increase in the opioid dose. This choice may give a temporary benefit that often disappears over time. Indeed, prolonged and continuous use of opioids, with a compensatory increase of dose, produces two types of neuroadaptation that interfere with opioid ability to provide analgesia [12]. The first neuroadaptation is tolerance, which is characterised by a progressive lack of response due to an adaptive mechanism that neutralises the drug effect by the opioid receptors desensitisation [13,14]. The second neuroadaptation is known as opioid-induced hyperalgesia, where opioids, paradoxically, cause pain hypersensitivity [15]. Hyperalgesia is a rare complication, dose dependent, mediated by the activation of specific pronociceptive processes, generally outside the opioidergic system [16,17]. Consequently, there is a need to establish a proper titration of opioids, aiming to achieve a defined optimal dose that could balance the benefits and harms of opioids in managing cancer pain. Important clinical parameters of adverse events (AEs) are prevalence, severity, and changes over time. The balance between opioid benefits and harms is fundamental in deciding the best management of pain in cancer patients.

We carried out this analysis with the aim of evaluating the analgesic responses in advanced-stage cancer patients treated with strong opioids over a period of treatment of three weeks and describe the course of the treatment in terms of analgesic effect, required doses, and AEs.

2. Material and Methods

This is a post-hoc analysis from a randomised, open-label, longitudinal, phase IV clinical trial [18,19] on advanced-stage cancer patients experiencing moderate to severe pain, randomised to receive one WHO Step III opioid (oral morphine, oxycodone, transdermal fentanyl, or buprenorphine), never administered previously. In this context, we considered patients allocated to the four opioids as a single group of patients.

The eligibility criteria and study details are described in the original study publication [18]. Briefly, the initial opioid doses were based on the recommendations of the European Association for Palliative Care [20], starting with 30 to 60 mg daily of oral morphine-equivalent daily dose (OMEDD), in respect of patient's general clinical condition, age, and previous analgesic therapy. During the follow-up, physicians (oncologists and palliative care or pain therapists) were allowed to modify doses, change the opioid, or discontinue the treatment, based on their experience and patient's clinical needs.

The study consisted of six visits, including the baseline visit and five follow-up visits at days 3, 7, 14, 21, and 28. At each visit, pain intensity (PI) was assessed as average pain intensity (API) experienced by the patient in the previous 24 hours by means of a numeric rating scale, from 0 (no pain) to 10 (worst imaginable pain). Moreover, at each visit, the prescribed opioid daily dose, expressed in OMEDD, was recorded. Moreover, the main opioid-induced AEs were also assessed using the Therapy Impact Questionnaire [21], where patients self-reported the presence and degree of six most frequent AEs (i.e., confusion, constipation, drowsiness, dry mouth, nausea, and vomiting) experienced over the previous week.

For this analysis, only the baseline visit and those at days 7, 14, and 21 were considered since we aimed to evaluate the role of the administered opioids with the associated dosages after one week of treatment. The visit at day 28 was not considered since 166 patients dropped-out for different reasons (36 of them, 22%, died). Pain intensity difference (PID) between baseline and each subsequent visit was calculated and used to classify patients as responders (i.e., ≥30% pain intensity reduction) or non-responders (i.e., <30% decrease in pain intensity), based on Farrar's criteria [6]. The Opioid

Escalation Index (OEI) was calculated [22], and patients were then grouped into high dose escalation; i.e., OEI >5% respect to initial dose) and low dose escalation (i.e., OEI ≤ 5%).

Original study approval was obtained by the review boards of each centre, and patients gave their written informed consent.

Statistical Analysis

Mean and standard deviation (SD) and absolute and percentage frequencies were used to describe continuous and categorical variables, respectively. Trends in API, PID, mean dose, and high dose escalation over time (from days 7 to day 21) were tested using linear regression models. Moreover, differences across responders and non-responders were evaluated by independent samples *t*-test. The profile of safety was analysed according to the combination of analgesic response (responders and non-responders) and dose escalation (low dose escalation and high dose escalation), and logistic regression models were used to estimate the odds ratio (OR) of AEs for high dose escalation patients as compared to low dose escalation patients, among responders and non-responders. The Breslow–Day test was used to detect heterogeneity of OR estimates between responders and non-responders. All the analyses were carried out with the SAS Software, version 9.4 (SAS Institute, Cary, North Carolina, USA).

3. Results

Table 1 shows the baseline demographic and clinical characteristics for the patients included in the study.

Table 1. Demographics and main clinical characteristics of 498 cancer patients at baseline.

	Cancer Patients (%)
Age (years), mean (SD)	66.9 (11.8)
Female	221 (44.4)
Primary site of tumour	
Lung/respiratory system	141 (28.3)
Breast	65 (13.1)
Genitourinary/Female reproductive system	65 (13.1)
Colon, rectum	57 (11.5)
Head and neck	42 (8.4)
Pancreas	39 (7.8)
Prostate	29 (5.8)
Stomach/Oesophagus	18 (3.6)
Other	42 (8.4)
Presence of metastasis	424 (85.1)
Ongoing anticancer therapy	191 (38.4)
Pain	
Average pain, mean (SD)	6.0 (1.4)
Worst pain, mean (SD)	8.0 (1.5)
Type of pain	
Nociceptive	412 (82.7)
Nociceptive /Neuropathic	80 (16.1)
Insufficient information to classify	6 (1.2)
Karnofsky Performance Status, mean (SD)	66.9 (17.0)
≤ 40	57 (11.5)
41–70	273 (54.8)
≥ 71	168 (33.7)
Concomitant diseases*	320 (64.3)
Therapies for concomitant disease°	294 (59.0)
Therapies for symptoms	187 (37.6)

SD: standard deviation. * Including metabolic/hormonal, cardiovascular, neurological/psychological, digestive system, and respiratory diseases. ° Including cardiovascular, antidiabetic, gastrointestinal, antibiotics, central nervous system, hormonal and respiratory drugs.

Table 2 reports API and PID at baseline and at days 7, 14, and 21, overall, and according to the analgesic response. Among all patients, overall, the API score decreased over time (from 6.0 at baseline to 2.4 at day 21), the API score decreased in the responders (from 2.1 to 1.9), while it was stable in non-responders (5.0 and 4.9). Corresponding changes in PID were from −3.1 at day 7 to −3.6 at day 21 in all patients (p-value for trend: 0.002), from −4.0 to −4.2 in responders (p-value for trend: 0.063), and from −0.8 to −0.9 in non-responders (p-value for trend: 0.575).

Table 2. Average pain intensity and pain intensity difference over time overall and by analgesic response among 498 cancer patients.

	Baseline	Day 7	Day 14	Day 21
All patients				
N	498	445	416	397
Average pain intensity (SD)	6.0 (1.36)	2.9 (1.9)	2.7 (1.9)	2.4 (1.8)
Pain intensity difference§ (SD)	-	−3.1 (2.2)	−3.3 (2.4)	−3.6 (2.2)
		P-value for trend = 0.002*		
Responders				
N (%)	−	329 (73.9)	323 (77.6)	323 (81.4)
Average pain intensity (SD)	−	2.1 (1.4)	2.0 (1.4)	1.9 (1.3)
Pain intensity difference§ (SD)	−	−4.0 (1.7)	−4.1 (1.7)	−4.2 (1.8)
		P-value for trend = 0.063*		
Non-responders				
N (%)	−	116 (26.1)	93 (22.4)	74 (18.6)
Average pain intensity (SD)	−	5.0 (1.6)	5.1 (1.4)	4.9 (1.6)
Pain intensity difference§ (SD)	−	−0.8 (1.5)	−0.7 (1.2)	−0.9 (1.2)
		P-value for trend = 0.575*		
P-value°		<0.001	<0.001	<0.001

SD: standard deviation. § Compared to baseline. * A linear regression model was used to detect the trend in pain intensity difference values over time. The t-test was performed to compare PID values between responders and non-responders.

Table 3 shows the distribution of low dose escalation and high dose escalation patients and their respective opioid daily doses over time. Opioid daily dose increased over time, overall (from 63.4 mg at day 7 to 79.6 mg at day 21; p-value for trend <0.001) and according to dose escalation status (from 52.3 to 65.3 mg in low dose escalation patients, p-value for trend <0.001; and from 94.1 to 146.7 mg in high dose escalation patients, p-value for trend <0.001; p-value: < 0.001 for the difference between low dose escalation and high dose escalation at day 21).

Table 3. Opioid daily dose prescribed over time overall and by dose escalation among 498 cancer patients.

	Baseline	Day 7	Day 14	Day 21
All patients				
N	498	445	413	391
Mean Dose (mg; SD)	51.9 (16.2)	63.4 (30.3)	72.3 (44.9)	79.6 (54.5)
		P-value for trend <0.001*		
Low dose escalation				
N (%)	−	326 (73.3)	301 (72.9)	322 (82.4)
Mean Dose (mg; SD)	−	52.3 (16.4)	56.8 (20.29)	65.3 (28.6)
		P-value for trend <0.001*		
High dose escalation				
N (%)	−	119 (26.7)	112 (27.1)	69 (17.6)
Mean Dose (mg; SD)	−	94.1 (37.7)	113.9 (63.1)	146.7 (87.3)
		P-value for trend <0.001*		
P-value °		<0.001	<0.001	<0.001

SD: standard deviation. *A linear regression model was used to detect the trend for dosage over time. ° The t-test was performed to compare dosage values between low and high dose escalation. Note: at day 14, dosage was missing for three patients; at day 21, dosage was missing for six patients.

Mean dose and the prevalence of high dose escalation patients according to analgesic response (responders or non-responders) are reported in Table 4. Mean doses were higher in non-responders than responders at each visit (day 7: 68.2 vs. 61.8 mg, *p*-value: 0.049; day 14: 84.1 vs. 68.9 mg, *p*-value: 0.004; day 21: 93.5 vs. 76.4 mg, *p*-value: 0.015).

Table 4. Dose escalation according to analgesic response over time among 498 cancer patients.

	Day 7	Day 14	Day 21
Responders	329	321	318
Mean dose (mg; SD)	61.8 (29.3)	68.9 (37.0)	76.4 (48.1)
	P-value for trend <0.001*		
High dose escalation patients (%)	74 (22.5)	81 (25.2)	50 (15.7)
Non-responders	116	92	73
Mean dose (mg; SD)	68.2 (32.7)	84.1 (64.5)	93.5 (75.2)
	P-value for trend = 0.002*		
High dose escalation patients (%)	45 (38.8)	31 (33.7)	19 (26.0)
P-value °	0.049	0.004	0.015

SD: standard deviation. *A linear regression model was used to detect the trend for dosage values over time. ° The *t*-test was performed to compare dosage values between responders and non-responders.

The prevalence of the six most frequent AEs according to the analgesic response and dose escalation over time is reported in Table 5. High dose escalation patients had a higher risk of experiencing an AE in responders, particularly at day 7, except for vomiting. Significant ORs were found for confusion (OR: 2.09, 95% CI: 1.18–3.71, at day 7), constipation (OR: 2.35, 95% CI: 1.39–3.98, at day 7), drowsiness (OR: 1.88, 95% CI: 1.11–3.16, at day 7 and OR: 1.76, 95% CI: 1.06–2.92, at day 14), dry mouth (OR: 1.88, 95% CI: 1.13–3.13, at day 14 and OR: 1.99, 95% CI: 1.08–3.66, at day 21), and nausea (OR: 2.29, 95% CI: 1.32–3.97, at day 14).

Table 5. Adverse events over time according to analgesic response and dose escalation among 498 cancer patients.

	Day	Analgesic Response	High Dose Escalation (Events/Total)	Low Dose Escalation (Events/Total)	Odds Ratio (95% CI) *	*P*-value for heterogeneity#
Confusion	7	Responders	25/74	50/255	2.09 (1.18–3.71)°	0.074
		Non-responders	11/45	20/71	0.83 (0.35–1.94)	
	14	Responders	20/81	42/240	1.55 (0.84–2.83)	0.285
		Non-responders	7/31	5/61	3.27 (0.94–11.33)	
	21	Responders	9/50	38/268	1.33 (0.60–2.95)	0.947
		Non-responders	5/19	11/54	1.40 (0.41–4.72)	
Constipation	7	Responders	44/74	98/255	2.35 (1.39–3.98)°	0.036
		Non-responders	24/45	40/71	0.89 (0.42–1.88)	
	14	Responders	47/81	110/240	1.63 (0.98–2.72)	0.522
		Non-responders	16/31	29/61	1.18 (0.50–2.80)	
	21	Responders	27/50	125/268	1.34 (0.73–2.46)	0.389
		Non-responders	13/19	26/54	2.33 (0.77–7.04)	
Drowsiness	7	Responders	39/74	95/255	1.88 (1.11–3.16)°	0.446
		Non-responders	24/45	33/71	1.32 (0.62–2.78)	
	14	Responders	43/81	94/240	1.76 (1.06–2.92)°	0.774
		Non-responders	12/31	18/61	1.51 (0.61–3.74)	
	21	Responders	22/50	95/268	1.43 (0.78–2.64)	0.554
		Non-responders	8/19	23/54	0.98 (0.34–2.83)	

Table 5. *Cont.*

	Day	Analgesic Response	High Dose Escalation (Events/Total)	Low Dose Escalation (Events/Total)	Odds Ratio (95% CI) *	P-value for heterogeneity#
Dry mouth	7	Responders	30/74	83/255	1.41 (0.83–2.41)	0.723
		Non-responders	21/45	30/71	1.20 (0.56–2.54)	
	14	Responders	40/81	82/240	1.88 (1.13–3.13)°	0.461
		Non-responders	13/31	22/61	1.28 (0.53–3.10)	
	21	Responders	24/50	85/268	1.99 (1.08–3.66)°	0.039
		Non-responders	6/19	25/54	0.54 (0.18–1.62)	
Nausea	7	Responders	26/74	60/255	1.76 (1.01–3.08)°	0.689
		Non-responders	17/45	21/71	1.45 (0.66–3.18)	
	14	Responders	30/81	49/240	2.29 (1.32–3.97)°	0.068
		Non-responders	9/31	20/61	0.84 (0.33–2.15)	
	21	Responders	9/50	59/268	0.78 (0.36–1.69)	0.209
		Non-responders	9/19	18/54	1.80 (0.62–5.21)	
Vomiting	7	Responders	4/74	22/255	0.61 (0.20–1.82)	0.179
		Non-responders	8/45	8/71	1.70 (0.59–4.92)	
	14	Responders	8/81	23/240	1.03 (0.44–2.41)	0.180
		Non-responders	2/31	11/61	0.31 (0.06–1.51)	
	21	Responders	3/50	24/268	0.65 (0.19–2.24)	0.659
		Non-responders	2/19	12/54	0.41 (0.08–2.04)	

CI: confidence interval. * Odds ratio (OR) for high dose escalation versus low dose escalation, estimated from a logistic regression model. ° P-value < 0.05. #The Breslow–Day test was used to detect heterogeneity of OR estimates between responders and non-responders.

4. Discussion

The initial assumption of our study was that the assessment of the response to prolonged treatment with opioids was based on three variables: the achieved analgesia, the change of dose, and the opioid-induced AEs. Each of these variables was considered separately and then correlations between them were made. With reference to analgesia, the percentage of responders varied between 74% and 81% across the subsequent visits, and pain intensity in responders decreased by an average of 4 points. On the other hand, the percentage of non-responders ranged from 26% to 19% and pain intensity in non-responders diminished less than one point. From these data, it emerged, once again, that satisfactory analgesia was not always achieved [7,8], causing an important clinical problem especially in advance-stage cancer patients.

The daily dose of opioids on average tended to increase over time in the whole population. Low dose escalation patients were between 73% and 82% depending on the visit time. The difference in dose between low dose escalation and high dose escalation groups was quite impressive: at day 21, high dose escalation patients were prescribed a more than two-fold higher dose than low dose escalation ones. Responders received a significantly lower dose of opioids, their dose increased by an average of 50% in 21 days, and among them, the percentage of high dose escalation ranged from 16% to 22%. Conversely, non-responders were given higher opioid doses, with an increment of about 80%, and among them, high dose escalation proportion ranged from 26% to 39%. The trend was particularly critical in this last group of patients since the dose increase did not correspond to a better analgesic effect.

When we considered the prevalence of the six most common opioid-induced AEs according to the combination of opioid analgesic effect and dose escalation, we found that responders with high dose escalation experienced more frequently all AEs, except vomiting. In addition, AEs were significantly more frequent, especially at the beginning of treatment (at days 7 or 14). No substantial differences in the prevalence of AEs were observed over time in non-responders, regardless of dose increase.

The results that emerged in this analysis can provide useful indications for the clinical evaluations and therapeutic decisions for cancer patients with pain. First, in each patient, pain intensity should be measured at each visit, and the analgesic response should be considered positive if pain decreases by at least 30% compared to the baseline value [6]. Moreover, a satisfying result for the patient corresponds to the achievement of a pain intensity absolute value of 4 or more points [23]. The application of this double criterion allows us to know the level of achieved analgesia.

Second, the dose increase over time should also be measured. The opioid dose is often increased due to the failure of the analgesic effect. It is necessary to understand to what extent the increase can be considered normal. The cut-off between low dose escalation and high dose escalation is a daily increase of 5%. Although this value has been empirically calculated [22], it remains a method commonly used and its calculation can be done using a simple formula. Attention should be paid particularly to high dose escalation patients, who are in a worrying situation that suggests a likely onset of tolerance. More rarely, opioids induce hyperalgesia, which is normally associated with high doses and an increase in pain. In these cases, the continued administration of opioids is counterproductive, while the use of other drugs, such as ketamine, is a more appropriate choice [24]. Less frequently, high opioid doses are requested due to mechanisms generating pain as, for instance, the presence of neuropathic pain, or the involvement of central neuro-inflammation, sometimes observed in chronic pain [25]. In the case of high dose escalation patients, the best-known solution is to switch the opioid with another one [26]. Alternatively, several studies have suggested the use of low-dose methadone as an add-on to regular background opioid treatment, when this is not effective despite increasing doses [27,28]. Important pain relief was reached in about 70% of 410 cancer patients without significant modifications of AEs [28].

Third, AEs and safety profiles should be assessed along all the care path. A simple tool, like the Edmonton Symptom Assessment System [29], based on a list of symptoms/AEs measurable by a numeric rating scale, allows us to recognize the presence of symptoms, also giving a quantitative measure of their severity. The presence and severity of symptoms, however, must be considered after taking into consideration analgesia and dose. Intuitively, we may think that the higher the dose the more frequent and severe are the AEs. Indeed, our results suggest that things go differently: the dose affects the presence of undesirable effects only in non-responders. In these patients, it seems that the opioids do not really bind to their receptors, including both analgesic receptors and those producing AEs. Any additional dose increase is unnecessary in this situation, and the only possible solution is the change in the opioid. The situation is different in responders where effective analgesia, obtained at increasing doses, is also accompanied by more frequent undesired effects. In this case, the price to pay for maintaining analgesia can be heavy.

Fourth, a "time factor" should be considered. The response to opioid treatment is a dynamic and evolving process. Analgesia, dose, and tolerability change over time, differently in each patient. The speed of these changes is important and depends on the disease, the duration of treatment, and the prognosis. For example, a rapid dose increase can be accepted in a terminal patient where the primary goal is reducing suffering, but it becomes problematic when the disease is chronic, not advanced, and requires intercurrent cancer treatments other than long-term opioid treatment. In the latter case, frequent changes in a short time can be critical and require rapid and competent evaluation and decision-making processes. Possible solutions include the dose reduction of the opioid if analgesia does not worsen, or the co-treatment with non-opioid analgesic drugs, or, alternatively, an opioid switch [26].

The main strength of this study consists of the original idea of considering the response to opioids not only in terms of the obtained reduction in pain but also as the combination of various aspects relevant in determining the outcome and duration of the therapy. Previous studies that evaluated opioid treatment outcomes showed only a measure of positive responses, based on pain reduction by ≥30% [7]. Also, in a recent meta-analysis examining the risk factors for clinical response to opioids, the analgesic effect was the only parameter evaluated [30]. The second strength of this study is the large sample of patients with a homogeneous stage of disease. Among the limitations of our study, there is the quite-short period of observation (21 days), which can provide only an indication of the changes and interactions of the studied aspects. A more extended period of evaluation would have allowed a better understanding of the role played by the examined aspects in the long-term. Moreover, some patients dropped-off at day 21, with some difference in responders and non-responders (29 out of 329, 8.8%, in responders; and 19 out of 116, 16.4% in non-responders). Among responders, 62% died, 17% had a treatment withdrawal, 14% were transferred to other centres, and 2% dropped-out for other reasons; corresponding values in non-responders were 53%, 11%, 26% and 11%).

5. Conclusions

This analysis indicates that the clinical response to opioids results from the combination of three clinical aspects (the achieved analgesia, the change of dose, and the opioid-induced AEs), which are strongly interrelated, plus the "time factor". The time factor should be evaluated in pharmacological and clinical terms. Some changes in the opioid response are related to the adaptive behavior of the drug used, such as the onset of tolerance or opioid-induced hyperalgesia. In other cases, the variations of cancer pain and its multimorphic nature in the course of the disease influence the response [9]. Consequently, the clinician should evaluate all these clinical variables together at each patient visit. A balance between opioid benefits and harms is necessary. It ranges from a full positive balance of the three aspects, where treatment can continue with efficacy and safety, to a complete negative balance, which must lead to a drastic and rapid change of therapy. Intermediate situations require targeted interventions on the negative aspect.

Author Contributions: Conceptualization, O.C. and C.B.; formal analysis, L.P. and C.S.; methodology, L.P.; writing of original draft, O.C.; writing, review and editing, CB, L.P. and CS. All authors have read and agreed to the published version of the manuscript.

Abbreviations

AE: adverse events; API: Average Pain Intensity; OEI: Opioid Escalation Index; OMEDD: oral morphine-equivalent daily dose; OR: odds ratio; PID: pain intensity difference; SD: standard deviation; WHO: World Health Organization.

References

1.   World Health Organization. *Guidelines for the Pharmacological and Radiotherapeutic Management of Cancer Pain in Adults and Adolescents*; World Health Organization: Geneva, Switzerland, 2018.

2.   Fallon, M.; Giusti, R.; Aielli, F.; Hoskin, P.; Rolke, R.; Sharma, M.; ESMO Guidelines Committee. Management of cancer pain in adult patients: ESMO Clinical Practice Guidelines. *Ann. Oncol.* **2018**, *29*, iv166–iv191. [CrossRef] [PubMed]

3.   Paice, J.A.; Portenoy, R.; Lacchetti, C.; Campbell, T.; Cheville, A.; Citron, M.; Constine, L.S.; Coope, A.; Glare, P.; Koyyalagunta, L.; et al. Management of Chronic Pain in Survivors of Adult Cancers: American Society of Clinical Oncology Clinical Practice Guideline. *J. Clin. Oncol.* **2016**, *34*, 3325–3345. [CrossRef] [PubMed]

4.   Corli, O.; Roberto, A.; Greco, M.T.; Montanari, M. Assessing the response to opioids in cancer patients: A methodological proposal and the results. *Supportive Care Cancer* **2015**, *23*, 1867–1873. [CrossRef] [PubMed]

5.   Mun, C.J.; Suk, H.W.; Davis, M.C.; Karoly, P.; Finan, P.; Tennen, H.; Jensen, M.P. Investigating intraindividual pain variability: Methods, applications, issues, and directions. *Pain* **2019**, *160*, 2415–2429. [CrossRef] [PubMed]

6.   Farrar, J.T.; Portenoy, R.K.; Berlin, J.A.; Kinman, J.L.; Strom, B.L. Defining the clinically important difference in pain outcome measures. *Pain* **2000**, *88*, 287–294. [CrossRef]

7.   Mercadante, S.; Portenoy, R.K. Opioid poorly-responsive cancer pain. Part 1: Clinical considerations. *J. Pain Symptom Manag.* **2001**, *21*, 144–150. [CrossRef]

8.   Mercadante, S.; Maddaloni, S.; Roccella, S.; Salvaggio, L. Predictive factors in advanced cancer pain treated only by analgesics. *Pain* **1992**, *50*, 151–155. [CrossRef]

9.	Lemaire, A.; George, B.; Maindet, C.; Burnod, A.; Allano, G.; Minello, C. Opening up disruptive ways of management in cancer pain: The concept of multimorphic pain. *Supportive Care Cancer* **2019**, *27*, 3159–3170. [CrossRef] [PubMed]

10.	Corli, O.; Roberto, A.; Bennett, M.I.; Galli, F.; Corsi, N.; Rulli, E.; Antonione, R. Nonresponsiveness and Susceptibility of Opioid Side Effects Related to Cancer Patients' Clinical Characteristics: A Post-Hoc Analysis. *Pain Pract.* **2018**, *18*, 748–757. [CrossRef]

11.	Knudsen, A.K.; Brunelli, C.; Klepstad, P.; Aass, N.; Apolone, G.; Corli, O.; Montanari, M.; Caraceni, A.; Kaasa, S. Which domains should be included in a cancer pain classification system? Analyses of longitudinal data. *Pain* **2012**, *153*, 696–703. [CrossRef]

12.	Hayhurst, C.J.; Durieux, M.E. Differential Opioid Tolerance and Opioid-induced Hyperalgesia: A Clinical Reality. *Anesthesiology* **2016**, *124*, 483–488. [CrossRef] [PubMed]

13.	King, T.; Ossipov, M.H.; Vanderah, T.W.; Porreca, F.; Lai, J. Is paradoxical pain induced by sustained opioid exposure an underlying mechanism of opioid antinociceptive tolerance? *Neurosignals* **2005**, *14*, 194–205. [CrossRef] [PubMed]

14.	Williams, J.T.; Ingram, S.L.; Henderson, G.; Chavkin, C.; von Zastrow, M.; Schulz, S.; Koch, T.; Evans, C.J.; Christie, M.J. Regulation of mu-opioid receptors: Desensitization, phosphorylation, internalization, and tolerance. *Pharmacol. Rev.* **2013**, *65*, 223–254. [CrossRef] [PubMed]

15.	Angst, M.S.; Clark, J.D. Opioid-induced hyperalgesia: A qualitative systematic review. *Anesthesiology* **2006**, *104*, 570–587. [CrossRef] [PubMed]

16.	Ferrini, F.; Trang, T.; Mattioli, T.A.; Laffray, S.; Del'Guidice, T.; Lorenzo, L.E.; Castonguay, A.; Doyon, N.; Zhang, W.; Mohr, D.; et al. Morphine hyperalgesia gated through microglia-mediated disruption of neuronal Cl(-) homeostasis. *Nat. Neurosci.* **2013**, *16*, 183–192. [CrossRef] [PubMed]

17.	Ossipov, M.H.; Lai, J.; King, T.; Vanderah, T.W.; Porreca, F. Underlying mechanisms of pronociceptive consequences of prolonged morphine exposure. *Biopolymers* **2005**, *80*, 319–324. [CrossRef] [PubMed]

18.	Corli, O.; Floriani, I.; Roberto, A.; Montanari, M.; Galli, F.; Greco, M.T.; Luzzani, M. Are strong opioids equally effective and safe in the treatment of chronic cancer pain? A multicenter randomized phase IV 'real life' trial on the variability of response to opioids. *Ann. Oncol.* **2016**, *27*, 1107–1115. [CrossRef] [PubMed]

19.	Corli, O.; Santucci, C.; Corsi, N.; Radrezza, S.; Galli, F.; Bosetti, C. The Burden of Opioid Adverse Events and the Influence on Cancer Patients' Symptomatology. *J. Pain Symptom Manag.* **2019**, *57*, 899–908. [CrossRef]

20.	Caraceni, A.; Hanks, G.; Kaasa, S.; Bennett, M.I.; Brunelli, C.; Cherny, N.; Dale, P.O.; De Conno, F.; Fallon, M.; Haugen, D.F.; et al. Use of opioid analgesics in the treatment of cancer pain: Evidence-based recommendations from the EAPC. *Lancet Oncol.* **2012**, *13*, e58–e68. [CrossRef]

21.	Tamburini, M.; Rosso, S.; Gamba, A.; Mencaglia, E.; De Conno, F.; Ventafridda, V. A therapy impact questionnaire for quality-of-life assessment in advanced cancer research. *Ann. Oncol.* **1992**, *3*, 565–570. [CrossRef]

22.	Mercadante, S.; Fulfaro, F.; Casuccio, A.; Barresi, L. Investigation of an opioid response categorization in advanced cancer patients. *J. Pain Symptom Manag.* **1999**, *18*, 347–352. [CrossRef]

23.	Corli, O.; Montanari, M.; Greco, M.T.; Brunelli, C.; Kaasa, S.; Caraceni, A.; Apolone, G. How to evaluate the effect of pain treatments in cancer patients: Results from a longitudinal outcomes and endpoint Italian cohort study. *Eur. J. Pain* **2013**, *17*, 858–866. [CrossRef] [PubMed]

24.	Kapural, L.; Kapural, M.; Bensitel, T.; Sessler, D.I. Opioid-sparing effect of intravenous outpatient ketamine infusions appears short-lived in chronic-pain patients with high opioid requirements. *Pain Physician* **2010**, *13*, 389–394. [PubMed]

25.	Giron, S.E.; Griffis, C.A.; Burkard, J.F. Chronic Pain and Decreased Opioid Efficacy: An Inflammatory Link. *Pain Manag. Nurs.* **2015**, *16*, 819–831. [CrossRef] [PubMed]

26.	Quigley, C. Opioid switching to improve pain relief and drug tolerability. *Cochrane Database Syst. Rev.* **2004**, *3*, CD004847.

27.	Wallace, E.; Ridley, J.; Bryson, J.; Mak, E.; Zimmermann, C. Addition of methadone to another opioid in the management of moderate to severe cancer pain: A case series. *J. Palliat. Med.* **2013**, *16*, 305–309. [CrossRef]

28.	Furst, P.; Lundstrom, S.; Klepstad, P.; Strang, P. The Use of Low-Dose Methadone as Add-On to Regular Opioid Therapy in Cancer-Related Pain at End of Life: A National Swedish Survey in Specialized Palliative Care. *J. Palliat. Med.* **2020**, *23*, 226–232. [CrossRef]

29. Hui, D.; Bruera, E. The Edmonton Symptom Assessment System 25 Years Later: Past, Present, and Future Developments. *J. Pain Symptom Manag.* **2017**, *53*, 630–643. [CrossRef]

30. Lucenteforte, E.; Vagnoli, L.; Pugi, A.; Crescioli, G.; Lombardi, N.; Bonaiuti, R.; Aricò, M.; Giglio, S.; Messeri, A.; Vannacci, A.; et al. A systematic review of the risk factors for clinical response to opioids for all-age patients with cancer-related pain and presentation of the paediatric STOP pain study. *BMC Cancer* **2018**, *18*, 568. [CrossRef]

3

Efficacy and Safety of Ceftaroline for the Treatment of Community-Acquired Pneumonia

Shao-Huan Lan [1], Shen-Peng Chang [2], Chih-Cheng Lai [3], Li-Chin Lu [4] and Chien-Ming Chao [3,*]

[1] School of Pharmaceutical Sciences and Medical Technology, Putian University, Putian 351100, Fujian, China; shawnlan0713@gmail.com

[2] Department of Pharmacy, Chi Mei Medical Center, Liouying 73657, Taiwan; httremoon@ms.szmc.edu.tw

[3] Department of Intensive Care Medicine, Chi Mei Medical Center, Liouying 73657, Taiwan; dtmed141@gmail.com

[4] School of Management, Putian University, Putian 351100, Fujian, China; jane90467@gmail.com

[*] Correspondence: ccm870958@yahoo.com.tw

Abstract: This study aimed to compare the clinical efficacy and safety of ceftaroline with those of ceftriaxone for treating community-acquired pneumonia (CAP). The PubMed, Cochrane Library, Embase, and clinicalTrials.gov databases were searched until April 2019. This meta-analysis only included randomized controlled trials (RCTs) that evaluated ceftaroline and ceftriaxone for the treatment of CAP. The primary outcome was the clinical cure rate, and the secondary outcome was the risk of adverse events (AEs). Five RCTs were included. Overall, at the test of cure (TOC), the clinical cure rate of ceftaroline was superior to the rates of ceftriaxone for the treatment of CAP (modified intent-to-treat population (MITT) population, odds ratio (OR) 1.61, 95% confidence interval (CI) 1.31–1.99, $I^2 = 0\%$; clinically evaluable (CE) population, OR 1.38, 95% CI 1.07–1.78, $I^2 = 14\%$). Similarly, the clinical cure rate of ceftaroline was superior to that of ceftriaxone at the end of therapy (EOT) (MITT population, OR 1.57, 95% CI 1.16–2.11, $I^2 = 0\%$; CE population, OR 1.64, 95% CI 1.15–2.33, $I^2 = 0\%$). For adult patients, the clinical cure rate of ceftaroline remained superior to that of ceftriaxone at TOC (MITT population, OR 1.66, 95% CI 1.34–2.06, $I^2 = 0\%$; CE population, OR 1.39, 95% CI 1.08–1.80, $I^2 = 30\%$) and at EOT (MITT population, OR 1.64, 95% CI 1.20–2.24, $I^2 = 0\%$; CE population, OR 1.65, 95% CI 1.15–2.36, $I^2 = 0\%$). Ceftaroline and ceftriaxone did not differ significantly in the risk of serious AEs, treatment-emergent AEs, and discontinuation of the study drug owing to an AE. In conclusion, the clinical efficacy of ceftaroline is similar to that of ceftriaxone for the treatment of CAP. Furthermore, this antibiotic is as tolerable as ceftriaxone.

Keywords: ceftaroline; ceftriaxone; community-acquired pneumonia; safety

1. Introduction

Community-acquired pneumonia (CAP) is a common acute bacterial infection among adults and children and has become a significant global health problem [1–4]. Moreover, severe CAP is associated with high morbidity and mortality, particularly when prompt and appropriate treatment is not provided [5,6]. However, the emergence of antibiotic resistance in this era—with the increase in resistant bacteria not treatable with existing antibiotics—and the lack of development of novel antibiotics has complicated the use of antibiotics unlike before [3,7]. In addition to the most common CAP pathogen—*Streptococcus pneumoniae*, less than 8% of CAP can be caused by the so-called PES pathogens—*Pseudomonas aeruginosa*, extended-spectrum β-lactamase producing *Enterobacteriaceae*, and methicillin-resistant *Staphylococcus aureus* (MRSA), especially in intensive care unit (ICU) [8,9]. Among PES, MRSA is the most frequently reported, and it requires the use of specific antimicrobial agents for the treatment of typical CAP [10]. Currently, the antibiotics recommended for treating CAP when MRSA infection is suspected are vancomycin, teicoplanin, and linezolid [11–13].

Ceftaroline is a new cephalosporin with broad-spectrum activity against many commonly encountered pathogens causing CAP, including *S. pneumoniae, S. aureus, Moraxella catarrhalis, Haemophilus influenzae, and Klebsiella pneumonia* [14–16]. Moreover, several investigations have demonstrated the substantial in vitro activity of ceftaroline against MRSA from various clinical specimens, including skin/soft tissue and respiratory tract [15,17–19]. Global surveillance revealed that compared to ceftriaxone, ceftaroline showed superior in vitro activity against common CAP pathogens [17]. Subsequently, several randomized controlled trials (RCTs) [20–24] have investigated the efficacy and safety of ceftaroline for the treatment of CAP. In the present study, we conducted a comprehensive meta-analysis to provide high-quality evidence on the efficacy and safety of ceftaroline compared to those of ceftriaxone for treating CAP.

2. Methods

2.1. Study Search and Selection

All clinical studies were identified through a systematic review of the literature in the PubMed, Embase, ClinicalTrials.gov, and Cochrane databases until April 2019 using the following search terms: "ceftaroline", "Teflaro", "Zinforo", "pneumonia", and "RCT". Only RCTs that compared the clinical efficacy and adverse effects of ceftaroline and ceftriaxone were included. Two reviewers (Lan and Chang) searched and examined publications independently to avoid bias. When they disagreed, a third author (Lai) resolved the issue. The following data were extracted from each study included in the meta-analysis: year of publication, study design, duration, antibiotic regimens of ceftaroline and ceftriaxone, outcomes, and adverse events (AEs).

2.2. Definitions and Outcomes

The primary outcome was the overall clinical cure with the resolution of clinical signs and symptoms of pneumonia or improvement to the extent that no further antimicrobial therapy was necessary at the end of therapy (EOT) and test of cure (TOC) in the modified intent-to-treat population (MITT) and the clinically evaluable (CE) population. The EOT visit took place within 48 h after the last dose of oral study drug or within 24 h after the last dose of the IV study drug. The TOC visit was at 8–15 days after the last dose of the IV or oral study drug (whichever was given last). Patients in the MITT population who met minimal disease criteria and had ≥1 bacterial pathogen commonly associated with CAP identified at baseline were included in the microbiological modified MITT (mMITT) population, and those who met criteria for both the CE and mMITT populations were included in the microbiologically evaluable (ME) population. The secondary outcome was the risk of AEs, including mild, moderate, and severe degree and discontinuation because of AEs, relapse rate, and mortality.

2.3. Data Analysis

This study used the Cochrane risk-of-bias tool to assess the quality of enrolled RCTs and their risk of bias [25]. The Review Manager software program, version 5.3, was used to conduct statistical analyses. The degree of heterogeneity was evaluated using the Q statistic generated from the χ^2 test. The I^2 measure assessed the proportion of statistical heterogeneity. Heterogeneity was considered significant when the P value was less than 0.10 or the I^2 value was more than 50%. The random-effects model was used when data were significantly heterogeneous, and the fixed-effect model was used when the data were homogeneous. Pooled odds ratios (ORs) and 95% confidence intervals (CI) were calculated for outcome analyses.

3. Results

The search results yielded a total of 133 studies from the online databases, and 76 studies were excluded because of duplication. Additionally, 64 studies were found to be irrelevant after the title and abstract were screened (article type and language), and 7 studies were found to be irrelevant after the full text was screened. Eventually, five RCTs [20–24] were enrolled for the meta-analysis (Figure 1).

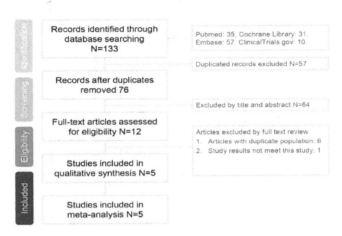

Figure 1. Flowchart of the study selection process.

3.1. Study Characteristics and Study Quality

All five RCTs [20–24] included were multinational and multicenter studies (Table 1). Three studies [20–22] focused on adult patients with CAP with Pneumonia Outcomes Research Term (PORT) [26] risk class III–IV, and two studies [23,24] enrolled pediatric patients only. Overall, the experimental group treated with ceftaroline and the control group treated with ceftriaxone comprised 1153 and 1050 patients, respectively. Almost all risks of basis in each study were low (Figure 2).

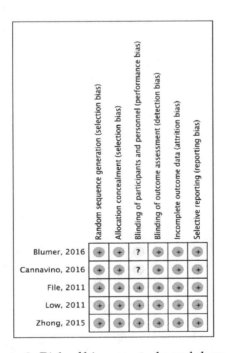

Figure 2. Risk of bias per study and domain.

Table 1. Characteristics of included studies.

Study, Published Year	Study Design	Study Period	Study Population	No of Patients		Dose Regimen		Comparator
				Ceftaroline	Comparator	Ceftaroline		
File et al., 2011 [20]	Multicenter, multinational, double-blinded, randomized trial	January 2008 to December 2008	Adult patients with PORT risk class III or IV CAP requiring hospitalization and IV therapy	304	309	600 mg q12 h		Ceftriaxone 1 g q24 h
Low et al., 2011 [21]	Multicenter, multinational, double-blinded, randomized trial	2007–2009	Patients (aged ≥18 years) with PORT risk class III or IV CAP requiring hospitalization and IV therapy	317	310	600 mg q12 h		Ceftriaxone 1 g q24 h
Zhong et al., 2015 [22]	Multicenter, multinational, double-blinded, randomized trial	2011–2013	Adult Asian patients with PORT risk class III–IV CAP	381	382	600 mg q12 h		Ceftriaxone 2 g q24 h
Cannavino et al., 2016 [23]	Multicenter, multinational, randomized	2012–2014	Ages of 2 months and <18 years with CAP requiring hospitalization and IV antibacterial therapy	121	39	Age < 6 m, 8 mg/kg q8 h; aged ≥ 6 m, 12 mg/kg q8 h for those weighing ≤ 33 kg or 400 mg q8 h for those weighing >33 kg		Ceftriaxone 75 mg/kg/d to a maximum 4g/d q12 h
Blumer et al., 2016 [24]	Multicenter, multinational randomized, observe-blinded	2012–2014	Pediatric patients between 2 months and 17 years of age with complicated CAP	30	10	15 mg/kg or 600 mg q8 h if weight > 40 kg if ≥6 m or 10 mg/kg q8 h if <6 m		Ceftriaxone, 75 mg/kg/d q12 h, and vancomycin 15 mg/kg q6 h

3.2. Clinical Efficacy

Notably, ceftaroline had a superior clinical cure rate at TOC compared with ceftriaxone for the treatment of CAP (MITT population, OR 1.61, 95% CI 1.31–1.99, I^2 = 0%; CE population, OR 1.38, 95% CI 1.07–1.78, I^2 = 14%; ME population, OR 1.98, 95% CI 1.20–3.25, I^2 = 0%; Figure 3). Similarly, at EOT, the clinical cure rate of ceftaroline was superior compared with that of ceftriaxone (MITT population, OR 1.57, 95% CI 1.16–2.11, I^2 = 0%; CE population, OR 1.64, 95% CI 1.15–2.33, I^2 = 0%).

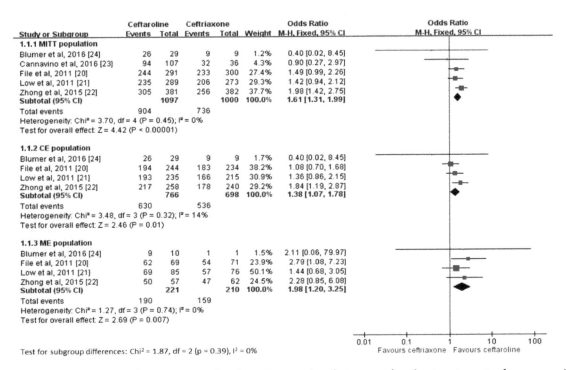

Figure 3. Overall clinical cure rates of ceftaroline and ceftriaxone for the treatment of community-acquired pneumonia. MITT, modified intent-to-treat population; CE, clinically evaluable; ME, microbiologically evaluable.

In the subgroup analysis of three studies [20–22] including adult patients, the clinical cure rate of ceftaroline remained superior to that of ceftriaxone at TOC (MITT population, OR 1.66, 95% CI 1.34–2.06, I^2 = 0%; CE population, OR 1.39, 95% CI 1.08–1.80, I^2 =30%) and at EOT (MITT population, OR 1.64, 95% CI 1.20–2.24, I^2 = 0%; CE population, OR 1.65, 95% CI 1.15–2.36, I^2 =0%). On the other hand, the pooled analysis of two studies showed that the clinical cure rates at TOC and EOT were similar between pediatric patients treated with ceftaroline or ceftriaxone (at TOC, OR 0.79, 95% CI 0.26–2.97, I^2 = 0%; at EOT, OR 1.02, 95% CI 0.38–2.75, I^2 = 0%)[23,24].

Figure 4 shows further analysis of the clinical cure rate (ceftaroline vs. ceftriaxone) at the TOC visit in various patient subgroups. Ceftaroline showed a superior clinical cure rate than ceftriaxone for patients with PORT risk III (OR 1.83, 95% CI 1.26–2.67, I^2 = 14%) but not for patients with PORT risk IV (OR 1.39, 95% CI 0.91–2.12, I^2 = 0%). The efficacy of ceftaroline was superior compared to that of ceftriaxone in patients who did not receive prior antibiotics (OR 1.90, 95% CI 1.22–2.95, I^2 = 37%) but not in those who received prior antibiotics (OR 1.18, 95% CI 0.75–1.87, I^2 = 0%). No differences were observed in the clinical cure rate between elderly patients (age ≥65 years) treated with ceftaroline or ceftriaxone (OR 1.72, 95% CI 0.95–3.11, I^2 = 58%) and between patients with bacteremia treated with ceftaroline or ceftriaxone (OR 1.62, 95% CI 0.46–5.72, I^2 = 0%).

We also assessed the clinical cure rate based on pathogens among the mMITT population, and we found that ceftaroline was superior to ceftriaxone in the overall population (OR 1.94, 95% CI 1.25–3.01, I^2 = 0%, Figure 5). Ceftaroline was superior to ceftriaxone in patients with gram-positive coccal (GPC) infection (OR 2.65, 95% CI 1.40–5.01, I^2 = 0%) but not in those with gram-negative bacterial

(GNB) infection (OR 1.26, 95% CI 0.65–2.42, $I^2 = 0\%$). No significant difference was noted between the ceftaroline and ceftriaxone groups for each of the following pathogens: *S. pneumoniae, S. aureus, H. influenzae, H. parainfluenzae, Escherichia coli,* and *K. pneumoniae.*

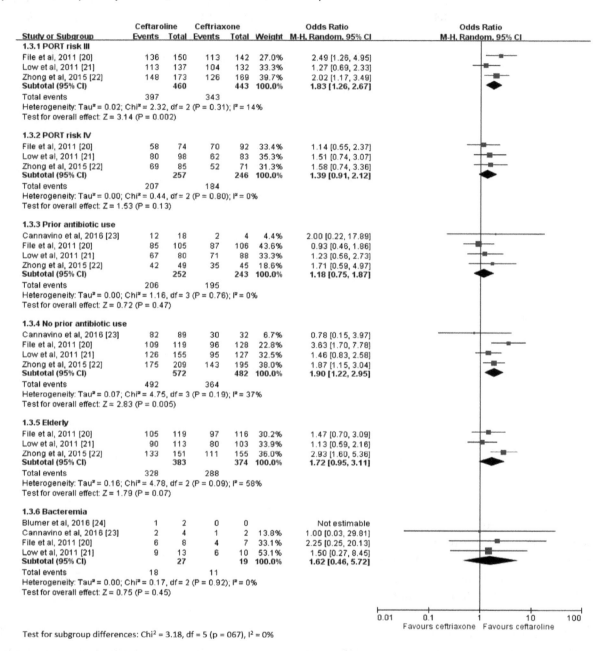

Figure 4. Overall clinical cure rates of ceftaroline and ceftriaxone for the treatment of community-acquired pneumonia based on patient group.

3.3. Adverse Events

No significant differences were observed in the risk of overall treatment-emergent adverse events (TEAEs) between the ceftaroline and ceftriaxone groups (OR 0.99, 95% CI 0.75–1.30, $I^2 = 43\%$), and the similarity was not changed by the degree of severity (Figure 6). The risks of serious AEs and discontinuation of the study drug were similar between the ceftaroline and ceftriaxone groups (Figure 5). In addition, no relapse was noted among all enrolled patients. Finally, the mortality rate was similar between the ceftaroline and ceftriaxone groups (OR 1.13, 95% CI 0.57–2.23, $I^2 = 0$), and none of the cases of mortality were related to the study drug.

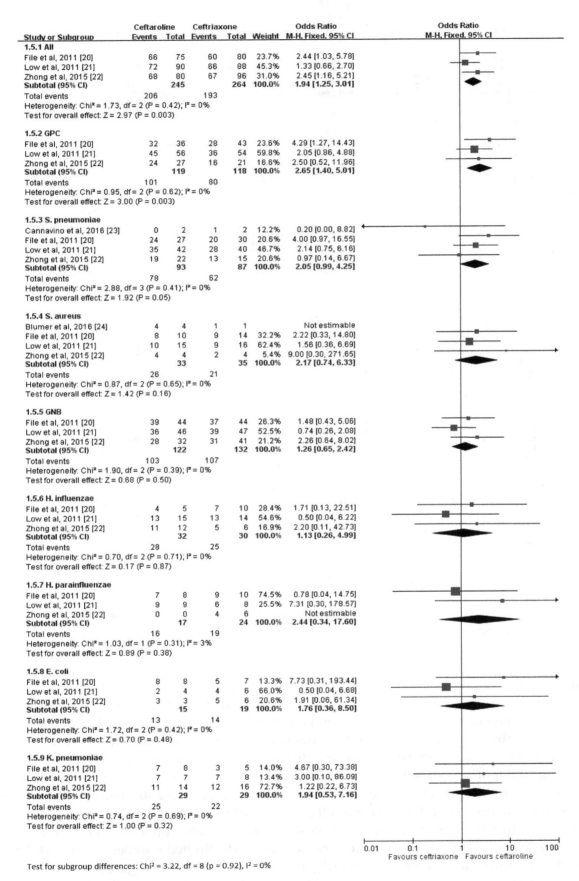

Figure 5. Overall clinical cure rates of ceftaroline and ceftriaxone for the treatment of community-acquired pneumonia based on pathogens.

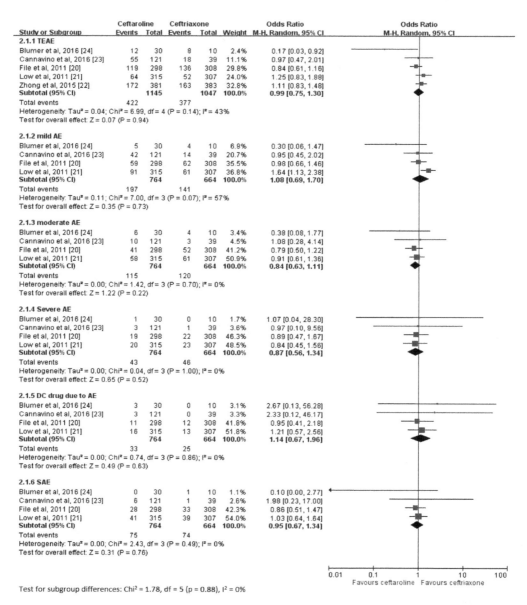

Figure 6. Risk of adverse events between ceftaroline and ceftriaxone for the treatment of community-acquired pneumonia.

4. Discussion

This meta-analysis of five RCTs determined that the clinical efficacy of ceftaroline was superior to that of ceftriaxone for the treatment of patients with CAP. First, the overall clinical cure rate of ceftaroline was superior to that of ceftriaxone for treating CAP in the pooled populations of the five RCTs, including pediatric and adult patients [20–24]. The superiority of ceftaroline compared to ceftriaxone remained significant at different times of outcome measurement, including EOT and TOC, and in different populations, including MITT, CE, and ME populations. Second, we found that ceftaroline had a higher clinical cure rate than ceftriaxone among adult patients in the subgroup analysis of three studies [20–22] including adult patients, but the pooled analysis of two studies [23,24] including pediatric patients showed similar clinical cure rates for ceftaroline and ceftriaxone. However, the two studies [23,24] that focused on pediatric patients had a limited number of patients. Therefore, more pediatric studies are warranted to clarify this issue. Third, the subgroup analysis of CAP in various populations demonstrated that ceftaroline was at least similar to ceftriaxone in patients with PORT risk IV, those who received previous antibiotics, those who were aged ≥65 years, and those with bacteremia but superior to ceftriaxone in patients with PORT risk III and those who did not receive previous antibiotics. In summary, the overall clinical efficacy of ceftaroline is similar to that of ceftriaxone for the treatment of CAP. For other populations, ceftaroline is at least similar to ceftriaxone in terms of the clinical cure rate. However, the case numbers of several subgroup analyses, such as bacteremia, PORT risk IV or different pathogens were limited, which may limit the significance of differences between ceftaroline and ceftriaxone. Therefore, a further large-scale study is warranted to prove our findings.

In the mMITT population, the present meta-analysis determined that the clinical cure rate of ceftaroline was superior to that of ceftriaxone for CAP caused by GPC, but no significant difference was found for CAP caused by GNB, *S. pneumoniae, S. aureus, H. influenzae, H. parainfluenzae, E. coli,* and *K. pneumoniae* between the ceftaroline and ceftriaxone groups. The effectiveness of ceftaroline for the treatment of CAP is supported by in vitro studies. In a surveillance study at a US medical center, ceftaroline was noted to be more potent against *S. pneumoniae* ($MIC_{50} \leq 0.015$ vs. ≤ 0.06 µg/mL; $MIC_{90} = 0.12$ vs. 1 µg/mL) and even remained active against strains nonsusceptible to ceftriaxone ($MIC_{90} = 0.25$ µg/mL) [18]. Similar findings were demonstrated in the analysis of bacterial isolates in pediatric patients [15]. Upon global surveillance, ceftaroline was noted to be more potent than ceftriaxone against MSSA and *S. pneumoniae,* and ceftaroline had similar efficacy to ceftriaxone against *H. influenzae* [17]. Overall, the in vitro activity of ceftaroline that is greater or at least equal to ceftriaxone against most commonly encountered pathogens causing CAP could largely explain the high in vivo clinical response in this meta-analysis. However, we can only see the trend of better efficacy of ceftaroline than the comparator in each subgroup; these differences do not reach statistical significance. This may be due to the limited case number of each pathogen, so further large-scale study is warranted.

Although this study demonstrated the clinical efficacy of ceftaroline in the treatment of CAP, antibiotics may have a limited effect on the outcome of CAP, particularly these severely affected cases. This could be due to the fact that pneumonia is caused by a variety of pathogens, including respiratory viruses, Mycoplasma pneumoniae, and bacteria. In addition, incidence of primary bacterial pneumonia may be very low and be far less than that of nonbacterial pneumonia in developed countries as well as in developing countries [27]. Incidences of each pathogen pneumonia may differ in children and adults (older persons) across the populations, but severe pneumonia of viral or nonpathogen origin can induce secondary bacterial infection caused by lung injuries from primary insults; hence, it is reasonable that any pneumonia patients could be treated with antibiotics. However, antibiotics have a limited effect on the natural course of infection-related extrapulmonary manifestations. Further, outcomes of severe pneumonia may be affected by underlying comorbidities or the immune status of the host, not only by antibiotic treatment. Moreover, the pattern of antimicrobial resistance may vary in different sites; therefore, the guidelines for antibiotic treatment for CAP may differ and could be changed in each country over time. In summary, although the appropriate use of antibiotics is essential for the successful treatment of pneumonia, many factors, including disease severity, underlying comorbidity, immune status, pathogens, and the timing of antibiotic use are also significantly associated with the outcome of pneumonia.

The risk of AEs is another major concern when treating CAP with this antimicrobial agent. The most common AEs are headache, diarrhea, and insomnia [28]. In this analysis, the pooled risks of TEAEs of all degrees and even serious AEs were similar between the ceftaroline and ceftriaxone groups. Additionally, ceftaroline is associated with the risk of discontinuation of the study drug that is similar to that of ceftriaxone; this risk is because of the development of AEs. Although the overall mortality of the ceftaroline group was only 1.81%—which was comparable to that of ceftriaxone group—none of the cases of mortality were associated with the study drug. Therefore, all these findings revealed that ceftaroline is as safe as ceftriaxone for the treatment of CAPs.

A major strength of this meta-analysis is that only RCTs were included, thereby reducing the risk of bias and providing strong evidence. However, this meta-analysis also has several limitations. First, the number of MRSA-associated pneumonia cases was limited in this study. Therefore, the anti-MRSA effect of ceftaroline, which is not owned by ceftriaxone, cannot be elucidated in this meta-analysis.

Second, this meta-analysis had a limited number of studies and patients in subgroup analyses, such as different pathogens among different age groups. Therefore, some differences between the ceftaroline and ceftriaxone groups did not reach statistical significance.

5. Conclusions

In conclusion, based on the findings of this meta-analysis of five RCTs, the clinical efficacy of ceftaroline is similar to that of ceftriaxone for the treatment of CAP. Additionally, ceftaroline was as tolerable as ceftriaxone. However, clinicians should cautiously use ceftaroline in the selected population at high risk of MRSA to avoid the unnecessary coverage of MRSA by ceftaroline. Overall, ceftaroline can be recommended as an appropriate antibiotic therapy for CAP.

Author Contributions: Conceptualization, S.-H.L., S.-P.C., C.-C.L., C.-M.C.; methodology: S.-H.L., S.-P.C., L.-C.L.; writing—original draft preparation, C.-C.L., C.-M.C.; writing—review and editing, C.-M.C.

References

1.   Le Roux, D.M.; Zar, H.J. Community-acquired pneumonia in children—A changing spectrum of disease. *Pediatr. Radiol.* **2017**, *47*, 1392–1398. [CrossRef] [PubMed]

2.   Musher, D.M.; Thorner, A.R. Community-acquired pneumonia. *N. Engl. J. Med.* **2014**, *37*, 1619–1628. [CrossRef] [PubMed]

3.   Peyrani, P.; Mandell, L.; Torres, A.; Tillotson, G.S. The burden of community-acquired bacterial pneumonia in the era of antibiotic resistance. *Expert Rev. Respir. Med.* **2019**, *13*, 139–152. [CrossRef] [PubMed]

4.   Cilloniz, C.; Dominedo, C.; Garcia-Vidal, C.; Torres, A. Community-acquired pneumonia as an emergency condition. *Curr. Opin. Crit. Care* **2018**, *24*, 531–539. [CrossRef] [PubMed]

5.   Leoni, D.; Rello, J. Severe community-acquired pneumonia: Optimal management. *Curr. Opin. Infect. Dis.* **2017**, *30*, 240–247. [CrossRef] [PubMed]

6.   Pereira, J.M.; Goncalves-Pereira, J.; Ribeiro, O.; Baptista, J.P.; Froes, F.; Paiva, J.A. Impact of antibiotic therapy in severe community-acquired pneumonia: Data from the Infauci study. *J. Crit. Care* **2018**, *43*, 183–189. [CrossRef] [PubMed]

7.   Wunderink, R.G.; Yin, Y. Antibiotic Resistance in Community-Acquired Pneumonia Pathogens. *Semin. Respir. Crit. Care Med.* **2016**, *37*, 829–838.

8.   Cilloniz, C.; Dominedo, C.; Nicolini, A.; Torres, A. PES Pathogens in Severe Community-Acquired Pneumonia. *Microorganisms* **2019**, *7*, 49. [CrossRef]

9.   Torres, A.; Chalmers, J.D.; Dela Cruz, C.S.; Dominedo, C.; Kollef, M.; Martin-Loeches, I.; Niederman, M.; Wunderink, R.G. Challenges in severe community-acquired pneumonia: A point-of-view review. *Intensiv. Care Med.* **2019**, *45*, 159–171. [CrossRef]

10.   Thomas, R.; Ferguson, J.; Coombs, G.; Gibson, P.G. Community-acquired methicillin-resistant Staphylococcus aureus pneumonia: A clinical audit. *Respirology* **2011**, *16*, 926–931. [CrossRef]

11.   Chou, C.C.; Shen, C.F.; Chen, S.J.; Chen, H.M.; Wang, Y.C.; Chang, W.S.; Chang, Y.T.; Chen, W.Y.; Huang, C.Y.; Kuo, C.C.; et al. Recommendations and guidelines for the treatment of pneumonia in Taiwan. *J. Microbiol. Immunol. Infect.* **2019**, *52*, 172–199. [CrossRef] [PubMed]

12.   Liu, C.; Bayer, A.; Cosgrove, S.E.; Daum, R.S.; Fridkin, S.K.; Gorwitz, R.J.; Kaplan, S.L.; Karchmer, A.W.; Levine, D.P.; Murray, B.E.; et al. Clinical practice guidelines by the infectious diseases society of America for the treatment of methicillin-resistant *Staphylococcus aureus* infections in adults and children. *Clin. Infect. Dis.* **2011**, *52*, e18–e55. [CrossRef] [PubMed]

13.   Lim, W.S.; Baudouin, S.V.; George, R.C.; Hill, A.T.; Jamieson, C.; Le Jeune, I.; Macfarlane, J.T.; Read, R.C.; Roberts, H.J.; Levy, M.L.; et al. BTS guidelines for the management of community acquired pneumonia in adults: Update 2009. *Thorax* **2009**, *64* (Suppl. 3), iii1–55. [CrossRef]

14.   Pfaller, M.A.; Mendes, R.E.; Duncan, L.R.; Flamm, R.K.; Sader, H.S. In Vitro Activities of Ceftaroline and Comparators against Streptococcus pneumoniae Isolates from U.S. Hospitals: Results from Seven Years of the AWARE Surveillance Program (2010 to 2016). *Antimicrob. Agents Chemother.* **2018**, *62*, e01555-17. [CrossRef] [PubMed]

15. Pfaller, M.A.; Mendes, R.E.; Castanheira, M.; Flamm, R.K.; Jones, R.N.; Sader, H.S. Ceftaroline Activity Tested Against Bacterial Isolates Causing Community-acquired Respiratory Tract Infections and Skin and Skin Structure Infections in Pediatric Patients From United States Hospitals: 2012–2014. *Pediatr. Infect. Dis. J.* **2017**, *36*, 486–491. [CrossRef]

16. Karlowsky, J.A.; Biedenbach, D.J.; Bouchillon, S.K.; Hackel, M.; Iaconis, J.P.; Sahm, D.F. In vitro activity of Ceftaroline against bacterial pathogens isolated from patients with skin and soft tissue and respiratory tract infections in African and Middle Eastern countries: AWARE global surveillance program 2012–2014. *Diagn. Microbiol. Infect. Dis.* **2016**, *86*, 194–199. [CrossRef]

17. Biedenbach, D.J.; Iaconis, J.P.; Sahm, D.F. Comparative in vitro activities of ceftaroline and ceftriaxone against bacterial pathogens associated with respiratory tract infections: Results from the AWARE surveillance study. *J. Antimicrob. Chemother.* **2016**, *71*, 3459–3464. [CrossRef]

18. Sader, H.S.; Farrell, D.J.; Mendes, R.E.; Flamm, R.K.; Castanheira, M.; Jones, R.N. Antimicrobial activity of ceftaroline tested against bacterial isolates causing respiratory tract and skin and skin structure infections in US medical centers in 2013. *Diagn. Microbiol. Infect. Dis.* **2015**, *82*, 78–84. [CrossRef]

19. Poon, H.; Chang, M.H.; Fung, H.B. Ceftaroline fosamil: A cephalosporin with activity against methicillin-resistant *Staphylococcus aureus*. *Clin. Ther.* **2012**, *34*, 743–765. [CrossRef]

20. File, T.M., Jr.; Low, D.E.; Eckburg, P.B.; Talbot, G.H.; Friedland, H.D.; Lee, J.; Llorens, L.; Critchley, I.A.; Thye, D.A.; Pullman, J.; et al. FOCUS 1: A randomized, double-blinded, multicentre, Phase III trial of the efficacy and safety of ceftaroline fosamil versus ceftriaxone in community-acquired pneumonia. *J. Antimicrob. Chemother.* **2011**, *66* (Suppl. 3), iii19–32. [CrossRef]

21. Low, D.E.; File, T.M., Jr.; Eckburg, P.B.; Talbot, G.H.; David Friedland, H.; Lee, J.; Llorens, L.; Critchley, I.A.; Thye, D.A.; Corral, J.; et al. FOCUS 2: A randomized, double-blinded, multicentre, Phase III trial of the efficacy and safety of ceftaroline fosamil versus ceftriaxone in community-acquired pneumonia. *J. Antimicrob. Chemother.* **2011**, *66* (Suppl. 3), iii33–44. [CrossRef] [PubMed]

22. Zhong, N.S.; Sun, T.; Zhuo, C.; D'Souza, G.; Lee, S.H.; Lan, N.H.; Chiang, C.-H.; Wilson, D.; Sun, F.; Iaconis, J.; et al. Ceftaroline fosamil versus ceftriaxone for the treatment of Asian patients with community-acquired pneumonia: A randomised, controlled, double-blind, phase 3, non-inferiority with nested superiority trial. *Lancet Infect. Dis.* **2015**, *15*, 161–171. [CrossRef]

23. Cannavino, C.R.; Nemeth, A.; Korczowski, B.; Bradley, J.S.; O'Neal, T.; Jandourek, A.; Friedland, H.D.; Kaplan, S.L. A Randomized, Prospective Study of Pediatric Patients with Community-acquired Pneumonia Treated with Ceftaroline Versus Ceftriaxone. *Pediatr. Infect. Dis. J.* **2016**, *35*, 752–759. [CrossRef] [PubMed]

24. Blumer, J.L.; Ghonghadze, T.; Cannavino, C.; O'Neal, T.; Jandourek, A.; Friedland, H.D.; Bradley, J. A Multicenter, Randomized, Observer-blinded, Active-controlled Study Evaluating the Safety and Effectiveness of Ceftaroline Compared with Ceftriaxone Plus Vancomycin in Pediatric Patients With Complicated Community-acquired Bacterial Pneumonia. *Pediatr. Infect. Dis. J.* **2016**, *35*, 760–766. [CrossRef] [PubMed]

25. Higgins, J.P.; Altman, D.G.; Gotzsche, P.C.; Juni, P.; Moher, D.; Oxman, A.D.; Savović, J.; Schulz, K.F.; Weeks, L.; Sterne, J.A.C.; et al. The Cochrane Collaboration's tool for assessing risk of bias in randomised trials. *BMJ* **2011**, *343*, d5928. [CrossRef] [PubMed]

26. Fine, M.J.; Auble, T.E.; Yealy, D.M.; Hanusa, B.H.; Weissfeld, L.A.; Singer, D.E.; Coley, C.M.; Marrie, T.J.; Kapoor, W.N. A prediction rule to identify low-risk patients with community-acquired pneumonia. *N. Engl. J. Med.* **1997**, *336*, 243–250. [CrossRef] [PubMed]

27. Rhedin, S.; Lindstrand, A.; Hjelmgren, A.; Ryd-Rinder, M.; Öhrmalm, L.; Tolfvenstam, T.; Örtqvist, Å.; Rotzén-Östlund, M.; Zweygberg-Wirgart, B.; Henriques-Normark, B.; et al. Respiratory viruses associated with community-acquired pneumonia in children: Matched case-control study. *Thorax* **2015**, *70*, 847–853. [CrossRef]

28. Sotgiu, G.; Aliberti, S.; Gramegna, A.; Mantero, M.; Di Pasquale, M.; Trogu, F.; Saderi, L.; Blasi, F. Efficacy and effectiveness of Ceftaroline Fosamil in patients with pneumonia: A systematic review and meta-analysis. *Respir. Res.* **2018**, *19*, 205. [CrossRef]

4

Patient Experience in Home Respiratory Therapies: Where we are and Where to Go

Cátia Caneiras [1,2,†,*], Cristina Jácome [3,4,†], Sagrario Mayoralas-Alises [5,6], José Ramon Calvo [6], João Almeida Fonseca [3,7,8], Joan Escarrabill [9,10,11] and João Carlos Winck [12]

[1] Institute of Environmental Health (ISAMB), Faculty of Medicine, Universidade de Lisboa, 1649-028 Lisboa, Portugal
[2] Healthcare Department, Praxair Portugal Gases, 2601-906 Lisboa, Portugal
[3] CINTESIS-Center for Health Technologies and Information Systems Research, Faculty of Medicine, University of Porto, 4200-450 Porto, Portugal; cjacome@med.up.pt (C.J.); fonseca.ja@gmail.com (J.A.F.)
[4] Respiratory Research and Rehabilitation Laboratory (Lab3R), School of Health Sciences (ESSUA), University of Aveiro, 3810-193 Aveiro, Portugal
[5] Service of Pneumology, Hospital Universitario Moncloa, 28008 Madrid, Spain; sarimayoralas@gmail.com
[6] Healthcare Department, Praxair Spain, 28020 Madrid, Spain; jose_ramon_calvo@praxair.com
[7] MEDCIDS-Department of Community Medicine, Health Information and Decision, Faculty of Medicine, University of Porto, 4200-450 Porto, Portugal
[8] Allergy Unit, Instituto and Hospital CUF, 4460-188 Porto, Portugal
[9] Hospital Clínic de Barcelona, 08036 Barcelona, Spain; ESCARRABILL@clinic.cat
[10] Master Plan for Respiratory Diseases (Ministry of Health) & Observatory of Home Respiratory Therapies (FORES), 08028 Barcelona, Spain
[11] REDISSEC Health Services Research on Chronic Patients Network, Instituto de Salud Carlos III, 28029 Madrid, Spain
[12] Faculty of Medicine, University of Porto, 4200-319 Porto, Portugal; jcwinck@mail.telepac.pt
*   Correspondence: ccaneiras@gmail.com
†   These authors contributed equally to this work.

Abstract: The increasing number of patients receiving home respiratory therapy (HRT) is imposing a major impact on routine clinical care and healthcare system sustainability. The current challenge is to continue to guarantee access to HRT while maintaining the quality of care. The patient experience is a cornerstone of high-quality healthcare and an emergent area of clinical research. This review approaches the assessment of the patient experience in the context of HRT while highlighting the European contribution to this body of knowledge. This review demonstrates that research in this area is still limited, with no example of a prescription model that incorporates the patient experience as an outcome and no specific patient-reported experience measures (PREMs) available. This work also shows that Europe is leading the research on HRT provision. The development of a specific PREM and the integration of PREMs into the assessment of prescription models should be clinical research priorities in the next several years.

Keywords: Long-term oxygen therapy; home mechanical ventilation; patient-reported experience measures; quality of care; healthcare; sustainability

1. Introduction

Long-term oxygen therapy (LTOT) and/or home mechanical ventilation (HMV) are well-established therapies for patients with chronic respiratory failure, such as those with chronic obstructive pulmonary disease (COPD), neuromuscular diseases, and obstructive sleep apnea (OSA), among others. These therapies represent key services in the home respiratory therapy (HRT) provided to these patients.

Increasing numbers of patients receiving HRT are reported not only in Europe but also worldwide [1–5]. Thus, HRT is imposing a major impact on clinical care and healthcare systems. Over the next several years, the main challenge will be to ensure a sustainable healthcare system to continue to guarantee access to HRT while maintaining the quality of care.

According to the World Health Organization, quality of care is defined as "the extent to which health care services provided to individuals and patient populations improve desired health outcomes. In order to achieve this, health care must be safe, effective, timely, efficient, equitable and people-centered" [6]. A necessary step in the process of maintaining and improving quality is to monitor and evaluate the quality of healthcare in routine clinical practice. Based on the reactive, disease-focused, and biomedical model, the indicators of quality have been mainly restricted to traditional clinical metrics. A number of studies conducted over the last few decades have addressed the beneficial effects of HRT on morbidity, mortality, and adverse outcomes, as well as the variations in HRT provision among countries [5,7,8]. However, these metrics alone do not provide a complete picture of HRT quality.

The patient's experience of treatment is a cornerstone of high-quality healthcare [9]. Only by analyzing the relational and functional aspects of the patient experience is it possible to assess the extent to which patients are receiving care that is in line with their preferences, needs, and values. The integration of the patient experience with healthcare delivery and quality evaluation are key steps in moving toward patient-centered and personalized care [10]. As Doyle et al. suggested, the patient's experience is the third pillar of quality, along with clinical safety and effectiveness [11]. However, it is only in recent years that patients' perceptions of healthcare provision have started to receive attention.

This review approaches the assessment of the patient experience in the clinical context of HRT while highlighting the European contribution to this emerging body of knowledge.

2. Patient Experience in the Context of HRT

The patient experience in the context of HRT is reviewed with a focus on two main areas: (1) HRT prescription models and the inclusion of the patient experience as an outcome of these models and (2) methods used to assess the patient experience. To address these two aims, a narrative review was conducted. The search, although not systematic in nature, included searches in electronic databases (PubMed, Medline, ISI Web of Knowledge and Google Scholar), as well as hand searches (expert consultation and a review of the reference lists in the included papers). The databases were searched between July and December 2018 using topic-related terms, such as oxygen therapy, home mechanical ventilation, noninvasive mechanical ventilation, home respiratory therapy, home treatment, chronic respiratory insufficiency, chronic respiratory failure, epidemiology, prescription, quality control, outcomes, patient experience, patient perspective, carers, caregivers, patient-reported experience measure, questionnaires, interviews, and focus groups. There was no time restriction in the literature search, although it was limited to English, Portuguese, or Spanish.

2.1. Prescription Models of HRT

There are a number of studies that have assessed the prescription of HRT. Table 1 summarizes 15 relevant studies on this topic. The majority of the studies ($n = 9$) were conducted from 2009 onward and primarily assessed the prescription of HMV ($n = 10$) [4,5,12–19], followed by LTOT ($n = 6$) [19–24]. The estimated prevalence of HMV (from 2.5 to 23/100,000 population) and of LTOT (from 31.6 to 102/100,000 population) were variable among distinct regions or countries. The estimated prevalence of HMV in Europe was 6.6 per 100,000 people, and Portugal was one of the countries with the highest prevalence [5].

Three studies reported the assessment of HRT prescription at a regional level (Catalan, Spain; Hong Kong, China; Tasmania, Australia), eight at a national level (Sweden, Canada, Poland, Denmark, England, Australia, France, Spain), and four at an international level (two countries, seven countries, 13 European countries, 16 European countries).

Table 1. Studies assessing the prescription of home respiratory therapies.

Author, Year	Region or Country, Years Analyzed	Aim	Method	Data Collection	Results
Ekström et al., 2017 [20]	Sweden, 1987–2015	Long-term oxygen therapy (LTOT): incidence, prevalence, and the quality of prescription and management	Data from the Swedevox registry between 1 January 1987 and 31 December 2015	Data: Birth date, Sex, Primary/secondary causes of LTOT, Follow-up, Stop date and stop cause, PaO_2 air and $PaCO_2$ air, PaO_2 oxygen and $PaCO_2$ oxygen, FEV_1 and VC, World Health Organization performance status, Height and weight, Never/Past/Current smoker, Maintenance treatment with oral corticosteroids, Oxygen dose, Oxygen duration.	23,909 patients on LTOT. 48 respiratory or medicine units. Incidence of LTOT increased from 3.9 to 14.7/100,000 inhabitants over the study time period. In 2015, 2596 patients had ongoing therapeutic LTOT in the registry, a prevalence of 31.6/100,000. Adherence to prescription recommendations and fulfilment of quality criteria were stable or improved over time. Of patients starting LTOT in 2015, 88% had severe hypoxemia and 97% had any degree of hypoxemia; 98% were prescribed oxygen for ≥15 hours/day; 76% had both stationary and mobile oxygen equipment; 75% had a mean $PaO_2 > 8.0$ kPa breathing oxygen; and 98% were non-smokers.
Rose et al., 2015 [12]	Canada, 2012–2013	Home mechanical ventilation (HMV): national data profiling	Survey administered via a web link from August 2012 to April 2013 to service providers delivering care/services to ventilator-assisted individuals requiring daily noninvasive ventilation (NIV) or invasive mechanical ventilation via tracheostomy at home.	Survey content: provider characteristics, including services and education provided; user characteristics (age, ventilation type, primary disorder, duration of ventilation); criteria for initiation and monitoring ventilation effectiveness; equipment (ventilators and interfaces used, ventilator servicing arrangements and backup); training and education (audience, structure, topics, ongoing competency assessment); liaisons and transitions (referral, barriers to transition); follow-up (structure, frequency, location).	Response rate 152/171 (89%). 4334 ventilator-assisted individuals: an estimated prevalence of 12.9/100,000 population. 73% receiving NIV and 18% receiving intermittent mandatory ventilation (9% not reported). Services were delivered by 39 institutional providers and 113 community providers. Various models of ventilator servicing were reported. 64% of providers stated that caregiver competency was a prerequisite for home discharge, but repeated competency assessment and retraining were offered by 45%. Barriers to home transition: insufficient funding for paid caregivers, equipment, and supplies; a shortage of paid caregivers; negotiating public funding arrangements.

Table 1. *Cont.*

Author, Year	Region or Country, Years Analyzed	Aim	Method	Data Collection	Results
Escarrabill et al., 2015 [13]	Catalan Health Service (Spain), 2008–2011	HMV: prevalence and variability in prescriptions	Catalan Health Service (CatSalut) billing database, between 2008 and 2011.	Not reported (NR)	240,760 patients received some type of HRT funded by the public system. 75.8% used continuous positive airway pressure equipment, 17.3% used various forms of oxygen supply, 4.2% used nebulized therapy, 2.5% used HMV, and 0.2% used miscellaneous treatments. 6,867 patients received HMV, 23 users per 100,000 population. Rates of HMV increased by 39% over the study period
Nasiłowski et al., 2015 [14]	Poland, 2000–2010	HMV: trends over the last decade	Questionnaire designed specifically for the study was sent to the heads of nine HMV centers	Survey Content: Center details: location, area of activity (uniregional/multiregional), and year of initiating HMV. Number of subjects treated with HMV in each consecutive year. Overall number of treated subjects, divided into five disease categories: (1) neuromuscular diseases, (2) lung diseases (chronic obstructive pulmonary disease (COPD), bronchiectasis, cystic fibrosis, interstitial diseases), (3) chest-wall diseases (scoliosis, thoracoplasty, ankylosing spondylitis, post-tuberculosis sequelae), (4) hypoventilation syndromes (due to obesity, central congenital hypoventilation syndrome, central sleep apnea), (5) other diseases. Technique of ventilation (invasive and noninvasive). Number of new cases; Overall number of subjects treated with NIV or tracheostomy. Age of the treated subjects, Site where ventilation was initiated: intensive care unit, respiratory department, neurology department, general medicine department, home, or other.	Nine HMV centers, 1495 subjects. Center experience 9 ± 3 years (6–13 years). One center was dedicated specifically to children, Two solely treated adults, and other centers treated subjects irrespective of age. In 2010, prevalence of HMV reached almost 2.5 subjects/100,000. The majority of subjects on HMV suffered from neuromuscular diseases (100% in 2000–2002 to 51% in 2010). Subjects with a diagnosis of respiratory failure due to pulmonary conditions appeared in 2004, and the number of subjects rapidly increased beginning in 2007. In 2010, they accounted for almost 25% of all HMV cases. Hypoventilation syndromes were the third main diagnostic group (4% until 2008, reaching 11% in 2010). Proportion of chest-wall diseases remained ~3%. In 2000 and 2001, ventilation via tracheostomy was exclusively used. The first subjects on NIV were treated in 2002. The number of subjects on NIV was 1/3 in 2004 and then leveled off for the following five years, followed by a rapid increase until 2010, when the proportions of subjects treated with NIV and tracheostomy equalized. Since 2008, the number of new cases treated noninvasively surpassed the number of new cases treated with invasive ventilation, and in 2010, the total number of subjects in both groups was virtually the same.

Table 1. *Cont.*

Author, Year	Region or Country, Years Analyzed	Aim	Method	Data Collection	Results
Garner et al., 2013 [15]	Australia and New Zealand, 2002–2004	HMV	HMV centers that had prescribed HMV for more than three months to more than five adult patients. A designed survey.	Survey Content: (1) Institutional details: location, type (e.g., tertiary), funding (e.g., government), patient catchment, years of service; (2) Criteria for HMV prescription by disease group (e.g., COPD); (3) HMV service details: number of patients receiving HMV, staffing levels, methods of implementation by location/tests utilized/staff involved, methods of follow-up by location/tests utilized/staff involved (0–3 grading from never to always), annual clinic attendances, presence of an outreach service; (4) Individual patient data (if available): age, gender, primary indication for HMV, duration of therapy, adherence to therapy, interface, machine settings (mode, inspiratory positive airway pressure, expiratory positive airway pressure, back-up rate); (5) Local database: current database for that center, data collected, what data should be collected, support for creation of a national database, center willing to participate; (6) Problems encountered with setting up an HMV service.	28 centers (82%) responded, providing data on 2725 patients. Prevalence of HMV was 9.9 patients/100,000 in Australia and 12.0 patients/100,000 in New Zealand. Variation existed among Australian states (range 4–13 patients/100,000) correlating with population density ($r = 0.82$, $p < 0.05$). The commonest indications for treatment were obesity hypoventilation syndrome (31%) and neuromuscular disease (30%). COPD was an uncommon indication (8%). No consensus on indications for commencing treatment was found.

Table 1. *Cont.*

Author, Year	Region or Country, Years Analyzed	Aim	Method	Data Collection	Results
Ringbaek et al., 2013 [21]	Denmark, 2001–2010	(LTOT: incidence, prevalence, treatment modalities, and survival in COPD.	Danish Oxygen Register in the period from 01 January 2001 to 31 December 2010: information on patients on home oxygen therapy, their prescriptions, and termination of therapy. National Health Services Central Register: information on diagnosis for LTOT and on vital status up to 31 December 2011.	NR	On 31 Dec 2001, a total of 2247 COPD patients (42.0/100,000) were receiving LTOT. The number of patients on LTOT had increased constantly to reach a prevalence of 48.1/100,000 in 2010. Incidence of oxygen therapy increased insignificantly from 30.5 to 32.2/100,000. The majority of COPD patients were women and older than 70 years of age. The mean age of patients who started LTOT during the study period increased from 73.4 ± 9 years to 74.8 ± 9.7 years. Most of the COPD patients were prescribed oxygen therapy by a hospital doctor immediately after an acute hospitalization, and the number of prescriptions from general practitioners was continuously declining toward zero during the study period. An increasing number of the COPD patients were prescribed oxygen at least 15 h daily and had delivered oxygen concentrator and mobile oxygen, whereas, in general, the oxygen flow remained low (≤ 1.5 L/minute). Compared with men, women started LTOT more often in connection with hospitalization and more often stopped LTOT within the first 6 months. Women were prescribed a lower oxygen flow than men and the treatment was more often specified to take place for 15–24 h per day.

Table 1. *Cont.*

Author, Year	Region or Country, Years Analyzed	Aim	Method	Data Collection	Results
Mandal et al., 2013 [16]	England, NA	HMV: prevalence of sleep and ventilation diagnostic and treatment services	A short survey delivered by email to 101 NHS Hospitals	Survey content: 10-item survey, focused on diagnostic services and HMV provision: (a) availability of diagnostics; (b) funding; (c) patient groups.	76 (68%) responses received; 42 (55%) trusts reported the provision of an HMV service. Only 65% of units charged for the delivery of an HMV service, with 12% of these services commissioned by an external provider. Median set-up frequency for the units charging was 42 patients per annum (interquartile range 23–73), whereas those units that failed to charge had a median of 11 (interquartile range 4–22). Of all the HMV set-ups, 67% were for obesity-related respiratory failure and COPD, with the other restrictive lung conditions forming the remainder
Serginson et al., 2009 [22]	Australia, 2004–2005	LTOT: prescription and costs	Data from all LTOT services in Australian Government's departments and health services (state and federal). Centralized departments managing state budgets for LTOT provided costs (for the financial year 2004–2005) and patient numbers (point prevalence in 2005). If centralized data were not available, regional departments administering LTOT services were contacted.	Data: Costs were defined as "equipment only" (fees paid to oxygen companies) or "equipment and administrative" (wages and non-labor costs of administering programs included).	20,127 patients (100/100,000) through 59 different services at a cost of over $31 million. Prescription rates for LTOT per 100,000 population within each state ranged from 44 to 133, a threefold difference. Costs of LTOT per patient prescribed per year funded by individual states and territories ranged from $1014 to $2574. The cost of oxygen concentrators averaged $85 per month (range, $29–$109), portable oxygen ranged from $16 to $35 per month without refills, and, with a conserver included, $55 (two refills) to $166 unlimited refills) per month. All services provided concentrators for home use. Portable oxygen was funded in all states, except one (where it was limited to children and patients waiting for heart or lung transplants).

Table 1. *Cont.*

Author, Year	Region or Country, Years Analyzed	Aim	Method	Data Collection	Results
Jones et al., 2007 [23]	Tasmania (Australia), 2002–2004	LTOT	Records of all patients receiving Tasmanian Government-funded LTOT between December 2002 and April 2004	Data: Recipient demographics, Indications for LTOT, Oxygen prescription, Time to follow-up. The service provider provided usage reports and costs.	April 2004: 490 patients receiving LTOT Rate of 102/100,000; Median age at prescription of LTOT was 71.5 (range 0.7–97.2) years, and 54% of patients were female. Oxygen was prescribed for 267 patients (54%) during hospitalization, although only 192 of these patients (72%) met criteria for oxygen use at this time. LTOT was prescribed by respiratory physicians for 248 patients (51%) and by other hospital physicians for most of the remaining patients (39%). Data on indications were available for 430 patients (88%), and COPD accounted for 48% of prescriptions, but this proportion varied regionally. Median time to reassessment was 5.5 (range, 0.1–116) months, but varied between regions. Usage data were available for 175 patients (41%) using oxygen concentrators in April 2004. Of these 175 patients, 122 (70%) were prescribed oxygen for COPD. In this group, the median use was 18.3 (range, 0.38–24) hours per day; however, 36 (30%) had a median use < 15 hours/day.

Table 1. *Cont.*

Author, Year	Region or Country, Years Analyzed	Aim	Method	Data Collection	Results
Lloyd-Owen et al., 2005 [5]	16 European countries (Austria, Belgium, Denmark, Finland, France, Germany, Greece, Ireland, Italy, Netherlands, Norway, Poland, Portugal, Spain, Sweden, UK), 2001–2002	HMV: patterns of use across Europe	Questionnaire of center details, HMV user characteristics and equipment choices sent to selected HMV centers	Survey Content: Center (type of institution and year of starting HMV), Number of HMV users on 01 July 2001, Users' characteristics (sex, age, and time on HMV). Users' causes for respiratory failure: (1) Lung: lung and airway diseases: COPD, cystic fibrosis, bronchiectasis, pulmonary fibrosis, and pediatric diseases, including bronchopulmonary dysplasia; (2) Thor: thoracic cage abnormalities: early-onset kyphoscoliosis, tuberculosis sequelae such as thoracoplasty, obesity hypoventilation syndrome, and sequelae of lung resection; (3) Neur: neuromuscular diseases: muscular dystrophy, motor neuron disease (including amyotrophic lateral sclerosis), post-polio kyphoscoliosis, central hypoventilation, spinal cord damage, and phrenic nerve paralysis. Type of ventilator and interface used.	329 centers completed surveys, 21,526 HMV users; Estimated prevalence of HMV was 6.6/100,000 in the 16 European countries. Differences between countries in the relative proportions of (1) lung and neuromuscular patients using HMV and (2) the use of tracheostomies in lung and neuromuscular HMV users. Lung users were linked to an HMV duration of <1 year, thoracic cage users with 6–10 years of ventilation and neuromuscular users with a duration of ≥6 years. Almost all of the HMV users had positive pressure ventilators, with only 0.005% (79 users) having other types. Volume preset positive pressure ventilators were used the least for lung problems and most frequently for neurological problems (% volume: Lung 15%; Thor 28%; Neur 41%). Overall, 13% of the survey population had ventilation via a tracheostomy with the highest percentage in neuromuscular patients (Neur 24%; Thor 5%; Lung 8%).
Chu et al., 2004 [17]	Hong Kong (China), 2002	HMV	Survey to consultants of respiratory medicine in all adult medical departments of Hong Kong Hospital Authority hospitals to report their adult patients (>18 years) who had ever been managed by HMV	Survey content: demographic data, mode of ventilation (non-invasive or tracheostomy ventilation), underlying disease, indications for HMV, time of starting ventilation, time and reason of stopping ventilation, if any, in the follow-up period.	249 cases reported to the survey from 14 centers of adult respiratory medicine; 156 males (62.7%) and 93 females (37.3%) with a mean age of 62.7 ± 13.8 years; 80% of HMV cases were under the care of six major centers. 197 cases were continuing with HMV, corresponding to ~2.9 HMV users per 100,000 population. The majority (n = 236, 94.8%) were treated by noninvasive ventilation (NIV), with the remaining 13 patients (5.2%) receiving tracheostomy ventilation. All NIVs were provided by bilevel pressure-support ventilators. All tracheostomized cases were put on HMV after repeated failures to wean. The disease conditions for which HMV was prescribed: COPD (121, 48.6%); Complicated obstructive sleep apnea/obesity hypoventilation syndrome (43, 17.2%); and Restrictive thoracic disorders (85, 34.1%).

Table 1. *Cont.*

Author, Year	Region or Country, Years Analyzed	Aim	Method	Data Collection	Results
Fauroux et al., 2003 [18]	France, 2000	Domiciliary non-invasive mechanical ventilation (NIMV) in children	Anonymous national cross-sectional Survey A postal questionnaire sent by the Paediatric Group of the National Home Care Organization (ANTADIR) in 1999 to all 64 senior pediatric respiratory, neurology, and intensive care physicians in France. Patients aged < 18 years and receiving home NIMV were included in the study.	All physicians taking care of children with NIMV were sent a second questionnaire in 2000. The specific information requested on each patient included: Sex and date of birth; Primary and secondary diagnosis; Symptoms that justified NIMV; Age at onset of NIMV; Type of nasal mask, ventilatory mode, and concurrent use of oxygen therapy; Investigations performed before initiating of NIMV and during follow-up.	102 patients from 15 centers: 4/15 centers cared for 84% of patients; 7% of patients were under 3 years; 35% were 4–11 years; and 58% were >12 years. Underlying diagnoses included neuromuscular disease (34%), obstructive sleep apnea and/or craniofacial abnormalities (30%), cystic fibrosis (17%), congenital hypoventilation (9%), scoliosis (8%), and other disorders (2%). NIMV was started because of nocturnal hypoventilation (67%), acute exacerbation (28%), and/or failure to thrive (21%). Volume-targeted ventilation was preferred in restrictive disorders (56%) and central hypoventilation (56%), while pressure support ventilation (PSV) was preferred in cystic fibrosis (71%). Patients with obstructive sleep apnea and/or craniofacial abnormalities were ventilated with continuous positive airway pressure (45%) or bilevel PSV (52%).

Table 1. *Cont.*

Author, Year	Region or Country, Years Analyzed	Aim	Method	Data Collection	Results
				Characteristics of the respirologists: Date of birth; How many years they had been practicing respiratory medicine; Number of patients for whom they prescribed oxygen for the first time or for renewal purposes over the previous month.	81% of respondents individualized the oxygen prescription at rest. Resting SaO_2 was most commonly targeted at 90–91%.
Wijkstra et al., 2001 [24]	Seven countries (Brazil, Canada, France, Italy, Spain, Netherlands, USA), NR	LTOT: prescription	Questionnaire mailed to 100 randomly selected respirologists from a list of respiratory specialists belonging to a professional organization in each country	Prescription of oxygen at rest; Whether they prescribed a standard oxygen flow rate for all their patients or whether they individualized flow rates with or without specific testing of each patient; How the recommended oxygen flow at rest was chosen (either tested at rest or tested during exercise); The position (sitting, semirecumbent, supine) in which the patients were tested, the target level of arterial oxygen saturation (SaO_2) used to establish an oxygen prescription and the percentage of time during the measure in which this target had to be achieved. Prescription of oxygen during sleep and exercise; How they prescribed oxygen during sleep and exercise; The type of exercise test (walking, laboratory testing) used to establish the exercise prescription; The target level of saturation during exercise and the percentage of time during the test in which this target had to be achieved.	The approach to night prescription varied. Respirologists in Canada and the USA increased the resting SaO_2 by 1–2 L/min during sleep, while those in Spain used the resting flow for the night prescription (62%). Respirologists in the Netherlands, France, and Italy individualized the night prescription more frequently. Although oxygen during exercise was individualized in most countries (74%), significant differences remained among countries. 62% of respirologists (62%) aimed to achieve an SaO_2 of 90–91% during exercise, while 70% of all respirologists tried to achieve the desired SaO_2 for 90% of the test.

Table 1. *Cont.*

Author, Year	Region or Country, Years Analyzed	Aim	Method	Data Collection	Results
de Lucas Ramos et al., 2000 [4]	Spain, 1998–1999	HMV: prescription	Questionnaire mailed to the respiratory medicine departments of 200 hospitals in the public health system	Survey Content: Center name, Year of initiation of the MV program, Number of patients in the first year, Number of patients in the current year. Diagnosis: Neuromuscular disease, Thoracic cage disease, Hypoventilation-obesity syndrome, COPD, Other. Ventilation type: Volumetric, BI-level Positive Airway Pressure, Interface, Nasal mask, Conventional, Personalized, Tracheostomy, Mouthpiece.	43 hospitals, 1821 patients; 813 patients had restrictive disease due to thoracic cage disease, 452 neuromuscular disease, 271 hypoventilation-obesity syndrome, 162 COPD, and 123 other diseases/conditions. 965 (53%) used pressure support devices and 856 (47%) used volumetric ventilators. 1320 conventional nasal mask, 336 personalized nasal mask, 118 tracheostomy, 41 facial mask, six mouthpiece.

Table 1. *Cont.*

Author, Year	Region or Country, Years Analyzed	Aim	Method	Data Collection	Results
					Information was easier to obtain for LTOT than for HMV. In all countries, both adults and children received LTOT at home for lung diseases and other less common problems, such as chest-wall deformities and sequelae of tuberculosis. Oxygen concentrators were used preferentially in all countries except Italy (80% of the patients received liquid oxygen), Denmark, Spain, and the Netherlands (cylinders were used by 80% of the patients).
	13 European countries (Belgium, Denmark, England, France,			Questionnaire content: Home treatments (LTOT, HMV); Prescribers; Practical organization of home care (supply of material, supervision of patients and equipment).	Both adults and children received HMV at home for chronic lung disease, neuromuscular disease, chest-wall deformities, and central
Fauroux et al., 1994 [19]	Germany, Ireland, Italy, Netherlands, Norway, Poland, Spain, Sweden, Switzerland), 1992	Home care of chronic respiratory insufficiency	Questionnaire at the end of 1992.	Information on patients: diagnostic information (either obstructive, restrictive, or mixed pulmonary disease); Age; Sex; Equipment supplied; Service provided; Therapeutic schedules.	hypoventilation in all countries, except in Denmark and Poland, where this treatment is almost unknown in the home. Home ventilator treatment was generally performed by volume-cycled ventilators. National prescription rules existed in some parts of Spain, Switzerland, and Belgium. In other countries, such as Germany, prescriptions relied on recommendations elaborated by specialists or international guidelines. Service and equipment were provided by national organizations, health services, commercial companies, or hospitals. Home supervision of the patient was performed by a nurse and/or a doctor and equipment maintenance by a technician.

Most studies included both children and adult patients in their analysis. Only one of the studies specifically focused on a pediatric population [18]. Questionnaires, having been used in 10 studies, were the preferred method of data collection. In five studies, existing databases from HRT registries or health services were used. Irrespective of the data collection method used, data on users (age, sex, and diagnosis), type and duration of respiratory therapy, and equipment and interfaces were the most commonly recorded. None of the 15 studies reported the patient's experience with HRT.

2.2. Assessment of Patient Experience

Assessing the patient experience has become a common approach to describing healthcare from the patient's point of view, evaluating the process of care, and measuring the outcome of care [25–27]. Both quantitative and qualitative methods are being used to assess patients' perception. Self-reported questionnaires, individual interviews, and focus groups are among the most frequently used methods of collecting data.

2.2.1. Patient-Reported Experience Measures

The development of self-reported questionnaires, namely, patient-reported experience measures (PREMs) and patient-reported outcome measures (PROMs), has exponentially increased in the last several years. These two types of questionnaires collect information about the patient's perspective but with distinct purposes. A PREM evaluates patients' perception of their personal experience of the healthcare received, while a PROM assesses the perception of their health status and health-related quality of life [10,28]. A combination of PROMs and PREMs is essential to fully understand the performance of healthcare systems. Moreover, both measures are useful to provide a patient-centered perspective of healthcare, but PREMs are more adequate to assess experience with healthcare.

Distinct instruments to assess the patient's experience with healthcare are available. Table 2 summarizes 14 instruments designed to assess the patient's experience with the provision of care in different clinical settings [29–34], hospital [35–38], primary care [39,40], intermediate care [41], and community [33,41]. The majority of such instruments are generic and designed to be used for a diverse range of health conditions. However, two of the described questionnaires were specifically developed for patients with chronic diseases [29,34], and one was intended particularly for patients with COPD [30]. The majority of PREMs were developed to target adult patients and tested in patients who were at least 15 years old. Only two developed instruments were tested with the carers of children [31,39]. English is the most common language used, with some instruments also in Norwegian [31,38,39], Italian [35,41], and Spanish [29]. Most instruments already had some of their psychometric properties explored, namely, their reliability and validity.

None of the instruments above were specifically designed to assess the patient's experience with HRT. However, a recent European Respiratory Society (ERS)/European Lung Foundation (ELF) survey was conducted across 11 European countries and assessed the attitudes and preferences of 687 patients on HMV and those of 100 carers [42]. A questionnaire was specifically developed for this study in eight languages (English, German, Dutch, Spanish, Italian, Portuguese, Greek, and French) and explored four areas: (1) patients' demographic and clinical characteristics; (2) issues influencing compliance, such as interface comfort, abilities to travel, sleep, and socialize with a ventilator, type and technical functioning of the ventilator (e.g., alarms, ability to operate and change settings, on/off switches, and electricity consumption); (3) support, training, and education; and (4) requests for improved devices and support.

Today, it is possible to evaluate a patient's perception of the HRT received using one of the described PREMs. Nevertheless, in the near future, the aim should be to develop a specific PREM to assess patients' personal experience with HRT.

Table 2. Instruments designed to assess patient's experience with the provision of care.

Instrument	Population	Setting	Language	Concepts	Structure	Measurement Properties
CEFIT: Care Experience Feedback Improvement Tool [36]	Tested in 802 patients (≥18 years) with healthcare experience.	Hospital	English	Safe, Timely, System navigation, Caring, Effective.	Five questions scored using a five-point scale, from 1 (never) to 5 (always).	Reliability Validity
COPD PREM9: disease-specific patient-reported experience measure in COPD [28,30]	Tested in 174 adult patients with COPD.	Clinical settings (e.g., pulmonary rehabilitation, nurse-led clinics, or GP annual reviews)	English	Everyday life with COPD, Everyday care in COPD, Self-management of COPD, exacerbations.	Nine questions scored using a six-point scale, from 0 (good experience) to 5 (bad experience).	Reliability Validity
GS-PEQ: Generic Short Patient Experiences Questionnaire [31]	Tested in 1324 patients (including outpatients undergoing rehabilitation and carers of children).	Services provided in a range of specialist healthcare (in- and out-patient)	Norwegian	Outcome, Clinician services, User involvement, Incorrect treatment, Information, Organization, Accessibility.	10 questions scored using a five-point scale, from 1 (Not at all/Not important) to 5 (To a very large extent/Of utmost importance).	Not reported
howRwe (how are we doing?)questionnaire: short generic patient experience questionnaire [32,43]	Tested in 828 patients in an orthopedic pre-operative assessment clinic [32] and in 90 adult patients (≥18 years) from general practices (10 with COPD) [43].	Generic, applicable without change across all patient categories and care settings, including primary, secondary, community, emergency, domiciliary, and social care.	English Dutch	Clinical care (kindness and communication), Organization of care (promptness and organization).	Four items scored using a four-point scale from 0 (poor) to 3 (excellent).	Reliability Validity

Table 2. *Cont.*

Instrument	Population	Setting	Language	Concepts	Structure	Measurement Properties
Health Services OutPatient Experience (HSOPE): global outcome measure of perceived patient-centeredness of the outpatient healthcare pathway [35]	Tested in 1532 adult outpatients (≥16 years) receiving care (including rehabilitation).	Hospital	Italian	Perceived technical effectiveness of the staff, Information on modalities of the outpatient visit, on the visit outcomes, and the course of the healthcare pathway, Relational aspects of outpatient–staff interaction, Involvement in decision making.	10 statements scored using a five-point Likert scale from 1 (never) to 5 (always) 1 item scored using a 10-point scale from 1 (very dissatisfied) to 10 (very satisfied). Three sociodemographic questions (sex, age, and residence). One question about suggestions to improve outpatient visits.	Reliability Validity
Intermediate care-IC-PREMs: Bed-Based Patient-Reported Experience Measure [41]	Tested in 1832 adult patients.	Bed-based IC services	English Italian	Goal Setting, Empowerment, Self-Management, Care-Planning, Transitions, Decision Making, Communication.	15 questions scored using two, three, or four response categories.	Reliability Validity
IC-PREMs: home-based (and reablement-based) Patient-Reported Experience Measure [41]	Tested in 4627 adult patients.	Home-based or reablement IC services	English Italian	Goal Setting, Empowerment, Self-Management, Care-Planning, Transitions, Decision Making, Communication.	15 questions scored using two, three, or four response categories.	Reliability Validity

Table 2. *Cont.*

Instrument	Population	Setting	Language	Concepts	Structure	Measurement Properties
IEXPAC, Instrument for Evaluation of the Experience of Chronic Patients [29]	Tested in 356 patients (≥16 years) with chronic diseases (20% with COPD).	Health and social services	Spanish	Type and scope of patient and professional interactions oriented to patient activation. Patient's self-management capacity of his/her wellbeing resulting from the interventions received. New relational model of the patient with the system through the internet or with partners in group intervention.	11 + 1 items scored using a five-point scale from 0 (never) to 10 (always). Since 2018, a new version with 11 + 4 items is used, with three additional items.	Reliability Validity
LifeCourse experience tool [33]	Tested in 607 adult patients with emergency department and in-patient utilization, advanced primary diagnosis of heart failure, cancer, or dementia.	Home, Nursing Homes, Assisted living	English	Care Team, Communication, Care Goals.	22 items scored using a four-point scale from 1 (Never or Strongly Disagree) to 4 (Always or Strongly Agree).	Reliability Validity
Multidimensional Semantic Patient Experience Measurement Questionnaire [37]	Tested in 60 patients (≥15 years) undergoing a magnetic resonance scan.	Hospital	English	Evaluation/valence, Potency/control, Activity/arousal, Novelty.	12 rating scales using a seven-point bipolar attribute rating scales: 'extremely', 'quite', 'slightly', 'neither', 'slightly', 'quite', and 'extremely'.	Reliability

Table 2. *Cont.*

Instrument	Population	Setting	Language	Concepts	Structure	Measurement Properties
PEQ: Patient experience questionnaire 2001 [39]	Tested in 1092 patients (1-91 years)/carers	Primary care	Norwegian	Communication, Emotions, Short-term outcome, Barriers, Relations with auxiliary staff.	Total 18 items: Four items using a five-point scale from 1 ('no more' or 'nothing') to 5 ('much more' or 'a lot'). 10 items using a five-point scale from 1 (disagree completely) to 5 (agree completely). Four items were formed on seven-point scales.	Reliability Validity
PEQ: Patient Experiences Questionnaire 2004 [38]	Tested in 19578 patients (≥16 years) with experience with surgical wards and wards of internal medicine	Hospital	Norwegian	Information on future complaints, Nursing services, Communication, Information examinations, Contact with next-of-kin, Doctor services, Hospital and equipment, Information medication, Organization, General satisfaction.	35 items with 10-point ordinal response scales from 1 (negative) to 10 (positive).	Reliability Validity
PACIC: Patient Assessment of Chronic Illness Care [34,44]	Tested in 4108 adult patients with diabetes, chronic pain, heart failure, asthma, coronary artery disease.	Chronic care management	English	Patient activation, Delivery system design, Goal setting, Problem solving, Follow-up/coordination. Focuses on the receipt of patient-centered care and self-management behaviors.	20 items using a five-point scale from 1 (Almost Never) to 5 (Almost Always).	Reliability Validity

Table 2. *Cont.*

Instrument	Population	Setting	Language	Concepts	Structure	Measurement Properties
ACES-SF: Ambulatory Care Experiences Survey [40]	Tested in 49,861 adult patients.	Primary care	English	Quality of physician–patient interaction, Health promotion support, Care coordination, Organizational access, Office staff interactions, An additional item to assess patients' willingness to recommend the physician to family and friends.	18 items using continuous responses: Never, Almost never, sometimes, Usually, Almost always, Always; or Yes, definitely, Yes, somewhat, No, definitely not; or Definitely yes, Probably yes, Not sure, Probably not, Definitely not.	Reliability Validity

2.2.2. Individual Interviews and Focus Groups

Qualitative studies that explore the experience of patients receiving HRT are still limited in the literature. Nevertheless, the literature review revealed some studies that explored the experience of patients living with COPD, pulmonary fibrosis, and OSA. These studies specifically focused on patients' needs and the adaptation process to respiratory therapies. Two studies explored the patient's experience with LTOT [45,46], and the others assessed the patient's experience with non-invasive ventilation [47–51]. These studies were conducted in the United States of America [45,47], New Zealand [48,49], the United Kingdom [50], Sweden [51], and Spain [46] and included both adult patients and carers. Two reviews were also found on the needs of patients with COPD and were also used in the present analysis [52,53].

From the analysis of these studies, it was possible to clearly identify education, training, support, and carer involvement as important key-points in facilitating a patient's treatment experience and subsequent adherence. Below, each one of these four key-points is described in detail.

Education: on the basis of the perspectives of patients, it is apparent that education is crucial for defining clear expectations about the treatment and motivating patient adherence. The main education topics raised by patients receiving respiratory therapies are related to disease self-management (e.g., COPD, OSA); physical effects and potential clinical benefits of the respiratory therapy; risks of not using the respiratory therapy; guidance on the use and function of equipment (e.g., continuous positive airway pressure (CPAP) devices, oxygen concentrators, how to use pulse oximeters and adjust flow with exertion); side effects and guidance on its management (skin protection, dry mouth, nasal congestion, irritated eyes); traveling with equipment; follow-up appointments; and assistance with financial elements (e.g., how to claim electricity costs) [45,46,49,50].

Training: formal training on appropriate equipment use has been suggested to be an important strategy for improving adherence [46–51]. Healthcare professionals need to introduce the device, explore possible practical problems, and give advice/help to solve these problems. In their initial experiences with respiratory therapy, patients should have a hands-on demonstration for setting up the device, trialing different masks/pressures, making mask adjustments, conquering different side-effects, and finding the best position for the tubing or machine (also considering the loudness of the device). Regular follow up visits or phone calls are important to assess practical problems being experienced (e.g., pressure from the mask, mask leakage, disturbing noise, and difficulties changing sleeping positions) and to discuss effective strategies to address them.

Support: establishing a trustworthy relationship with healthcare professionals after the initiation of respiratory therapy is perceived as helpful by patients, and these relationships positively influence their adherence [46]. Healthcare professionals need to foster a non-judgmental environment in which patients have opportunities to ask questions, share concerns and feelings, feel listened to, and feel understood. This is particularly important following the initiation of therapy [47], as questions or concerns are more likely to arise during the first days or weeks of treatment [49,52]. These opportunities can arise during regular follow-up visits, scheduled follow-up phone calls, and through access to a 24-h hotline [47].

Carer involvement: carers provide substantial care (emotional, physical) to the individual on a daily basis and, most of the time, live in the same house as the patient. On the basis of their important role in patients' lives, carer involvement has been found to be essential to patients receiving HRT [45–48,50–53]. Patients recognize that carers play a major role in their treatment by helping them manage the disease and adapt to the equipment (e.g., verbal reminders, encouragement, setting up the machine, making mask adjustments, reassurance of therapy benefits). Carers themselves recognize their need for information regarding aspects of the disease and benefits of the HRT [47]. Carer involvement is thus perceived by all stakeholders as an essential component of education and training from the beginning of treatment [45,47,48,50–53], and it is generally associated with positive results, namely, the patients' adoption and adherence to HRT [47,53].

3. Discussion

This comprehensive review is a first critical step toward the assessment of the patient experience in the clinical context of HRT. It demonstrates that research in this area is still limited, with no example of an HRT prescription model that incorporates the patient experience as an outcome and with no specific PREM available. This review also shows that European countries have been involved in HRT provision research from an early stage.

Most of the research on the assessment of HRT prescription models has been conducted within the last decade and mainly in European countries, highlighting the emergent interest and Europe's leading position in this area of health research. In addition, HMV has attracted more attention from the scientific community in comparison with LTOT. Questionnaires were found to be the preferred method for data collection, however, existing databases from HRT registries or health services have also been used. Databases in comparison with questionnaires have the advantage of generating more representative data and may be a method of choice in future studies. The patient experience has not been examined in the assessment of the prescription models presented. While this reality was expected from the oldest studies, it was quite a surprising result for those from the last decade. These results show that, until now, the assessment of patients' perceptions has not been seen as a priority in the assessment of prescription models. Unfortunately, this is also a reality in other health contexts and settings [10]. The Organisation for Economic Co-operation and Development (OECD) and Europe in "Health at a Glance: Europe 2018" reported critical gaps in the data on patient-reported experience, and they recommended collecting data on the patient experience from any doctor in ambulatory care settings [10]. Thus, future studies on the provision of HRT should address this important gap in the literature.

To address this gap, we need to be aware of the current methods being used to assess the patient experience. Different instruments used at distinct levels of healthcare are available and described in this review. These instruments were developed to be completed by adult patients and, in some cases, by carers of children. In our opinion, although the carers' perspective is, of course, incredibly valuable, it should do not replace the children's experience. The development of PREMs for pediatric populations is crucial to the collection of information on the experience and outcome of children's care. Additionally, as previously mentioned, none of the instruments have been specifically designed to assess the patient's experience with HRT. The development of a specific PREM for this health context should be a research priority in the upcoming years. The most commonly assessed domains in the described instruments, including the ERS/ELF survey, together with the key facilitators of the patient's treatment experience, can be used as important sources of data to inform the development of a comprehensive instrument. Access to information and support, implementation of effective and clear communication, active participation in shared decision making, enhanced accessibility and navigability across the healthcare system for patients and families, particularly across transitional care, and management of polypharmacy are known to influence the patient experience in other healthcare settings and could be topics of interest to be included in future PREMs for patients on HRT [54]. Future studies should explore which of these raised topics are indeed meaningful for patients and carers.

On the basis of qualitative studies, it was found that education, training, support, and carer involvement were important key-points in facilitating the patient's treatment experience and adherence. This knowledge comes mainly from the perspective of adult patients with COPD, pulmonary fibrosis, and OSA receiving CPAP and from their carers. These studies were conducted in five countries (three from Europe) [45–53]. Thus, this evidence may not completely apply to the experience of younger patients (including children) and that of their carers or to patients with other diseases and other treatment modalities (e.g., Bilevel Positive Pressure Airway, LTOT) and from other countries/continents. Considering these identified gaps, the experience of other patients receiving HRT could be explored in future studies. The identified key-points may inform the development process of semi-structured guides of focus groups or individual interviews to be used in these exploratory studies.

4. Conclusions

To the authors' best knowledge, this is the first published work to review the emerging topic of the patient experience in the clinical context of HRT and give important insights into the status of this clinical research area while also pointing out possible directions in which to move to realize patient-centered care. The assessment of the patient experience is in its early stages, and further research is needed to integrate these measures with routine healthcare delivery and the core set of healthcare quality indicators, as well as and to drive quality improvements in HRT.

Author Contributions: Conceptualization, C.C., C.J., J.A.F., J.E., and J.C.W.; writing—original draft preparation, C.C. and C.J.; writing-review and editing, S.M.A., J.R.C., J.A.F., J.E., and J.C.W.; project administration, C.C., S.M.A., J.R.C., and J.C.W.

References

1. Cranston, J.; Crockett, A.; Moss, J.; Alpers, J. Domiciliary oxygen for chronic obstructive pulmonary disease. *Cochrane Database Syst. Rev.* **2005**, *4*, CD001744. [CrossRef] [PubMed]
2. Annane, D.; Orlikowski, D.; Chevret, S. Nocturnal mechanical ventilation for chronic hypoventilation in patients with neuromuscular and chest wall disorders. *Cochrane Database Syst. Rev.* **2014**, *12*, CD001941. [CrossRef] [PubMed]
3. Melo, I. Alguns dados sobre a Assistência Respiratória Domiciliária em Portugal. *Rev. Port. Pneumol.* **1997**, *3*, 481–492. [CrossRef]
4. De Lucas Ramos, P.; Rodríguez González-Moro, J.M.; Santa-Cruz Siminiani, A.; Cubillo Marcos, J.M.; Paz González, L. Estado actual de la ventilación mecánica domiciliaria en España: Resultados de una encuesta de ámbito nacional. *Arch. Bronconeumol.* **2000**, *36*, 545–550. (In Spanish) [CrossRef]
5. Lloyd-Owen, S.J.; Donaldson, G.C.; Ambrosino, N.; Escarabill, J.; Farre, R.; Fauroux, B.; Robert, D.; Schoenhofer, B.; Simonds, A.K.; Wedzicha, J.A. Patterns of home mechanical ventilation use in Europe: Results from the Eurovent survey. *Eur. Respir. J.* **2005**, *25*, 1025–1031. [CrossRef] [PubMed]
6. World Health Organization. What is Quality of Care and Why Is It Important? Available online: http://www.who.int/maternal_child_adolescent/topics/quality-of-care/definition/en/ (accessed on 11 April 2019).
7. Simonds, A.K. Home Mechanical Ventilation: An Overview. *Ann. Am. Thorac. Soc.* **2016**, *13*, 2035–2044. [CrossRef]
8. Dogan, O.T.; Turkyilmaz, S.; Berk, S.; Epozturk, K.; Akkurt, I. Effects of long-term non-invasive home mechanical ventilation on chronic respiratory failure. *Curr. Med. Res. Opin.* **2010**, *26*, 2229–2236. [CrossRef]
9. NHS Department of Health. *High Quality Care for All: NHS Next Stage Review Final Report*; Norwich, UK, 2008. Available online: https://assets.publishing.service.gov.uk/government/uploads/system/uploads/attachment_data/file/228836/7432.pdf (accessed on 11 April 2019).
10. OECD/EU. Health at a Glance: Europe 2018: State of Health in the EU Cycle. OECD Publishing: Paris, France, 2018. Available online: https://doi.org/10.1787/health_glance_eur-2018-en (accessed on 11 April 2019).
11. Doyle, C.; Lennox, L.; Bell, D. A systematic review of evidence on the links between patient experience and clinical safety and effectiveness. *BMJ Open* **2013**, *3*, e001570. [CrossRef]
12. Rose, L.; McKim, D.A.; Katz, S.L.; Leasa, D.; Nonoyama, M.; Pedersen, C.; Goldstein, R.S.; Road, J.D. Home mechanical ventilation in Canada: A national survey. *Respir. Care* **2015**, *60*, 695–704. [CrossRef]
13. Escarrabill, J.; Tebe, C.; Espallargues, M.; Torrente, E.; Tresserras, R.; Argimon, J. Variability in home mechanical ventilation prescription. *Arch. Bronconeumol.* **2015**, *51*, 490–495. [CrossRef]
14. Nasilowski, J.; Wachulski, M.; Trznadel, W.; Andrzejewski, W.; Migdal, M.; Drozd, W.; Pytel, A.; Suchanke, R.; Czajkowska-Malinowska, M.; Majszyk, T.; et al. The evolution of home mechanical ventilation in poland between 2000 and 2010. *Respir. Care* **2015**, *60*, 577–585. [CrossRef] [PubMed]

15. Garner, D.J.; Berlowitz, D.J.; Douglas, J.; Harkness, N.; Howard, M.; McArdle, N.; Naughton, M.T.; Neill, A.; Piper, A.; Yeo, A.; et al. Home mechanical ventilation in Australia and New Zealand. *Eur. Respir. J.* **2013**, *41*, 39–45. [CrossRef] [PubMed]

16. Mandal, S.; Suh, E.; Davies, M.; Smith, I.; Maher, T.M.; Elliott, M.W.; Davidson, A.C.; Hart, N. Provision of home mechanical ventilation and sleep services for England survey. *Thorax* **2013**, *68*, 880–881. [CrossRef]

17. Chu, C.M.; Yu, W.C.; Tam, C.M.; Lam, C.W.; Hui, D.S.; Lai, C.K. Home mechanical ventilation in Hong Kong. *Eur. Respir. J.* **2004**, *23*, 136–141. [CrossRef]

18. Fauroux, B.; Boffa, C.; Desguerre, I.; Estournet, B.; Trang, H. Long-term noninvasive mechanical ventilation for children at home: A national survey. *Pediatr. Pulmonol.* **2003**, *35*, 119–125. [CrossRef] [PubMed]

19. Fauroux, B.; Howard, P.; Muir, J.F. Home treatment for chronic respiratory insufficiency: The situation in Europe in 1992. The European Working Group on Home Treatment for Chronic Respiratory Insufficiency. *Eur. Respir. J.* **1994**, *7*, 1721–1726. [CrossRef]

20. Ekstrom, M.; Ahmadi, Z.; Larsson, H.; Nilsson, T.; Wahlberg, J.; Strom, K.E.; Midgren, B. A nationwide structure for valid long-term oxygen therapy: 29-year prospective data in Sweden. *Int. J. Chron. Obstruct. Pulmon. Dis.* **2017**, *12*, 3159–3169. [CrossRef] [PubMed]

21. Ringbaek, T.J.; Lange, P. Trends in long-term oxygen therapy for COPD in Denmark from 2001 to 2010. *Respir. Med.* **2014**, *108*, 511–516. [CrossRef]

22. Serginson, J.G.; Yang, I.A.; Armstrong, J.G.; Cooper, D.M.; Matthiesson, A.M.; Morrison, S.C.; Gair, J.M.; Cooper, B.; Zimmerman, P.V. Variability in the rate of prescription and cost of domiciliary oxygen therapy in Australia. *Med. J. Aust.* **2009**, *191*, 549–553.

23. Jones, A.; Wood-Baker, R.; Walters, E.H. Domiciliary oxygen therapy services in Tasmania: Prescription, usage and impact of a specialist clinic. *Med. J. Aust.* **2007**, *186*, 632–634. [PubMed]

24. Wijkstra, P.J.; Guyatt, G.H.; Ambrosino, N.; Celli, B.R.; Güell, R.; Muir, J.F.; Préfaut, C.; Mendes, E.S.; Ferreira, I.; Austin, P.; et al. International approaches to the prescription of long-term oxygen therapy. *Eur. Respir. J.* **2001**, *18*, 909–913. [CrossRef] [PubMed]

25. Sitzia, J.; Wood, N. Patient satisfaction: A review of issues and concepts. *Soc. Sci. Med.* **1997**, *45*, 1829–1843. [CrossRef]

26. Donabedian, A. Evaluating the Quality of Medical Care. *Milbank Q.* **2005**, *83*, 691–729. [CrossRef] [PubMed]

27. Tarlov, A.R.; Ware, J.E., Jr.; Greenfield, S.; Nelson, E.C.; Perrin, E.; Zubkoff, M. The Medical Outcomes Study. An application of methods for monitoring the results of medical care. *JAMA* **1989**, *262*, 925–930. [CrossRef] [PubMed]

28. Hodson, M.; Andrew, S.; Michael Roberts, C. Towards an understanding of PREMS and PROMS in COPD. *Breathe* **2013**, *9*, 358–364. [CrossRef]

29. Mira, J.J.; Nuno-Solinis, R.; Guilabert-Mora, M.; Solas-Gaspar, O.; Fernandez-Cano, P.; Gonzalez-Mestre, M.A.; Contel, J.C.; Del Rio-Camara, M. Development and Validation of an Instrument for Assessing Patient Experience of Chronic Illness Care. *Int. J. Integr. Care* **2016**, *16*, 13. [CrossRef] [PubMed]

30. Hodson, M. Development of a Patient Reported Experience Measure in Chronic Obstructive Pulmonary Disease (COPD). Ph.D. Thesis, University of Portsmouth, Hampshire, UK, 2018.

31. Sjetne, I.S.; Bjertnaes, O.A.; Olsen, R.V.; Iversen, H.H.; Bukholm, G. The Generic Short Patient Experiences Questionnaire (GS-PEQ): Identification of core items from a survey in Norway. *BMC Health Serv. Res.* **2011**, *11*, 88. [CrossRef]

32. Benson, T.; Potts, H.W. A short generic patient experience questionnaire: howRwe development and validation. *BMC Health Serv. Res.* **2014**, *14*, 499. [CrossRef]

33. Fernstrom, K.M.; Shippee, N.D.; Jones, A.L.; Britt, H.R. Development and validation of a new patient experience tool in patients with serious illness. *BMC Palliat. Care* **2016**, *15*, 99. [CrossRef]

34. Schmittdiel, J.; Mosen, D.M.; Glasgow, R.E.; Hibbard, J.; Remmers, C.; Bellows, J. Patient Assessment of Chronic Illness Care (PACIC) and improved patient-centered outcomes for chronic conditions. *J. Gen. Intern. Med.* **2008**, *23*, 77–80. [CrossRef]

35. Coluccia, A.; Ferretti, F.; Pozza, A. Health Services OutPatient Experience questionnaire: Factorial validity and reliability of a patient-centered outcome measure for outpatient settings in Italy. *Patient Relat. Outcome Meas.* **2014**, *5*, 93–103.

36. Beattie, M.; Shepherd, A.; Lauder, W.; Atherton, I.; Cowie, J.; Murphy, D.J. Development and preliminary psychometric properties of the Care Experience Feedback Improvement Tool (CEFIT). *BMJ Open* **2016**, *6*, e010101. [CrossRef]

37. Kleiss, J.A. Preliminary Development of a Multidimensional Semantic Patient Experience Measurement Questionnaire. *Herd* **2016**, *10*, 52–64. [CrossRef]

38. Pettersen, K.I.; Veenstra, M.; Guldvog, B.; Kolstad, A. The Patient Experiences Questionnaire: Development, validity and reliability. *Int. J. Qual. Health Care* **2004**, *16*, 453–463. [CrossRef]

39. Steine, S.; Finset, A.; Laerum, E. A new, brief questionnaire (PEQ) developed in primary health care for measuring patients' experience of interaction, emotion and consultation outcome. *Fam. Pract.* **2001**, *18*, 410–418. [CrossRef]

40. Rodriguez, H.P.; von Glahn, T.; Grembowski, D.E.; Rogers, W.H.; Safran, D.G. Physician effects on racial and ethnic disparities in patients' experiences of primary care. *J. Gen. Intern. Med.* **2008**, *23*, 1666–1672. [CrossRef]

41. Teale, E.A.; Young, J.B. A Patient Reported Experience Measure (PREM) for use by older people in community services. *Age Ageing* **2015**, *44*, 667–672. [CrossRef]

42. Masefield, S.; Vitacca, M.; Dreher, M.; Kampelmacher, M.; Escarrabill, J.; Paneroni, M.; Powell, P.; Ambrosino, N. Attitudes and preferences of home mechanical ventilation users from four European countries: An ERS/ELF survey. *ERJ Open Res.* **2017**, *3*, 00015–02017. [CrossRef]

43. Hendriks, S.H.; Rutgers, J.; van Dijk, P.R.; Groenier, K.H.; Bilo, H.J.G.; Kleefstra, N.; Kocks, J.W.H.; van Hateren, K.J.J.; Blanker, M.H. Validation of the howRu and howRwe questionnaires at the individual patient level. *BMC Health Serv. Res.* **2015**, *15*, 447. [CrossRef]

44. Glasgow, R.E.; Wagner, E.H.; Schaefer, J.; Mahoney, L.D.; Reid, R.J.; Greene, S.M. Development and validation of the Patient Assessment of Chronic Illness Care (PACIC). *Med. Care* **2005**, *43*, 436–444. [CrossRef]

45. Holm, K.E.; Casaburi, R.; Cerreta, S.; Gussin, H.A.; Husbands, J.; Porszasz, J.; Prieto-Centurion, V.; Sandhaus, R.A.; Sullivan, J.L.; Walsh, L.J.; et al. Patient Involvement in the Design of a Patient-Centered Clinical Trial to Promote Adherence to Supplemental Oxygen Therapy in COPD. *Patient* **2016**, *9*, 271–279. [CrossRef]

46. Clèries, X.; Solà, M.; Chiner, E.; Escarrabill, J. Aproximación a la experiencia del paciente y sus cuidadores en la oxigenoterapia domiciliaria. *Arch. Bronconeumol.* **2016**, *52*, 131–137. (In Spanish) [CrossRef] [PubMed]

47. Luyster, F.S.; Dunbar-Jacob, J.; Aloia, M.S.; Martire, L.M.; Buysse, D.J.; Strollo, P.J. Patient and partner experiences with obstructive sleep apnea and CPAP treatment: A qualitative analysis. *Behav. Sleep Med.* **2016**, *14*, 67–84. [CrossRef] [PubMed]

48. Ward, K.; Gott, M.; Hoare, K. Making choices about CPAP: Findings from a grounded theory study about living with CPAP. *Collegian* **2017**, *24*, 371–379. [CrossRef]

49. Gibson, R.; Campbell, A.; Mather, S.; Neill, A. From diagnosis to long-term treatment: The experiences of older New Zealanders with obstructive sleep apnoea. *J. Prim. Health Care.* **2018**, *2*, 140–149. [CrossRef] [PubMed]

50. Gale, N.K.; Jawad, M.; Dave, C.; Turner, A.M. Adapting to domiciliary non-invasive ventilation in chronic obstructive pulmonary disease: A qualitative interview study. *Palliat. Med.* **2015**, *29*, 268–277. [CrossRef] [PubMed]

51. Brostrom, A.; Nilsen, P.; Johansson, P.; Ulander, M.; Stromberg, A.; Svanborg, E.; Fridlund, B. Putative facilitators and barriers for adherence to CPAP treatment in patients with obstructive sleep apnea syndrome: A qualitative content analysis. *Sleep Med.* **2010**, *11*, 126–130. [CrossRef]

52. Gardener, A.C.; Ewing, G.; Kuhn, I.; Farquhar, M. Support needs of patients with COPD: A systematic literature search and narrative review. *Int. J. Chron. Obstruct. Pulmon. Dis.* **2018**, *13*, 1021–1035. [CrossRef] [PubMed]

53. Katsenos, S.; Constantopoulos, S.H. Long-Term Oxygen Therapy in COPD: Factors Affecting and Ways of Improving Patient Compliance. *Pulm. Med.* **2011**, *2011*, 325362. [CrossRef]

54. Fujisawa, R.; Klazinga, N.S. Measuring patient experiences (PREMS): Progress made by the OECD and its member countries between 2006 and 2016. *OECD Health Work. Pap.* **2017**. [CrossRef]

Comparison of Oncologic Outcomes in Laparoscopic versus Open Surgery for Non-Metastatic Colorectal Cancer: Personal Experience in a Single Institution

Chong-Chi Chiu [1,2,3], Wen-Li Lin [4], Hon-Yi Shi [5,6,7], Chien-Cheng Huang [8,9], Jyh-Jou Chen [10], Shih-Bin Su [11,12,13], Chih-Cheng Lai [14], Chien-Ming Chao [14], Chao-Jung Tsao [15], Shang-Hung Chen [16] and Jhi-Joung Wang [17,18,*]

[1] Department of General Surgery, Chi Mei Medical Center, Liouying 73657, Taiwan; chiuchongchi@yahoo.com.tw

[2] Department of General Surgery, Chi Mei Medical Center, Tainan 71004, Taiwan

[3] Department of Electrical Engineering, Southern Taiwan University of Science and Technology, Tainan 71005, Taiwan

[4] Department of Cancer Center, Chi Mei Medical Center, Liouying 73657, Taiwan; wenlilin2012@gmail.com

[5] Department of Healthcare Administration and Medical Informatics, Kaohsiung Medical University, Kaohsiung 80708, Taiwan; hshi@kmu.edu.tw

[6] Department of Business Management, National Sun Yat Sen University, Kaohsiung 80424, Taiwan

[7] Department of Medical Research, Kaohsiung Medical University Hospital, Kaohsiung 80708, Taiwan

[8] Department of Emergency Medicine, Chi-Mei Medical Center, Tainan 71004, Taiwan; chienchenghuang@yahoo.com.tw

[9] Department of Senior Services, Southern Taiwan University of Science and Technology, Tainan 71005, Taiwan

[10] Department of Gastroenterology and Hepatology, Chi Mei Medical Center, Liouying 73657, Taiwan; jjchen@mail.chimei.org.tw

[11] Department of Occupational Medicine, Chi Mei Medical Center, Liouying 73657, Taiwan; shihbin.su@msa.hinet.net

[12] Department of Occupational Medicine, Chi Mei Medical Center, Tainan 71004, Taiwan

[13] Department of Leisure, Recreation and Tourism Management, Southern Taiwan University of Science and Technology, Tainan 71005, Taiwan

[14] Department of Intensive Care Medicine, Chi Mei Medical Center, Liouying 73657, Taiwan; dtmed141@gmail.com (C.-C.L.); ccm870958@yahoo.com.tw (C.-M.C.)

[15] Department of Oncology, Chi Mei Medical Center, Liouying 73657, Taiwan; m961193@mail.chimei.org.tw

[16] National Institute of Cancer Research, National Health Research Institutes, Tainan 70403, Taiwan; bryanchen@nhri.edu.tw

[17] Department of Medical Research, Chi Mei Medical Center, Tainan 71004, Taiwan

[18] AI Biomed Center, Southern Taiwan University of Science and Technology, Tainan 71005, Taiwan

* Correspondence: 400002@mail.chimei.org.tw

Abstract: The oncologic merits of the laparoscopic technique for colorectal cancer surgery remain debatable. Eligible patients with non-metastatic colorectal cancer who were scheduled for an elective resection by one surgeon in a medical institution were randomized to either laparoscopic or open surgery. During this period, a total of 188 patients received laparoscopic surgery and the other 163 patients received the open approach. The primary endpoint was cancer-free five-year survival after operative treatment, and the secondary endpoint was the tumor recurrence incidence. Besides, surgical complications were also compared. There was no statistically significant difference between open and laparoscopic groups regarding the average number of lymph nodes dissected, ileus, anastomosis leakage, overall mortality rate, cancer recurrence rate, or cancer-free five-year survival. Even though performing a laparoscopic approach used a significantly longer operation time, this technique was more effective for colorectal cancer treatment in terms of shorter hospital stay and less blood loss. Meanwhile, fewer patients receiving the laparoscopic approach developed postoperative urinary tract infection, wound infection, or pneumonia, which reached statistical significance. For non-metastatic colorectal cancer patients, laparoscopic surgery resulted in better short-term outcomes, whether in several surgical complications and intra-operative blood loss. Though there was no significant statistical difference in terms of cancer-free five-year survival and tumor recurrence, it is strongly recommended that patients undergo laparoscopic surgery if not contraindicated.

Keywords: laparoscopic; open surgery; non-metastatic colorectal cancer; surgical complication; oncologic outcome; single surgeon experience

---

1. Introduction

Since the first laparoscopic-assisted colon resection introduced in 1991 by Jacobs et al., it has gradually become popular [1]. Increasingly more colorectal surgeons admit that the laparoscopic technique leads to quicker functional recovery [2–5] and improved short-term results when compared with the open approach [6–12]. However, the laparoscopic technique has not previously been proven to gain significant benefits in colorectal surgeries [13–17]. Recently, oncologic outcomes of colorectal cancer resection, in terms of lymph node harvest number and excision safety margin lengths, achieved under laparoscopy could be comparable to those obtained using the conventional open technique. However, the curability of colorectal cancer under the laparoscopic technique remains controversial because of the uncertainty about the overall recurrence rate [18]. Besides, three principal, randomized clinical trials have proven that the laparoscopic technique can lead to the same oncological outcomes related to an open approach, but did not distinguish a survival benefit favoring laparoscopy [2,4,6].

It is believed that the role of the laparoscopic technique for advanced non-metastatic colorectal cancer management will be clarified through this study. The aim of this research was a comparison of surgical complications and five-year oncologic results of non-metastatic colorectal cancer patients receiving laparoscopic resection (LR) or open resection (OR) by one surgeon in a medical institution.

2. Materials and Methods

2.1. Ethics Statement

The institutional Ethics of Research Committee of Chi Mei Medical Center, Taiwan permitted this study. The protocol conformed to ethical standards according to the Declaration of Helsinki published in 1964. Moreover, written or verbal consent from patients was acquired for this study.

2.2. Study Population

From January 2008 to December 2013, a total of 375 consecutive colorectal cancer patients scheduled for resection by Dr. Chiu in a regional hospital with LR or OR were assessed (Figure 1). The treatment protocol was based on the National Comprehensive Cancer Network (NCCN) Guidelines®. The exclusion criteria included patients with cancer distant metastasis, synchronous tumors, adjacent organ invasion, intestinal obstruction, combined operations for other disease, history of trans-abdominal or trans-anal colorectal surgery, history of inflammatory bowel disease, polyposis, past episode of ileus related to severe intra-abdominal adhesions, morbid obesity, severe medical disease, pregnancy, emergent surgeries, patient unwilling to participate in the study, or conversion to open approach. Conversion to open approach was defined as an abdominal incision larger than necessary for specimen retrieval. Written informed consent was obtained from all patients in this study. This study divided patients into several groups according to the tumor locations. Patients of each tumor location group were randomly allocated to receive LR or OR using the random numbers belonging to that location group in the envelopes, blindly selected by the surgeon before the operation. In the LR group, all patients needed to pay for the extra fee of the harmonic scalpel and wound retractor.

Data were collected in a prospectively maintained database that was supplemented by a retrospective chart review.

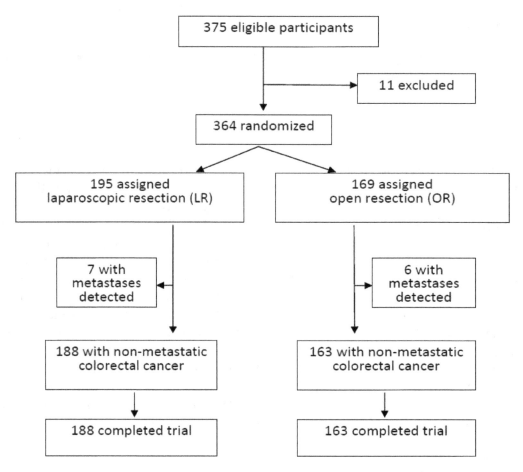

Figure 1. The flowchart of the study design.

2.3. Pre-Operative Staging Work-Up

The evaluation included physical examination, colonoscopy with biopsy, abdominal, and pelvic computed tomography (CT) scan. Pelvic magnetic resonance imaging was routinely performed for rectal cancer patients. Serum level of carcinoembryonic antigen (CEA) was sampled before the operation. The pre-operative clinical oncologic staging was classified by tumor node metastasis (TNM) system of the American Joint Committee on Cancer (AJCC)/International Union Against Cancer (UICC).

2.4. Surgical Techniques

All LR and OR procedures proceeded with a standardized medial-to-lateral approach and non-touch technique. During LR surgery, the surgeon and camera operator stood on the opposite side of the colorectal lesion, while the first assistant positioned to the same side of the lesion. Briefly, the right hemicolectomy including the range extended to the mid-transverse colon with lymphadenectomy about the ileocolic, right colic, and middle colic vessel origin was selected for proximal lesions (those sited proximal to the flexure of the spleen). The left hemicolectomy with lymphadenectomy at the level of the left colic and the left branch of the middle colic vessel origins was selected for lesions at the descending colon. The omentum was transected to allow entry into the omental bursa and mobilization of the liver flexure (right hemicolectomy) or splenic flexure (left hemicolectomy). As lesions of the sigmoid colon or rectosigmoid junction, the sigmoid colectomy with upper rectum resection and lymphadenectomy extended to the inferior mesenteric vessel origin were selected. At least 5 cm safety surgical clearance margin was mandatory for all patients. As for rectal cancer, the technique was standardized as follows: (1) for upper third rectal lesions, a 5 cm mesorectal resection with end-to-end colorectal anastomosis was done; (2) for mid and low rectal lesions, total mesorectal excision with pouch supra-anal or anal anastomosis was performed; and (3) abdominoperineal excision was indicated once the levator muscle was involved by tumor. According to the principle of the non-touch technique, high ligation of the inferior mesenteric artery and mobilization of the splenic flexure were first systematically performed, whether the procedures were performed in LR or OR group. Dissected tissue was pulled out via a wound retractor at the extended umbilical wound for abdominal wall protection. For proximal lesions, anastomosis was routinely performed extra-corporeally. We routinely performed trans-anally intra-corporeal circular stapled anastomosis after the descending colon, sigmoid colon, or rectum lesion resection, because the residual distal intestine stump after resection was hardly managed extra-corporeally. In the OR group, the procedures were performed through a midline laparotomy with the same rules, and the wound was protected by gauze covering. The harmonic scalpel was generally used for soft tissue dissection in the LR group, but not in the OR group. Besides, in cases with difficult tumor localization by vision or palpation, an intra-operative colonoscopy would be routinely used to locate the actual tumor site instead of using other methods. However, no one in the OR group needed an intra-operative colonoscopy, but only three patients in the other group needed one.

2.5. Post-Operative Management

Post-operative treatment was the same for both groups. Patients were discharged when they had sufficient oral intake, well-controlled complications, or no complications. Complications designated as more severe than grade I according to the Clavien–Dindo classification system were categorized as ileus, urinary tract infection, wound infection, pneumonia, anastomotic leakage, and so on. Besides, most patients with stage III colorectal cancer would receive post-operative chemotherapy (oral or intravenous form), except six patients of the LR group and three of the OR group owing to general weakness or intolerance to chemotherapy.

2.6. Post-Operative Follow-Up

One specialized pathologist assessed all specimens. All patients were followed up with clinical examination, serum CEA assay, chest X-ray exam every three months, and liver ultrasound every six months for the first two years, and then annually. An abdominal CT exam was arranged annually. A colonoscopy was performed at one year after the operation, then every three years.

2.7. Statistical Analysis

The main endpoint of this study was cancer-free five-year survival. The secondary endpoint was the incidence of tumor recurrence. Predefined baseline variables are listed in Tables 1 and 2. Variables for the univariate analysis were gender, age, American Society of Anesthesiologists (ASA) class, tumor location, TNM stage, histopathology, pre-surgery serum CEA level, type of intervention, postoperative complications, and tumor recurrence. Categorical variables were compared using the χ^2 test. Continuous variables (e.g., number of lymph nodes removed, hospitalization period, intra-operative blood loss, and operation time) were compared using Student's t-test. Survival period was evaluated from the day of surgery to the last visit or death. For cancer-free survival, patients dying from other causes were censored at the time of death. Probability curves were constructed according to the Kaplan–Meier method and compared with the log-rank test (Table 3) (Figure 2). A p-value less than 0.05 was regarded as statistically significant. All calculations were performed using the SPSS software package version 20 (SPSS Inc., Chicago, IL, USA).

Table 1. Comparison of baseline characteristics between laparoscopic resection (LR) versus open resection (OR).

Items	LR (n = 188)	OR (n = 163)	p-Value
Gender			0.435
Male	102	87	
Female	86	76	
Age (mean ± SD)	68.6 ± 12.7	71.5 ± 12.1	0.23
ASA class			0.698
I	113	92	
II	75	71	
TNM stage (clinical/radiologic)			0.345
0	3	0	
I	70	55	
II	26	26	
III	89	82	
TNM stage (pathologic)			0.344
0	3	0	
I	68	53	
II	30	29	
III	87	81	
Histopathology			0.624
Well differentiated	92	79	
Moderate differentiated	71	65	
Poorly differentiated	25	19	
Tumor location			0.431
Cecum	29	20	
Ascending colon	41	36	
Transverse colon	12	15	
Descending colon	21	18	
Sigmoid colon	52	45	
Rectum	33	29	
Intervention			0.720
Right hemicolectomy	65	56	
Left hemicolectomy	24	21	
Transverse colectomy	14	10	
Sigmoid colectomy	50	44	
Protectomy	32	27	
Abdominal perineal resection	3	5	
Protective diversional stoma	13	15	
Pre-surgery serum CEA level			1.000
<5	24	13	
≥5	164	150	

ASA—American Society of Anesthesiologists; TNM—tumor node metastasis; CEA—carcinoembryonic antigen.

Table 2. Comparison of surgical outcomes between laparoscopic resection (LR) versus open resection (OR).

Items	LR (n = 188)	OR (n = 163)	p-Value
Tumor recurrence	17 (9.0%)	22 (13.5%)	0.186
Lymph nodes removed	16.0 ± 9.2	19.2 ± 13.7	0.07
Hospitalization (days)	13.2 ± 4.2	18.8 ± 9	<0.001 **
Blood loss (mL)	23.5 ± 14.6	162.2 ± 63.4	<0.001 **
Operation time (min)	191.4 ± 71.1	150.8 ± 46.3	<0.001 **
Postoperative complications			
Total	8	25	
Ileus	3	5	0.273
Urinary tract infection	1	5	<0.001 **
Wound infection	2	7	<0.001 **
Pneumonia	2	6	0.048 *
Anastomosis leakage	0	2	0.140

* $p \leq 0.05$ ** $p \leq 0.001$. LR Tumor recurrence: liver metastasis ×13, lung metastasis ×5, carcinomatosis ×4, anastomotic recurrence ×1, local recurrence ×3; OR Tumor recurrence: liver metastasis ×19, lung metastasis ×8, carcinomatosis ×6, anastomotic recurrence ×3, local recurrence ×2.

Table 3. Cancer-free survival rates between laparoscopic resection (LR) versus open resection (OR).

Stage	Group	n	Death		Survival 1st Year	2nd Year	3rd Year	4th Year	5th Year	p-Value
			n	%	% (n)	% (n)	% (n)	% (n)	% (n)	
0	LR	3	0	0	100 (3)	100 (3)	100 (3)	100 (3)	100 (3)	-
	OR	0	-	-	-	-	-	-	-	
I	LR	68	0	0	100 (68)	100 (68)	100 (68)	100 (68)	100 (68)	0.206
	OR	53	4	7.5	100 (53)	100 (53)	98.1 (52)	96.2 (51)	92.5 (49)	
II	LR	30	3	10.0	100 (30)	100 (30)	100 (30)	93.3 (28)	90.0 (27)	0.713
	OR	29	5	17.2	100 (29)	93.1 (27)	93.1 (27)	89.7 (26)	82.8 (24)	
III	LR	87	18	20.7	100 (87)	97.7 (85)	88.5 (77)	86.2 (75)	79.3 (69)	0.426
	OR	81	23	28.4	97.5 (79)	93.8 (76)	88.9 (72)	82.7 (67)	71.6 (58)	
Total	LR	188	21	11.2	100 (188)	98.9 (186)	94.7 (178)	92.6 (174)	88.8 (167)	0.328
	OR	163	32	19.6	98.8 (161)	95.7 (156)	92.6 (151)	88.3 (144)	80.3 (131)	

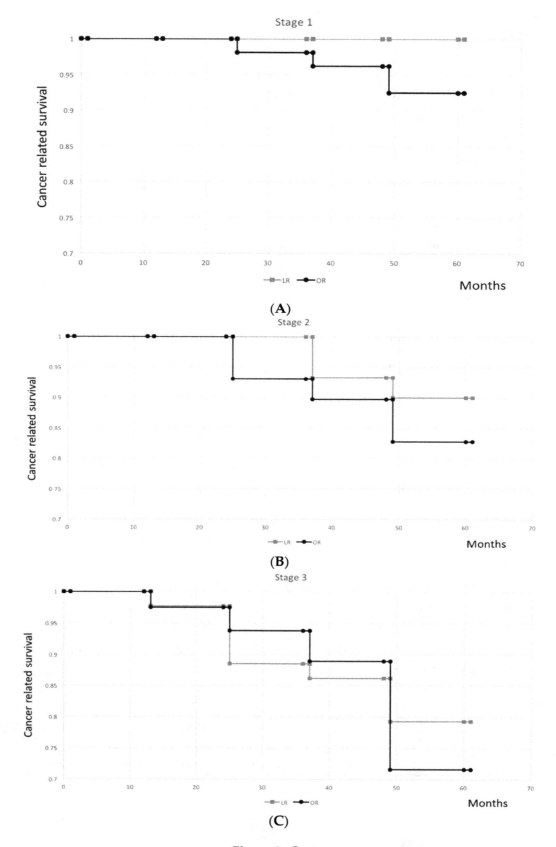

Figure 2. *Cont.*

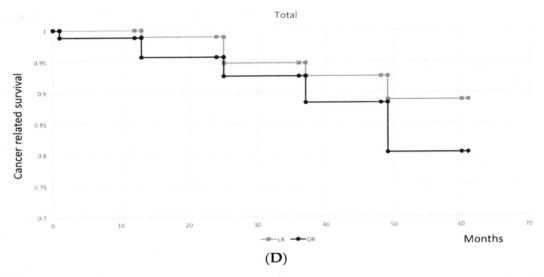

Figure 2. (**A**) Kaplan–Meier curve of cancer-free five-year survival in stage I patients ($p = 0.206$); (**B**) Kaplan–Meier curve of cancer-free five-year survival in stage II patients ($p = 0.713$); (**C**) Kaplan–Meier curve of cancer-free five-year survival in stage III patients ($p = 0.426$); (**D**) Kaplan–Meier curve of cancer-free five-year survival in all stage patients ($p = 0.328$).

3. Results

3.1. Baseline Characteristics of Patients

The basic profile of this study is shown in Figure 1. Initially, 375 colorectal cancer patients under Dr. Chiu's service were sorted. Of these, 11 were excluded from the study. A total of 364 patients receiving curative resection were assessed in this study; 195 received LR and 169 received OR. Carcinomatosis was detected intra-operatively in seven patients of LR and six patients of OR, which were excluded. The remaining patients were compliant with the follow-up protocol. The median surveillance period was about 60 months.

In Table 1, both groups of patients were well matched in terms of demographic and clinicopathologic parameters. During this study period, 188 patients of the LR group were compared with the data obtained from the other 163 patients of the OR group. In the LR group, the mean age was 68.6 ± 12.7 years, and 102 (54.3%) patients were male. According to the final pathology report, three patients were classified in stage 0, 68 in stage I, 30 in stage II, and 87 in stage III. In the OR group, the mean age was 71.5 ± 12.1 years, and 87 (53.4%) patients were male; none were affected by tumors in stage 0, 53 in stage I, 29 in stage II, and 81 in stage III. There was a little disparity between clinical/radiologic staging and pathological staging in this study. Other characteristics of tumors and patients were summarized, and there was no statistical difference between these two groups.

3.2. Surgical Outcomes

In Table 2, the rate of tumor recurrence was 9.0% (17/188) in the LR group and 13.5% (22/163) in the OR group. Although the difference was not statistically significant, tumor recurrence seemed to be lower in the LR group ($p = 0.186$). The average number of lymph nodes removed in LR was 16.0 ± 9.2 and 19.2 ± 13.7 in OR ($p = 0.07$). Tumor margins were non-involved in patients of both groups. However, this study demonstrated that LR was more effective for the treatment of colorectal cancer in terms of hospital stay ($p < 0.001$) and blood loss ($p < 0.001$). Conversely, operation time was significantly longer in LR than in OR (191.4 ± 71.1 min vs. 150.8 ± 46.3 min, $p < 0.001$). Compared with the LR group, more patients in the OR group encountered postoperative urinary tract infection, wound infection, and pneumonia, which reached statistical significance. Only two patients in the OR group were found with mild anastomosis leakage from the drainage tube clinically. Abdominal CT confirmed the diagnosis and that the degree was mild. These two patients received conservative treatment, including intravenous fluid supply and nil per os. However, further surgical intervention was not necessary.

3.3. Cancer-Free Survival Rates and Tumor Recurrence Incidence

In Table 3, twenty-one patients (11.2%) of the LR group and 32 patients (19.6%) of the OR group expired. There was a trend of higher overall mortality in the OR group, with 4 in stage I, 5 in stage II, and 23 in stage III, but it was not statistically different. In stage 0, there were only three patients in the LR group and none in the other. All three patients survived more than five years after surgery. In stage I, all four deaths of the OR group were non-cancer related. All patients survived for at least 30 months after surgery. In stage II, two patients in the OR group died within the second year after surgery, but they were non-cancer related. Others in both groups who died were all cancer-related. In stage III patients, all eighteen deaths in the LR group and twenty-three deaths in the OR group were cancer-related. In the OR group, two patients died fewer than six months after a second oncologic surgery for cancer recurrence, about three years after previous surgery.

There was a phenomenon of a higher cancer-free five-year survival in stage I (p = 0.206, Figure 2A), stage II (p = 0.713, Figure 2B), stage III (p = 0.426, Figure 2C), and all stages (p = 0.328, Figure 2D) in the LR group when compared with those in the OR group, although the difference was not statistically significant.

The median time for tumor recurrence was 57.0 months (range 25–68 months) in LR and 53.5 months (range 25–63 months) in OR. Importantly, no difference was observed in the cumulative incidence of recurrence between these two groups (p = 0.186) (Figure 3). Besides, there was no incidence of port-site recurrence in the LR group or wound recurrence in the OR group.

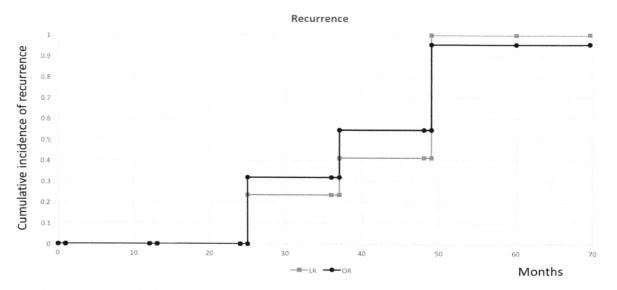

Figure 3. Cumulative incidence curve of tumor recurrence in all stage patients (p = 0.186).

4. Discussion

Previously, randomized controlled studies demonstrated that LR had favorable operative outcomes with less wound pain, earlier functional return of the gastrointestinal tract, a shorter hospital stay, and better cosmetics when compared with OR [19–22]. Moreover, a meta-analysis [23] and two large retrospective studies [24,25], which included a large number of patients, also showed a significant reduction in the mortality rate and lowered the morbidity after LR.

However, survival is the most crucial concern for assessing success for malignant disease treatment. This study included a 60-month follow-up and compared LR and OR for non-metastatic colorectal cancer. The results of cancer-related survival and incidence of tumor recurrence favored the LR group, despite that there was no statistically significant difference regarding the oncological results.

The Clinical Outcome of Surgical Therapy study, which was the largest randomized controlled trial conducted so far, also showed the same results as ours and even overall survival between the two groups after a median four-year follow-up [2]. However, in a single institution randomized study, Lacy et al. advocated that there was a cancer-related survival advantage after LR for stage III colon cancer patients [26]. Capussotti et al. also demonstrated that LR was related to significantly better disease-free and cancer-related survival stage III colon cancer patients [27]. Other studies have reported better survival for patients undergoing LR, even for those with stage II colorectal cancer [28].

One of the assumptions about better survival might be the number difference in dissected lymph nodes between the LR and OR groups. Laparoscopy provides better visualization of intra-abdominal conditions [29], including a more comprehensive, more precise, and brighter image to allow surgeons to perform a more radical and precise resection of the mesocolon and mesorectum, while facilitating an accurate and complete lymphadenectomy [30,31]. Complete lymphadenectomy for colorectal cancer is essential for the patient's oncological prognosis because of a reduced risk of residual nodal disease, as well as accurate nodal staging (achieving a better stratification of tumor staging) [19]. However, there was no statistical difference in the lymph node retrieval number between these two groups. Similarly, the retrieved and assessed lymph node number in many patients of both groups was higher than the threshold of 12 lymph nodes recommended by the American Joint Committee on Cancer (AJCC) in our study. Lymphadenectomy of colorectal cancer was a decisive factor for the prognostic and therapeutic staging of the patient. Different variables could affect the retrieval number of lymph nodes. Some, like the surgeon, the surgery, and the pathology exam, were without question modifiable; however, other both patient- and disease-related variables were non-modifiable and posed the question of whether the minimum number of examined lymph nodes must be individually assigned. However, since 2010, the AJCC classification subdivided patients treated for colorectal cancer into prognostic categories according to the number of metastatic lymph nodes [32]. The accuracy of the staging was influenced by the number of retrieved lymph nodes as the relationship between positive nodes divided by the total number of retrieved nodes. With regard to the prognosis prediction, this "lymph nodal ratio" is also effective in cases of reduced lymph nodal sampling [33–36]. Besides, the sentinel lymph nodes were thought to find valid application in this field in the future [37]. Of course, improvement of these modifiable factors is the only aspect that our team could strive for at this moment, as well as the opportunity to gain a better oncologic outcome of cancer remission or recurrence after reducing the risk of residual nodal disease.

Other proven benefits in oncologic results about LR include its effect on cellular immunity, intra-operative tumor manipulation, related stress response and subsequent cytokine release, surgical complication rate, and blood transfusion amount [26]. Conclusively, one of the most essentially beneficial theories of LR is regarded as the preservation of the patient's immunological response against cancer from the first postoperative days [38]. There has been significant evidence suggesting that surgical stress interferes with immunity, and this phenomenon is more apparent in OR than in LR [39]. The role of immunosuppression has been advocated because immunologic response mediators (e.g., C-reactive protein, interleukin 1–6, and tumor necrosis factor alpha) are decreased after LR in colorectal surgery compared with the OR approach. On the other hand, immunosuppression deteriorates both sepsis and cancer cell proliferation [40]. Lacy et al. have also pointed out that the post-LR stress response of colorectal cancer is less pronounced and finally leads to better preservation of cellular immune function, and attenuates inflammatory mediator interference [41,42]. Correlation of the stress response degree after the trauma of surgery with the host resistance to cancer has been proven in an animal model [26]. Immunity is a critical barrier against tumor progression and metastatic spread [39]. LR could, therefore, theoretically increase either overall or cancer-free survival. However, we should routinely examine these immunologic response mediators after surgery to improve the quality of our further study.

Tumor manipulation has been proven to contribute to cancer cell spread. There is some evidence that tumor mobilization is related to cancer cells' exfoliation into the peritoneal cavity and portal vein bloodstream migration, which might be alleviated by non-touch surgical techniques or the avoidance of tumor manipulation. Preliminary reports have shown that cancer cell spread is not worsened [43], and dissemination of cancer cells is reduced by LR [39]. However, this phenomenon is difficult evaluated in this study based on the safety issue of blood sampling from portal vein bloodstream. Under the laparoscopic vision, limited access inside the abdominal cavity leads to minimal tumor handling and compliance of non-touch technique, both favoring the important oncology principle to avoid tumor cell spread during surgery. In this study, all patients received non-touch isolation techniques in both the LR and OR groups, which should cause no difference in prognosis. In the future, we could also perform intra-operative abdominal cavity normal saline irrigation after tumor resection to compare the difference of possible exfoliated cancer cells into the peritoneal cavity by two surgical techniques.

There is an evident statistical difference in fewer complication rates and the amount of blood loss in the LR group compared with the OR group. These factors theoretically contribute to better prognosis of tumor recurrence and cancer-free survival in LR patients. Despite that the differences regarding the oncological results did not reach the statistical significance of both groups, other better short-term outcomes, including smaller incisions, less postoperative pain, quicker functional recovery, shorter hospital stays, and earlier return to regular activity, suggested colorectal cancer patients should receive LR if not contraindicated. Meanwhile, although the operation length was longer in our LR group, the benefit of this minimally invasive technique on peri-operative care (quicker functional recovery and shorter hospital stays) further overcame this disadvantage. Besides, this benefit in shorter peri-operative care would significantly lower the total medical cost, especially in Western countries. Meanwhile, it is believed that we could set up some standard protocols and guidelines for routine use to decrease the operation time in the OR group in the future.

There are many debates about the effect of wound size. Several experienced colorectal surgeons pointed out that most colectomies could be performed with an abdominal wound of less than 7 cm, and thus opposed the wound benefits of LR [44]. However, the advantages of LR for colorectal cancer not only include a comparatively smaller wound size, but also relate to the properties of laparoscopy, especially the operation field magnification, more precise tumor resection, and its minimal invasiveness [5]. One meta-analysis including 3863 patients even showed that single-incision laparoscopic surgery (SILS) had comparable outcomes to LR in terms of operating time, conversion rate, reoperations, postoperative complications, and mortality, but only shorter mean hospital stay. There was no difference in the oncological results regarding average lymph node retrieval, adequate resection margins, survival rates, and local recurrence [45].

Application of LR for colorectal cancer encountered much criticism in the early 1990s as a result of several case reports about port site recurrence and suspicion of the adverse effect of oncologic outcome [25]. However, many surgeons advocated that LR did not aggravate cancer cell spillage intra-corporeally when surgeons strictly followed the oncologic principles [5]. However, the routine practice of the laparoscopic technique in colorectal cancer treatment is only performed in a few experienced centers in Taiwan. Localization of the tumors remains a major limiting factor of LR popularity among most surgeons, despite that there are several techniques, including conventional colonoscopy and colonoscopic tattooing, colonoscopic clip placement, radio-guided colorectal lesion localization, and the application of magnetic colonoscopic imaging [46]. Besides, some specialists are still quite hesitant about laparoscopy because of the lack of "direct" physical and visual contact of the lesion. Particularly during the LR process, the intestinal color is more difficult to assess, and direct palpation of blood vessels to the anastomosis is not possible [47]. The phenomenon of the slow popularity of this minimally invasive technique further reflects its complexity, especially at the initial stage of the learning curve; the lack of three-dimensional visualization, the absence of safe laparoscopic instruments, and the paucity of tactile feedback are still usually the causes of barriers to popularity and the causes of conversion during surgery [48].

Moreover, practicing a new or pioneer surgical technique on patients with a malignant disease is not permitted in the ethical aspect. However, inreasingly more improved new techniques of LR are being explored [47]. For the majority of cases, pioneers feel confident to employ LR. If further efforts are made to achieve standardization of these minimally invasive procedures and improvement of the related educational system, LR will undoubtedly become the standard and mainstay therapy for many bowel diseases, besides colorectal cancer. Furthermore, it is expected that other new techniques such as reduced port surgery and robotic surgery will be confirmed efficient and safe in the future [49].

Many experts pointed out that the learning curve for laparoscopic colorectal surgery is about greater than twenty cases [50]. In 2013, one meta-analysis by Comité de l'évolution des pratiques en oncologie (CEPO) recommended that LR be considered an option for the curative treatment of colon and rectal cancer in consideration of surgeon experience, tumor stage, potential contraindications, and patient expectations. Instead, CEPO also suggested only competent experts with sufficient annual surgeon volume should perform LR for rectal cancer patients [51]. However, safety control, quality monitor, and technique standardization applied to the surgical aspects of the study would provide a solution to the learning curve issues by the collaboration of interested experts to set up safe and reproducible experiment steps even in the setting of new technology [52]. As for the surgeon on our team, he had experience with LR of more than 100 cases before this study. Thus, the learning curve effect of our study series was not discussed.

Compared with previously published randomized studies in the literature, there were some weak points of this study that needed to be further addressed. Our hospital was an 800-bed regional hospital with a total of around 120 colorectal cancer operations per year. Admittedly, the number of patients included in this study was too small (only 351 patients) for comparison of the oncological outcomes; we should increase the sample size to make a reliable comparison between these two groups and to avoid the related bias in the future. Second, our surgeon excluded morbidly obese patients in this study because our surgeon preferred them to receive LR to lower the incidence of possible abdominal wound herniation in the future, which might cause a potential bias. However, only one morbidly obese patient was encountered during the study period, and he was excluded because he encountered the problem of severe intestinal adhesion and received conversion from LR to the OR approach. Third, recently developed and popular trans-anal surgery for patients with rectal lesions was not discussed in this study because we could not compare traditional OR and LR techniques. Fourth, some patients might encounter the problem of their retrieved and assessed lymph node number being lower than the threshold of twelve, which might cause inaccurate TNM staging and select inappropriate minor treatment in their protocol.

In Table 2, the result of our anastomosis leakage rate (0.57%) compared favorably to those of the published literature (0.9%–3.5%). Higher leak rates were typically reported for low pelvic anastomoses or anastomoses to the anal canal [53]. There were three reasons for this comparatively "better" result in our study. First, we largely selected surgical patients with good pre-operative nutrition status (Subjective Global Assessment of Nutritional Status class A or B). Second, we preferred to perform protective diversional stoma for patients with a higher risk of anastomosis leakage, especially those having pre-operative concurrent chemoradiotherapy. We believed nearly all small contained leaks of the anastomosis site would heal after fecal diversion for about six months. Third, the true incidence of anastomosis leakage was underestimated. We only performed post-operative CT for patients when turbid or stool-like discharge was noted from the drainage tube near the anastomosis site. Pickleman et al. advocated that some colorectal surgical patients ultimately found to have an anastomosis leakage developed a more insidious presentation, often with low-grade fever, prolonged ileus, or failure to thrive [54]. In these patients, confirmation of the diagnosis might be much more difficult, as the clinical course was often similar to other postoperative infectious complications. Radiologic imaging was usually required; even then, the definitive diagnosis might be elusive or at least uncertain [53]. Although there have been many studies that specify a rate of anastomotic leakage, it is seldom possible to know what constitutes a "leak". Bruce et al. performed a systematic review of studies measuring the incidence of anastomotic leaks after gastrointestinal surgery; in the 97 studies reviewed, there was a total of 56 separate definitions of the anastomotic leak [55]. A leak may be defined by the need for reoperation, clinical findings, or radiologic criteria (CT scanning or contrast enema), making "accurate" comparisons between these studies difficult or impossible [53].

Meanwhile, colorectal cancers at different sites were included for analysis of oncologic outcomes and functional results in our study. This study design was debatable because the lymphatic drainage route, range of dissection during tumor resection, operation techniques, and even the biologic behavior were different in various colorectal locations [5]. However, all patients of the LR and OR groups were treated by a single surgeon, and this could avoid the related bias when patients were treated by multiple surgeons. Besides, if we could increase the patient number (sample size) in the future, we could analyze and discuss the tumor located at one specific site to decrease this bias.

Patients with liver metastasis (a common metastasis area of colorectal cancer) were excluded in our study because we thought these terminal patients (defined by current TNM staging system) should receive systemic treatment if no evident clinical lumen obstruction. However, in China, the attitudes of therapeutic approaches in these patients seem to vary among areas [56]. Specific guidelines regarding liver metastasis were revised in 2018 in order to improve the diagnosis and treatment strategy, including the overall clinical evaluation, personalized treatment goals, and comprehensive treatment protocol, in order to prevent the occurrence of liver metastases, and improve the resection rate of liver metastases and survival [57]. Although experts of different countries have investigated their treatment strategy for colorectal cancer thoroughly for many years, the TNM staging system is still commonly regarded as an essential tool to predict oncologic outcomes [58]. It has made an essential contribution to the clinical management of cancer patients over the past 50 years [59], but are we sure it delivers what is needed to provide adequate advice in the 21st century? Would patients face different oncologic outcomes despite that they have been labeled with the same TNM stage clinically?

Nowadays, the degree of cancer infiltration, the number of lymph nodes involved, and distant metastasis have generally been accepted as the most paramount items to predict outcomes [60]. Nevertheless, some patients in the same clinicopathological stage might exhibit unique variation in outcomes with different rates of cancer recurrence and mortality when merely evaluated with the current TNM staging system [60,61]. Specialists conducted intensive studies about the possible causes of this discrepancy. Maguire et al. pointed out that the classification of peritoneal involvement was different in TNM 5 and TNM 7. The Royal College of Pathologists in the United Kingdom still recommended the use of the TNM 5 staging system, while TNM 7 had been adopted in many other jurisdictions. In TNM 5, a tumor directly invading other organs was staged as pT4a, while a tumor involving the visceral peritoneum was staged as pT4b [60]. However, the reported incidence of peritoneal involvement ranged from 5% to 43% in studies of stage II colorectal cancer, which led to a wide statistical variation and an unreliable result [62–69]. Besides, Puppa et al. also advocated that identification and classification of morphologic features encountered in the pathologic examination of colorectal cancer specimens might be difficult and a source of subjective variability. They suggested that enhanced pathologic analysis, agreed-upon standard protocols, and standardization should improve the completeness and accuracy of pathology reports. In other words, the optimal staging system of colorectal cancer should encompass both anatomic and nonanatomic factors, the latter including molecular and treatment factors [61]. Some oncologists also advocated that cancer development and progression might depend partly on "changes" in several histological features, which might lead to this discrepancy clinically. These previously unrecognized features were closely related to the way cancerous cells interact with the surrounding stroma and obtain their potential for invasiveness [70]. These characteristics included tumor budding, poorly differentiated clusters, extramural vascular (vein) invasion, perineural invasion, tumor deposits, and mucin pools [58]. This discrepancy in the molecular signature of colorectal cancer has also revealed differences in phenotypic aggressiveness and therapeutic response rates [58]. Thus, we should remind colorectal cancer patients of the potential risk of having a disappointing result when choosing inappropriate minor post-operative treatment.

The discrepancy in staging colorectal cancer has critical effects on management, outcomes, and survival rates of the patients. Accurate predictions of the final pathological disease stage using high quality, accurate pre-operative clinical-radiological staging techniques enables multidisciplinary teams to plan prompt optimal management strategies for patients with colorectal neoplasms [71]. As cancer clinicians strive to improve survival by increasingly smaller steps, the accuracy of TNM staging becomes even more critical in the interpretation of reports of further clinical trials [59]. More importantly, it is essential to introduce effective preventive measures to this increasing global disease [72].

5. Conclusions

Within the limitations of this study, the results showed better short-term outcomes in terms of postoperative urinary tract infection, wound infection, pneumonia, and blood loss in LR versus OR for non-metastatic colorectal cancer. Although the differences regarding cancer-free five-year survival and tumor recurrence did not reach the statistical significance of both groups, it is strongly recommended that patients undergo laparoscopic surgery if not contraindicated.

Author Contributions: C.-C.C. performed the operations, cared the patients, designed the study, obtained IRB approval, collected clinical records, and wrote the first and final draft; W.-L.L. analyzed the statistical data; H.-Y.S. assisted with the statistical data analysis; C.-C.H. managed patients in the emergency room; J.-J.C. performed pre-operative colonoscopy exams; S.-B.S. performed stool occult blood screening; C.-C.L. and C.-M.C. cared some patients in the intensive care unit post-operatively; C.-J.T. and S.-H.C. performed chemotherapy or concurrent chemoradiotherapy for patients; J.-J.W. provided critical feedback, supervision, and opinion of this study.

Acknowledgments: This study was approved by the institutional review board of Chi Mei Medical Center, 10410-L03.

References

1. Guo, D.Y.; Eteuati, J.; Nguyen, M.H.; Lloyd, D.; Ragg, J.L. Laparoscopic assisted colectomy: Experience from a rural centre. *ANZ J. Surg.* **2007**, *77*, 283–286. [CrossRef] [PubMed]
2. Clinical Outcomes of Surgical Therapy Study Group. A comparison of laparoscopically assisted and open colectomy for colon cancer. *N. Engl. J. Med.* **2004**, *350*, 2050–2059. [CrossRef] [PubMed]
3. Leung, K.L.; Kwok, S.P.; Lam, S.C.; Lee, J.F.; Yiu, R.Y.; Ng, S.S.; Lai, P.B.; Lau, W.Y. Laparoscopic resection of rectosigmoid carcinoma: Prospective randomised trial. *Lancet* **2004**, *363*, 1187–1192. [CrossRef]
4. Guillou, P.J.; Quirke, P.; Thorpe, H.; Walker, J.; Jayne, D.G.; Smith, A.M.; Heath, R.M.; Brown, J.M.; MRC CLASICC Trial Group. Short-term endpoints of conventional versus laparoscopic-assisted surgery in patients with colorectal cancer (MRC CLASICC trial): Multicentre, randomised controlled trial. *Lancet* **2005**, *365*, 1718–1726. [CrossRef]
5. Liang, J.T.; Huang, K.C.; Lai, H.S.; Lee, P.H.; Jeng, Y.M. Oncologic results of laparoscopic versus conventional open surgery for stage II or III left-sided colon cancers: A randomized controlled trial. *Ann. Surg. Oncol.* **2007**, *14*, 109–117. [CrossRef] [PubMed]
6. Veldkamp, R.; Kuhry, E.; Hop, W.C.; Jeekel, J.; Kazemier, G.; Bonjer, H.J.; Haglind, E.; Påhlman, L.; Cuesta, M.A.; Msika, S.; et al. Laparoscopic surgery versus open surgery for colon cancer: Short-term outcomes of a randomised trial. *Lancet Oncol.* **2005**, *6*, 477–484. [PubMed]
7. Jayne, D.G.; Guillou, P.J.; Thorpe, H.; Quirke, P.; Copeland, J.; Smith, A.M.; Heath, R.M.; Brown, J.M.; UK MRC CLASICC Trial Group. Randomized trial of laparoscopic-assisted resection of colorectal carcinoma: 3-year results of the UK MRC CLASICC Trial Group. *J. Clin. Oncol.* **2007**, *25*, 3061–3068. [CrossRef]
8. Colon Cancer Laparoscopic or Open Resection Study Group; Buunen, M.; Veldkamp, R.; Hop, W.C.; Kuhry, E.; Jeekel, J.; Haglind, E.; Påhlman, L.; Cuesta, M.A.; Msika, S.; et al. Survival after laparoscopic surgery versus open surgery for colon cancer: Long-term outcome of a randomised clinical trial. *Lancet Oncol.* **2009**, *10*, 44–52.

9. Hemandas, A.K.; Abdelrahman, T.; Flashman, K.G.; Skull, A.J.; Senapati, A.; O'Leary, D.P.; Parvaiz, A. Laparoscopic colorectal surgery produces better outcomes for high risk cancer patients compared to open surgery. *Ann. Surg.* **2010**, *252*, 84–89. [CrossRef]

10. Bagshaw, P.F.; Allardyce, R.A.; Frampton, C.M.; Frizelle, F.A.; Hewett, P.J.; McMurrick, P.J.; Rieger, N.A.; Smith, J.S.; Solomon, M.J.; Stevenson, A.R.; et al. Long-term outcomes of the australasian randomized clinical trial comparing laparoscopic and conventional open surgical treatments for colon cancer: The Australasian Laparoscopic Colon Cancer Study trial. *Ann. Surg.* **2012**, *256*, 915–919. [CrossRef]

11. Cummings, L.C.; Delaney, C.P.; Cooper, G.S. Laparoscopic versus open colectomy for colon cancer in an older population: A cohort study. *World J. Surg. Oncol.* **2012**, *10*, 31. [CrossRef] [PubMed]

12. Hinoi, T.; Kawaguchi, Y.; Hattori, M.; Okajima, M.; Ohdan, H.; Yamamoto, S.; Hasegawa, H.; Horie, H.; Murata, K.; Yamaguchi, S.; et al. Laparoscopic versus open surgery for colorectal cancer in elderly patients: A multicenter matched case-control study. *Ann. Surg. Oncol.* **2015**, *22*, 2040–2050. [CrossRef] [PubMed]

13. Hutter, M.M.; Randall, S.; Khuri, S.F.; Henderson, W.G.; Abbott, W.M.; Warshaw, A.L. Laparoscopic versus open gastric bypass for morbid obesity: A multicenter, prospective, risk-adjusted analysis from the National Surgical Quality Improvement Program. *Ann. Surg.* **2006**, *243*, 657–662. [CrossRef] [PubMed]

14. Weeks, J.C.; Nelson, H.; Gelber, S.; Sargent, D.; Schroeder, G.; Clinical Outcomes of Surgical Therapy (COST) Study Group. Short-term quality-of-life outcomes following laparoscopic-assisted colectomy vs open colectomy for colon cancer: A randomized trial. *JAMA* **2002**, *287*, 321–328. [CrossRef] [PubMed]

15. Tong, D.K.; Law, W.L. Laparoscopic versus open right hemicolectomy for carcinoma of the colon. *JSLS* **2007**, *11*, 76–80. [PubMed]

16. Steele, S.R.; Brown, T.A.; Rush, R.M.; Martin, M.J. Laparoscopic vs open colectomy for colon cancer: Results from a large nationwide population-based analysis. *J. Gastrointest. Surg.* **2008**, *12*, 583–591. [CrossRef] [PubMed]

17. Kennedy, G.D.; Heise, C.; Rajamanickam, V.; Harms, B.; Foley, E.F. Laparoscopy decreases postoperative complication rates after abdominal colectomy: Results from the national surgical quality improvement program. *Ann. Surg.* **2009**, *249*, 596–601. [CrossRef] [PubMed]

18. Liang, Y.; Li, G.; Chen, P.; Yu, J. Laparoscopic versus open colorectal resection for cancer: A meta-analysis of results of randomized controlled trials on recurrence. *Eur. J. Surg. Oncol.* **2008**, *34*, 1217–1224. [CrossRef]

19. Cianchi, F.; Trallori, G.; Mallardi, B.; Macrì, G.; Biagini, M.R.; Lami, G.; Indennitate, G.; Bagnoli, S.; Bonanomi, A.; Messerini, L.; et al. Survival after laparoscopic and open surgery for colon cancer: A comparative, single-institution study. *BMC Surg.* **2015**, *15*, 33. [CrossRef]

20. Neudecker, J.; Klein, F.; Bittner, R.; Carus, T.; Stroux, A.; Schwenk, W.; LAPKON II Trialists. Short-term outcomes from a prospective randomized trial comparing laparoscopic and open surgery for colorectal cancer. *Br. J. Surg.* **2009**, *96*, 1458–1467. [CrossRef]

21. Biondi, A.; Grosso, G.; Mistretta, A.; Marventano, S.; Toscano, C.; Gruttadauria, S.; Basile, F. Laparoscopic-assisted versus open surgery for colorectal cancer: Short- and long-term outcomes comparison. *J. Laparoendosc. Adv. Surg. Tech. A* **2013**, *23*, 1–7. [CrossRef] [PubMed]

22. Małczak, P.; Mizera, M.; Torbicz, G.; Witowski, J.; Major, P.; Pisarska, M.; Wysocki, M.; Strzałka, M.; Budzyński, A.; Pędziwiatr, M. Is the laparoscopic approach for rectal cancer superior to open surgery? A systematic review and meta-analysis on short-term surgical outcomes. *Wideochir. Inne Tech. Maloinwazyjne* **2018**, *13*, 129–140. [CrossRef] [PubMed]

23. Tjandra, J.J.; Chan, M.K. Systematic review on the short-term outcome of laparoscopic resection for colon and rectosigmoid cancer. *Colorectal. Dis.* **2006**, *8*, 375–388. [CrossRef] [PubMed]

24. Senagore, A.J.; Stulberg, J.J.; Byrnes, J.; Delaney, C.P. A national comparison of laparoscopic vs. open colectomy using the National Surgical Quality Improvement Project data. *Dis. Colon Rectum* **2009**, *52*, 183–186. [CrossRef]

25. Law, W.L.; Poon, J.T.; Fan, J.K.; Lo, S.H. Comparison of outcome of open and laparoscopic resection for stage II and stage III rectal cancer. *Ann. Surg. Oncol.* **2009**, *16*, 1488–1493. [CrossRef] [PubMed]

26. Lacy, A.M.; Delgado, S.; Castells, A.; Prins, H.A.; Arroyo, V.; Ibarzabal, A.; Pique, J.M. The long-term results of a randomized clinical trial of laparoscopy-assisted versus open surgery for colon cancer. *Ann. Surg.* **2008**, *248*, 1–7. [CrossRef] [PubMed]

27. Capussotti, L.; Massucco, P.; Muratore, A.; Amisano, M.; Bima, C.; Zorzi, D. Laparoscopy as a prognostic factor in curative resection for node positive colorectal cancer: Results for a single-institution nonrandomized prospective trial. *Surg. Endosc.* **2004**, *18*, 1130–1135. [CrossRef]

28. Law, W.L.; Poon, J.T.; Fan, J.K.; Lo, O.S. Survival following laparoscopic versus open resection for colorectal cancer. *Int. J. Colorectal. Dis.* **2012**, *27*, 1077–1085. [CrossRef]

29. Li, J.; Guo, H.; Guan, X.D.; Cai, C.N.; Yang, L.K.; Li, Y.C.; Zhu, Y.H.; Li, P.P.; Liu, X.L.; Yang, D.J. The impact of laparoscopic converted to open colectomy on short-term and oncologic outcomes for colon cancer. *J. Gastrointest. Surg.* **2015**, *19*, 335–343. [CrossRef]

30. Patankar, S.K.; Larach, S.W.; Ferrara, A.; Williamson, P.R.; Gallagher, J.T.; DeJesus, S.; Narayanan, S. Prospective comparison of laparoscopic vs. open resections for colorectal adenocarcinoma over a ten-year period. *Dis. Colon Rectum* **2003**, *46*, 601–611. [CrossRef]

31. Lujan, H.J.; Plasencia, G.; Jacobs, M.; Viamonte, M., III; Hartmann, R.F. Long-term survival after laparoscopic colon resection for cancer: Complete five-year follow-up. *Dis. Colon Rectum* **2002**, *45*, 491–501. [CrossRef] [PubMed]

32. Edge, S.B.; Compton, C.C. The American Joint Committee on Cancer: The 7th edition of the AJCC cancer staging manual and the future of TNM. *Ann. Surg. Oncol.* **2010**, *17*, 1471–1474. [CrossRef] [PubMed]

33. Qiu, H.B.; Zhang, L.Y.; Li, Y.F.; Zhou, Z.W.; Keshari, R.P.; Xu, R.H. Ratio of metastatic to resected lymph nodes enhances to predict survival in patients with stage III colorectal cancer. *Ann. Surg. Oncol.* **2011**, *18*, 1568–1574. [CrossRef] [PubMed]

34. Huh, J.W.; Kim, Y.J.; Kim, H.R. Ratio of metastatic to resected lymph nodes as a prognostic factor in node-positive colorectal cancer. *Ann. Surg. Oncol.* **2010**, *17*, 2640–2646. [CrossRef]

35. Wang, J.; Hassett, J.M.; Dayton, M.T.; Kulaylat, M.N. Lymph node ratio: Role in the staging of node-positive colon cancer. *Ann. Surg. Oncol.* **2008**, *15*, 1600–1608. [CrossRef] [PubMed]

36. Greenberg, R.; Itah, R.; Ghinea, R.; Sacham-Shmueli, E.; Inbar, R.; Avital, S. Metastatic lymph node ratio (LNR) as a prognostic variable in colorectal cancer patients undergoing laparoscopic resection. *Tech. Coloproctol.* **2011**, *15*, 273–279. [CrossRef] [PubMed]

37. Li Destri, G.; Di Carlo, I.; Scilletta, R.; Scilletta, B.; Puleo, S. Colorectal cancer and lymph nodes: The obsession with the number 12. *World J. Gastroenterol.* **2014**, *20*, 1951–1960.

38. Novitsky, Y.W.; Litwin, D.E.; Callery, M.P. The net immunologic advantage of laparoscopic surgery. *Surg. Endosc.* **2004**, *18*, 1411–1419. [CrossRef]

39. Lacy, A.M.; García-Valdecasas, J.C.; Delgado, S.; Castells, A.; Taurá, P.; Piqué, J.M.; Visa, J. Laparoscopy-assisted colectomy versus open colectomy for treatment of non-metastatic colon cancer: A randomised trial. *Lancet* **2002**, *359*, 2224–2229. [CrossRef]

40. Laurent, C.; Leblanc, F.; Wütrich, P.; Scheffler, M.; Rullier, E. Laparoscopic versus open surgery for rectal cancer: Long-term oncologic results. *Ann. Surg.* **2009**, *250*, 54–61. [CrossRef]

41. Whelan, R.L.; Franklin, M.; Holubar, S.D.; Donahue, J.; Fowler, R.; Munger, C.; Doorman, J.; Balli, J.E.; Glass, J.; Gonzalez, J.J.; et al. Postoperative cell mediated immune response is better preserved after laparoscopic vs open colorectal resection in humans. *Surg. Endosc.* **2003**, *17*, 972–978. [CrossRef] [PubMed]

42. Wichmann, M.W.; Hüttl, T.P.; Winter, H.; Spelsberg, F.; Angele, M.K.; Heiss, M.M.; Jauch, K.W. Immunological effects of laparoscopic vs open colorectal surgery: A prospective clinical study. *Arch. Surg.* **2005**, *140*, 692–697. [CrossRef] [PubMed]

43. Bessa, X.; Castells, A.; Lacy, A.M.; Elizalde, J.I.; Delgado, S.; Boix, L.; Piñol, V.; Pellisé, M.; García-Valdecasas, J.C.; Piqué, J.M. Laparoscopic-assisted vs. open colectomy for colorectal cancer: Influence on neoplastic cell mobilization. *J. Gastrointest. Surg.* **2001**, *5*, 66–73. [CrossRef]

44. Hsu, T.C. Feasibility of colectomy with mini-incision. *Am. J. Surg.* **2005**, *190*, 48–50. [CrossRef] [PubMed]

45. Hoyuela, C.; Juvany, M.; Carvajal, F. Single-incision laparoscopy versus standard laparoscopy for colorectal surgery: A systematic review and meta-analysis. *Am. J. Surg.* **2017**, *214*, 127–140. [CrossRef] [PubMed]

46. Acuna, S.A.; Elmi, M.; Shah, P.S.; Coburn, N.G.; Quereshy, F.A. Preoperative localization of colorectal cancer: A systematic review and meta-analysis. *Surg. Endosc.* **2017**, *31*, 2366–2379. [CrossRef] [PubMed]

47. Nishigori, N.; Koyama, F.; Nakagawa, T.; Nakamura, S.; Ueda, T.; Inoue, T.; Kawasaki, K.; Obara, S.; Nakamoto, T.; Fujii, H.; et al. Visualization of Lymph/Blood Flow in Laparoscopic Colorectal Cancer Surgery by ICG Fluorescence Imaging (Lap-IGFI). *Ann. Surg. Oncol.* **2016**, *23*, S266–S274. [CrossRef] [PubMed]

48. Chung, C.C.; Ng, D.C.; Tsang, W.W.; Tang, W.L.; Yau, K.K.; Cheung, H.Y.; Wong, J.C.; Li, M.K. Hand-assisted laparoscopic versus open right colectomy: A randomized controlled trial. *Ann. Surg.* **2007**, *246*, 728–733. [CrossRef] [PubMed]

49. Sato, T.; Watanabe, M. Present laparoscopic surgery for colorectal cancer in Japan. *World J. Clin. Oncol.* **2016**, *7*, 155–159. [CrossRef] [PubMed]

50. Tekkis, P.P.; Senagore, A.J.; Delaney, C.P.; Fazio, V.W. Evaluation of the learning curve in laparoscopic colorectal surgery: Comparison of right-sided and left-sided resections. *Ann. Surg.* **2005**, *242*, 83–91. [CrossRef] [PubMed]

51. Morneau, M.; Boulanger, J.; Charlebois, P.; Latulippe, J.F.; Lougnarath, R.; Thibault, C.; Gervais, N.; Comité de l'Évolution des Pratiques en Oncologie. Laparoscopic versus open surgery for the treatment of colorectal cancer: A literature review and recommendations from the Comité de l'évolution des pratiques en oncologie. *Can. J. Surg.* **2013**, *56*, 297–310. [CrossRef] [PubMed]

52. Fleshman, J.; Sargent, D.J.; Green, E.; Anvari, M.; Stryker, S.J.; Beart, R.W., Jr.; Hellinger, M.; Flanagan, R., Jr.; Peters, W.; Nelson, H.; et al. Laparoscopic colectomy for cancer is not inferior to open surgery based on 5-year data from the COST Study Group trial. *Ann. Surg.* **2007**, *246*, 655–662. [CrossRef] [PubMed]

53. Hyman, N.; Manchester, T.L.; Osler, T.; Burns, B.; Cataldo, P.A. Anastomotic leaks after intestinal anastomosis: it's later than you think. *Ann. Surg.* **2007**, *245*, 254–258. [CrossRef] [PubMed]

54. Pickleman, J.; Watson, W.; Cunningham, J.; Fisher, S.G.; Gamelli, R. The failed gastrointestinal anastomosis: An inevitable catastrophe? *J. Am. Coll. Surg.* **1999**, *188*, 473–482. [CrossRef]

55. Bruce, J.; Krukowski, Z.H.; Al-Khairy, G.; Russell, E.M.; Park, K.G. Systematic review of the definition and measurement of anastomotic leak after gastrointestinal surgery. *Br. J. Surg.* **2001**, *88*, 1157–1168. [CrossRef] [PubMed]

56. Zhang, Y.; Chen, Z.; Li, J. The current status of treatment for colorectal cancer in China: A systematic review. *Medicine* **2017**, *96*, e8242. [CrossRef] [PubMed]

57. Xu, J.; Ren, L. China Guideline for Diagnosis and Comprehensive Treatment of Colorectal Liver Metastases (Version 2018). *Zhonghua Wei Chang Wai Ke Za Zhi* **2018**, *21*, 601–626. [PubMed]

58. Athanasakis, E.; Xenaki, S.; Venianaki, M.; Chalkiadakis, G.; Chrysos, E. Newly recognized extratumoral features of colorectal cancer challenge the current tumor-node-metastasis staging system. *Ann. Gastroenterol.* **2018**, *31*, 525–534. [CrossRef]

59. Quirke, P.; Williams, G.T.; Ectors, N.; Ensari, A.; Piard, F.; Nagtegaal, I. The future of the TNM staging system in colorectal cancer: Time for a debate? *Lancet Oncol.* **2007**, *8*, 651–657. [CrossRef]

60. Maguire, A.; Sheahan, K. Controversies in the pathological assessment of colorectal cancer. *World J. Gastroenterol.* **2014**, *20*, 9850–9861. [CrossRef]

61. Puppa, G.; Sonzogni, A.; Colombari, R.; Pelosi, G. TNM staging system of colorectal carcinoma: A critical appraisal of challenging issues. *Arch. Pathol. Lab. Med.* **2010**, *134*, 837–852. [PubMed]

62. Lennon, A.M.; Mulcahy, H.E.; Hyland, J.M.; Lowry, C.; White, A.; Fennelly, D.; Murphy, J.J.; O'Donoghue, D.P.; Sheahan, K. Peritoneal involvement in stage II colon cancer. *Am. J. Clin. Pathol.* **2003**, *119*, 108–113. [CrossRef] [PubMed]

63. Kojima, M.; Nakajima, K.; Ishii, G.; Saito, N.; Ochiai, A. Peritoneal elastic laminal invasion of colorectal cancer: The diagnostic utility and clinicopathologic relationship. *Am. J. Surg. Pathol.* **2010**, *34*, 1351–1360. [CrossRef] [PubMed]

64. Burdy, G.; Panis, Y.; Alves, A.; Nemeth, J.; Lavergne-Slove, A.; Valleur, P. Identifying patients with T3-T4 node-negative colon cancer at high risk of recurrence. *Dis. Colon Rectum* **2001**, *44*, 1682–1688. [CrossRef] [PubMed]

65. Merkel, S.; Wein, A.; Günther, K.; Papadopoulos, T.; Hohenberger, W.; Hermanek, P. High-risk groups of patients with stage II colon carcinoma. *Cancer* **2001**, *92*, 1435–1443. [CrossRef]

66. Morris, M.; Platell, C.; de Boer, B.; McCaul, K.; Iacopetta, B. Population-based study of prognostic factors in stage II colonic cancer. *Br. J. Surg.* **2006**, *93*, 866–871. [CrossRef] [PubMed]

67. Newland, R.C.; Dent, O.F.; Chapuis, P.H.; Bokey, L. Survival after curative resection of lymph node negative colorectal carcinoma. A prospective study of 910 patients. *Cancer* **1995**, *76*, 564–571. [CrossRef]

68. Petersen, V.C.; Baxter, K.J.; Love, S.B.; Shepherd, N.A. Identification of objective pathological prognostic determinants and models of prognosis in Dukes' B colon cancer. *Gut* **2002**, *51*, 65–69. [CrossRef]

69. Grin, A.; Messenger, D.E.; Cook, M.; O'Connor, B.I.; Hafezi, S.; El-Zimaity, H.; Kirsch, R. Peritoneal elastic lamina invasion: Limitations in its use as a prognostic marker in stage II colorectal cancer. *Hum. Pathol.* **2013**, *44*, 2696–2705. [CrossRef]

70. Grizzi, F.; Celesti, G.; Basso, G.; Laghi, L. Tumor budding as a potential histopathological biomarker in colorectal cancer: Hype or hope? *World J. Gastroenterol.* **2012**, *18*, 6532–6536. [CrossRef]

71. Elfaedy, O.; Owens, P.; Aakif, M.; Mansour, E. Discrepancy in Colorectal Cancer Staging: A Single Center Experience. Available online: http://www.surgeryresearchjournal.com/full-text/wjssr-v1-id1054.php (accessed on 1 March 2019).

72. Gong, Y.; Peng, P.; Bao, P.; Zhong, W.; Shi, Y.; Gu, K.; Zheng, Y.; Wu, C.; Cai, S.; Xu, Y.; et al. The Implementation and First-Round Results of a Community-Based Colorectal Cancer Screening Program in Shanghai, China. *Oncologist* **2018**, *23*, 928–935. [CrossRef] [PubMed]

6

Relationship between Morbidity and Health Behavior in Chronic Diseases

Munjae Lee [1,2], Sewon Park [1,2] and Kyu-Sung Lee [2,3,*]

[1] Research Institute for Future Medicine, Samsung Medical Center, Seoul 06351, Korea; emunjae@skku.edu (M.L.); se10919@g.skku.edu (S.P.)

[2] Department of Medical Device Management and Research, SAIHST, Sungkyunkwan University, Seoul 06355, Korea

[3] Department of Urology, Samsung Medical Center, Sungkyunkwan University School of Medicine, Seoul 06351, Korea

* Correspondence: ksleedr@skku.edu

Abstract: This study aimed to analyze the demographic characteristics and health behaviors related to chronic diseases and to identify factors that may affect chronic diseases. Data from the Seventh Korea National Health and Nutrition Examination Survey were used, and 3795 adults aged above 40 years were included. The following demographic variables were obtained: sex, age, education, income, type of health insurance, and private insurance. The following health behavior factors were also analyzed: medical checkup, drinking, smoking, exercise, obesity, and hypercholesterolemia. Participants with lower socioeconomic status had a higher risk of developing chronic diseases. Meanwhile, those with private health insurance had a lower risk of developing chronic diseases. In addition, participants who underwent medical checkups and performed exercises had a lower risk, while those with obesity and hypercholesterolemia had a higher risk of developing chronic diseases. It is necessary to manage chronic diseases through comprehensive programs, rather than managing these diseases individually, and through community primary care institutions to improve health behaviors.

Keywords: chronic disease; health behavior; socioeconomic status; primary care; Korea

1. Introduction

An individual's behavior related to health may have an effect on their physical health or ability to recover from illness. In particular, health-related behavior, such as a lack of exercise, smoking, and drinking, are some of the main factors that can contribute to morbidity and mortality [1–3]. Health behavior affects 40% of premature deaths; in order to reduce premature mortality, improving health behaviors is more cost-effective than improving the social and physical environments or health-care systems [4]. These health behaviors are important in maintaining good health, which is influenced by biological and socioeconomic factors, among others [5,6]. Rapid economic growth, high health-care costs, lifestyle changes, and population aging have been associated with an increased prevalence of chronic diseases worldwide. Chronic diseases may cause complications, and thus, require continuous care and are among the types of diseases with high health-care costs due to their long disease duration [7–9].

Chronic diseases, one of the leading causes of death worldwide, especially cardiocerebrovascular diseases, diabetes, and hypertension, have a high mortality rate. However, the mortality rate of chronic diseases can be reduced through prevention [10–12]. Chronic disease is closely related to changes in health behaviors; the main health behaviors affecting the development of chronic diseases include health risk behavioral factors, such as smoking, drinking, and physical activities, and clinicopathologic factors, including obesity, hypertension, and hypercholesterolemia [13,14]. In particular, since health-related lifestyles have increased the risk of mortality, the significance of managing health risk behavioral factors has also been increasing. Thus, it is necessary to prevent chronic diseases and delay the aggravation of symptoms by improving individual lifestyles [15–17]. In addition, individual health behaviors may differ according to sociodemographic characteristics including age and sex [18]. In the identification of the individual physical condition, sociodemographic and socioeconomic factors are known to act as important factors, and prevalence rates vary in accordance with the individual's income level, education level, and socioeconomic factors [19].

Previous studies have analyzed the relationship between chronic diseases and health promotion behaviors, but were only conducted in predetermined age groups, such as in older patients, or examined the relationship between chronic diseases and health behaviors while only targeting certain chronic diseases [20–24]. As the number of polychronic patients has increased, a comprehensive analysis of chronic diseases is required. To date, the number of studies evaluating patients with chronic diseases is limited. Accordingly, in this study, we aimed to analyze the sociodemographic characteristics and health behaviors related to the development of chronic diseases and to identify factors that may have an effect on the morbidity of chronic diseases. Through this and by suggesting measures to contribute to the effective management and prevention of chronic diseases, we intend to promote the health of the people.

2. Experimental Section

2.1. Data Source and Research Participants

In this study, we utilized the source data from the 2nd year (2017) of the 7th period of the Korea National Health and Nutrition Examination Survey, performed by the Korea Centers for Disease Control and Prevention. The Korea National Health and Nutrition Examination Survey (KNHANES) is a nationwide national survey, conducted to determine health-related parameters including the prevalence of chronic diseases and health behaviors based on Article 16 of the National Health Promotion Act. A total of 10,430 individuals from 3580 households were surveyed, but only 8127 participated in the study. Of them, 5159 aged above 40 years were extracted. In addition, 658 individuals whose answers were not related to chronic diseases were excluded; hence, only 3795 participants were analyzed, after further excluding 706 who did not respond to the questions related to health behaviors. The KNHANES is approved by the ethical committee of the Korea Centers for Disease Control and Prevention. The requirement for informed consent was waived because data in the KNHANE database are anonymized in adherence to strict confidentiality guidelines. The flowchart is shown in Figure 1.

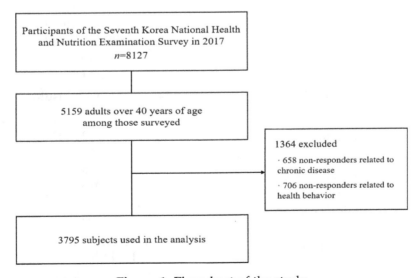

Figure 1. Flowchart of the study.

2.2. Description of Variables

In this study, questions related to sociodemographic characteristics, morbidity, and presence of chronic diseases, and health behaviors were utilized. Sex, age, education level, level of income, type of health insurance, and private insurance policy were used as sociodemographic variables. In terms of age, participants aged 19 years or older were divided into two groups: adults and older adults (aged 65 years and above). The education level was stratified into middle school graduates or less and high school graduates or more. Income status was determined by the monthly mean household gross income and was classified based on 3 million won as the cut-off point. The patients with health insurance were classified as health insurance subscribers and medical care beneficiaries [23,25–28].

Hypertension and diabetes are the main causes of cardiovascular disease, and the number of patients continues to rise due to the increase in obesity rate. In addition, the cost of medical care is proliferating more rapidly than the number of patients. Therefore, it is significant to prevent it by analyzing the factors influencing chronic diseases. Hitherto, chronic disease was defined as hypertension, dyslipidemia, stroke, myocardial infarction, and diabetes. The presence of chronic disease was determined based on a response of "Yes" to the question related to a doctor's diagnosis. Health behaviors included health checkups, drinking, smoking, exercise, obesity, and hypercholesterolemia [28–31]. Health checkup status was classified as patients who underwent health checkups and those who did not undergo health checkups. Drinking status was classified as non-drinkers and drinkers based on the monthly drinking rate; smoking status was classified as non-smokers and smokers using the current smoking rate. Exercise history was stratified as those who performed exercises and those who did not perform exercises based on the aerobic physical activity practice rate [32,33]. Furthermore, the prevalence of obesity was determined and obesity was stratified based on the following indices: a body mass index of 18.5 kg/m^2 or higher or a body mass index of 23 kg/m^2 or lower indicates normal weight, while a body mass index of 25 kg/m^2 or higher indicates obesity [34–36]. Hypercholesterolemia was stratified based on its prevalence (Table 1).

Table 1. Classification and definition of variables.

Variable	Definition
Sex	0 = Female 1 = Male
Age	0 = Adult 1 = Senior
Education	0 = ≤Middle school 1 = ≥Middle school
Income	0 = <300 1 = ≥300
Type of insurance	0 = National Health Insurance 1 = Assistance
Private insurance	0 = No 1 = Yes
Chronic disease	0 = No 1 = Yes
Medical checkup	0 = No 1 = Yes
Drinking	0 = Non-drinker 1 = Drinker
Smoking	0 = Non-smoker 1 = Smoker

Table 1. *Cont.*

Variable	Definition
Exercise	0 = No 1 = Yes
Obesity	0 = Obesity 1 = Normal
Hypercholesterolemia	0 = No 1 = Yes

2.3. Statistical Analysis

In order to analyze the relationship among sociodemographic characteristics, health behaviors, and the presence of chronic diseases, statistical analyses were conducted using the SPSS (version 25.0, https://www.ibm.com/kr-ko/analytics/spss-statistics-software).

First, cross-analysis was performed to analyze the relationship between chronic diseases and sociodemographic characteristics and between health behaviors and chronic diseases. In order to determine the relationship between sociodemographic characteristics and health behaviors and the risk for developing chronic diseases, a logistic regression analysis was performed.

3. Results

3.1. Participants' Demographic Characteristics

Of the total participants, 56% were women and the proportion of women was higher than that of men; older adults aged 65 years or higher accounted for 33% of the total study population. Most of the participants were middle school graduates or had obtained higher education (2269 persons, 59.8%) and had an income of more than 3 million won (2107 persons, 55.5%). With regard to the type of health insurance, national health insurance subscribers accounted for 95.7% of the total participants according to the characteristics of health insurance in Korea. Meanwhile, private insurance subscribers accounted for 74.2%, even though the proportion of health insurance subscribers corresponded to a majority; this finding indicates that most of the patients took a private medical insurance policy due to the lack of coverage by the national health insurance. A total of 857 patients (22.6%) underwent medical checkups, which suggests that only a few patients were able to undergo medical checkups. A total of 1762 patients (46.4%) developed chronic diseases, of whom 21.4% had two or more chronic diseases (Table 2).

Table 2. Demographic characteristics (n = 3795).

Characteristic	Type	N	%
Sex	Female	2126	56.0
	Male	1669	44.0
Age	40–65	2544	67.0
	≥65	1251	33.0
Education	<Middle school	1526	40.2
	≥Middle school	2269	59.8
Income	<300	1688	44.5
	≥300	2107	55.5
Type of insurance	National health insurance	3632	95.7
	Assistance	163	4.3
Private insurance	Y	2814	74.2
	N	981	25.8

Table 2. *Cont.*

Characteristic	Type	N	%
Medical checkup	Y	857	22.6
	N	2938	77.4
Chronic disease	0	2033	53.6
	1	950	25.0
	<2	812	21.4

3.2. Relationship between Demographic Characteristics and Chronic Diseases

In this study, we intended to analyze the relationship between sociodemographic characteristics and chronic diseases, and the results are shown in Table 3. Among chronic disease patients, 955 (44.9%) were women, this proportion being higher than that of men. Meanwhile, 807 (48.4%) of 862 male participants had chronic diseases, which indicates that men had a higher rate of chronic disease morbidity. Approximately 71.3% of the participants aged 65 years or higher had chronic diseases. In addition, most of the patients with a lower educational level and lower-income level had chronic diseases (981 patients (64.3%)and 1008 patients (59.7%), respectively). A total of 1648 (45.4%) health insurance subscribers were chronic disease patients, while 114 (69.9%) medical care recipients were chronic disease patients. Furthermore, 1128 (40.1%) chronic disease patients were private insurance subscribers.

Table 3. Relationship between demographic characteristics and chronic diseases.

Characteristic	Type	Chronic Disease				p-Value
		N	%	Y	%	
Sex **	Female	1171	55.1	955	44.9	0.019
	Male	862	51.6	807	48.4	
Age ***	40–65	1674	65.8	870	34.2	0.001
	≥65	359	28.7	892	71.3	
Education ***	<Middle school	545	35.7	981	64.3	0.001
	≥Middle school	1488	65.6	781	34.4	
Income ***	<300	680	40.3	1008	59.7	0.001
	≥300	1353	64.2	754	35.8	
Type of insurance ***	NHI	1984	54.6	1648	45.4	0.001
	Assistance	49	30.1	114	69.9	
Private insurance ***	Y	1686	59.9	1128	40.1	0.001
	N	347	35.4	634	64.6	

** $p < 0.05$, *** $p < 0.001$.

3.3. Relationship between Health Behavior and Chronic Diseases

We analyzed the relationship between health behaviors and chronic diseases; the results are shown in Table 4. Of the total chronic disease patients, 944 (50.6%) were alcohol drinkers, 1503 (47%) were smokers, and 605 (40.1%) performed exercises, which is less than the number of patients who did not perform exercises (1157, 50.6%). Moreover, 1263 (52.7%) and 823 (73.9%) patients with obesity and hypercholesterolemia, respectively, had chronic diseases.

Table 4. Relationship between health behavior and chronic diseases.

Characteristic	Type	Chronic Disease				p-Value
		N	%	Y	%	
Medical checkup	Y	453	52.9	404	47.1	0.331
	N	1580	53.8	1358	46.2	
Drinking ***	Y	923	49.4	944	50.6	0.001
	N	1110	57.6	818	42.4	
Smoking *	Y	1696	53.0	1503	47.0	0.062
	N	337	56.5	259	43.5	
Exercise ***	Y	904	59.9	605	40.1	0.001
	N	1129	49.4	1157	50.6	
Obesity ***	Y	1132	47.3	1263	52.7	0.001
	N	901	64.4	499	35.6	
Hypercholesterolemia ***	Y	291	26.1	823	73.9	0.001
	N	1742	65.0	939	35.0	

* $p < 0.1$, *** $p < 0.001$.

3.4. Factors Affecting Chronic Diseases

In order to determine the factors that may affect the development of chronic diseases, logistic regression analysis was performed, and the results are shown in Table 5. The factors with statistically significant effects in patients with chronic disease included sex, age, education, income, types of health insurance, decision to take a private insurance policy, health checkups, exercise, obesity, and hypercholesterolemia.

Table 5. Factors affecting the development of chronic diseases.

Dependent Variable	Independent Variable	Exp(B)	p-Value
Chronic disease	Sex ***	1.498	0.001
	Age ***	3.145	0.001
	Education ***	0.535	0.001
	Income **	0.773	0.004
	Type of insurance **	1.727	0.008
	Private insurance **	0.803	0.036
	Medical checkup **	0.782	0.009
	Drinking	1.101	0.252
	Smoking	1.061	0.606
	Exercise *	0.861	0.060
	Obesity ***	0.544	0.001
	Hypercholesterolemia ***	5.444	0.001

* $p < 0.1$, ** $p < 0.05$, *** $p < 0.001$.

In men, the risk of developing chronic diseases was higher by 1.498 times. Further, as age increased, the risk of developing chronic diseases also increased by 3.145 times. In participants with a higher education level, the risk of developing chronic diseases increased by 0.535 times. In participants with higher income, the risk of developing chronic disease reduced by 0.773 times. With regard to the type of health insurance, the risk of developing chronic diseases increased by 1.727 times among medical care beneficiaries. In addition, for those who took a private insurance policy, the risk of developing chronic diseases increased by 0.782 times. Meanwhile, the risk of developing chronic diseases decreased by 0.782 times and 0.861 times among those who underwent medical checkups and who performed exercises, respectively. In normal-weight people, the risk of developing chronic diseases reduced by 0.544 times. In patients with hypercholesterolemia, the risk increased by 5.444 times.

4. Discussion

In this study, we analyzed the factors affecting the development of chronic diseases through logistic regression analysis using the data from the Korea National Health and Nutrition Examination Survey (2017). Of the sociodemographic characteristics, sex, age, education and income level, types of health insurance, and private insurance were found to have an effect on chronic diseases. In terms of sex, the proportion of women with chronic diseases was higher than that of men. Compared with women, men had a higher rate of chronic disease morbidity and the risk of developing chronic diseases. These results are inconsistent with those of previous studies, which reported that the prevalence of chronic diseases is higher among women than in men because men can maintain their economic level for longer than women. Women who have a lower income level than men have relatively low medical accessibility and find it difficult to manage their chronic diseases [37]. The number of chronic disease patients is increasing due to the lack of physical activity and the increasing prevalence of hypercholesterolemia and obesity, and considering that previous studies have shown that the prevalence of chronic disease was lower among men who received management, managing chronic diseases according to sex seems to be of utmost importance [38]. In addition, the number of patients aged 65 years or older who had chronic diseases was higher; therefore, the higher the age, the higher the risk of developing chronic diseases. This finding is consistent with those of a previous study, which reported that as age increases, the prevalence of chronic diseases also increases due to the decreased amount of physical activities and habit-based health risk behaviors [8,39].

It was also found that the higher the income and education levels, the lower the risk of chronic diseases. This finding is consistent with those of previous studies reporting that socioeconomic status, including income, education, and occupation levels, affects the health-related lifestyles and risk of chronic diseases [40]. Because of the low rates of physical activity and exercise practice and as the provision of medical services for managing chronic diseases has still not been ensured owing to lower educational levels or living standards, the prevalence of chronic diseases is increasing. Among medical care beneficiaries, the risk of developing chronic diseases was high, which was similar to the results of a previous study reporting that the incidence of chronic disease increased among individuals who belonged to the lower social class, like those in the low-income bracket. Social determinants, such as income, education, and social class, may cause health-related inequality but create an environment in which quality medical care can be provided for the treatment of chronic diseases. In addition, non-medical factors, such as social determinants, play a more substantial role in the management of chronic diseases than medical factors. It seems that medical care beneficiaries with low income may have more difficulty in managing chronic diseases [41–43]. There were many chronic disease patients who obtained a private medical insurance policy; the results showed that patients with private medical insurance had a lower risk of developing chronic diseases. These findings are similar to those of a previous study, which indicated that those who have private medical insurance policies tend to receive outpatient and inpatient treatments. In line with these findings, among patients with chronic diseases who require continuous health care, those with private medical insurance have a reduced burden in terms of medical expenses, leading to better health-care outcomes [44–46]. Considering these results, there are limitations in managing chronic diseases with national health insurance only. Furthermore, it is estimated that people obtain commercial medical insurance policies due to the burden of medical expenses caused by the recent increase in polychronic diseases. Therefore, since health-related inequalities in the low-income group patients, who find it difficult to pay the private medical insurance premiums, will become a serious problem if we only rely on private medical insurance for the management of chronic diseases, the coverage of the national health insurance should be reinforced for the management of chronic diseases.

Among health behaviors, the factors affecting the risk of developing chronic diseases included health checkups, exercise, obesity, and hypercholesterolemia. Those who underwent periodic health checkups had a risk of developing chronic diseases, which is similar to previous findings showing that periodic health checkups promote health and help prevent chronic diseases [8,47]. In addition, considering the results of previous studies reporting that those who benefit from health insurance are more likely to receive health checkups depending on the nature of the health insurance system in Korea, chronic diseases could be effectively managed through modifying the nature of the insurance provided. Previous studies have shown that health behavior factors related to chronic diseases include smoking, drinking, exercise, body mass index, and regular life and eating habits [7,29,36,48,49]. However, in this study, drinking and smoking did not have a statistically significant effect on the prevalence of chronic diseases, and these results are different from those of existing research. Furthermore, exercise, obesity, and hypercholesterolemia were associated with the risk of developing chronic diseases, consistent with existing research. Among those who performed exercises, the risk of developing chronic diseases was lower, while among those with obesity and hypercholesterolemia, the risk of developing chronic diseases was higher. Weight loss via exercise programs reduces the risk of developing chronic diseases. Maintaining a standard body weight can prevent chronic diseases by alleviating hypercholesterolemia. Management of chronic diseases should be comprehensively performed with weight management through exercise; however, there seems to be a limitation in this regard according to patients' behavioral changes [50,51]. In order to overcome this limitation, wearable medical devices, which use ICT (Information & Communication Technology), have recently been developed for chronic disease management. Prevention and management of chronic diseases can be ensured through exercise [52–55]. The use of medical devices to promote physical activity leads to obesity and hypercholesterolemia management, and through the linkage between these medical devices and local clinic-centered, effective management of chronic diseases can be achieved through periodic monitoring. The results of this study also suggest that gender, age, education, and income levels have impacts on chronic disease, and it is significant to add these as risk factors and to continue monitoring in local clinic-centered facilities. Through this, a personalized chronic disease management system could be established.

This study has some limitations. First, chronic disease patients aged 40 years or below were not included. Recently, the number of younger chronic disease patients has increased owing to changes in lifestyle, therefore, further studies to analyze the factors influencing the risk of developing chronic diseases in this age group will be required, with the patients stratified as follows: youth, middle-aged, and older adults. Second, analyses according to the number of chronic diseases were not performed. In this study, only the presence or absence of chronic diseases in patients was assessed. Further studies to determine the influencing factors according to the number of chronic diseases are required. Third, there was no analysis of factors affecting chronic disease according to the residential area. Accessibility to medical services varies depending on where you live; therefore, chronic disease management may be different. Hence, it is necessary to analyze the factors affecting chronic diseases according to urban and rural areas. Despite these limitations, we comprehensively analyzed the factors influencing the prevalence of chronic diseases. Our study is significant as we were able to determine the risk factors for chronic diseases, which can be used as a basis for developing policies for the comprehensive management of chronic diseases, based on sex, age, and social factors.

5. Conclusions

In order to manage chronic diseases, the management approach should be based on patients' socioeconomic characteristics to address the differences related to sex, education, income, and medical care. The management should also include approaches to improve health behaviors, including the use of wearable medical devices and digital healthcare products. Based on our findings, we presume that chronic diseases develop due to a combination of factors. Age, socioeconomic factors, obesity, and hypercholesterolemia are factors that can be controlled to prevent and manage chronic diseases through comprehensive programs rather than through individual management. Moreover, those who belong to the lower social class, are more likely to require chronic disease management via primary healthcare institutions in the community. In order to improve health behaviors, continuous observation is required, and local clinic-centered chronic disease management can help improve health behaviors. It is significant to establish a comprehensive management system and promote efficient medical delivery systems for chronic diseases focused on local clinic-centered facilities. However, Korea's medical delivery system urgently needs reorganization due to the concentration of university hospitals and the weakening of a local clinic-centered structure. Therefore, in order to expand the role of local clinic-centered facilities and to efficiently manage chronic diseases, the integrated local clinic-centered care chronic disease management project is being implemented. Through this, medical treatment for chronic disease management and education for improving lifestyle, are applied to lower the patient's copayment. If the burden reduction of chronic disease management is expanded, the dependency on private health insurance will be reduced, which will prevent excessive medical expenses for chronic patients. In addition, strengthening the role of local clinic-centered facilities will lead to strengthening medical access for low-income people, thereby relieving health inequalities. For older adults, when included in the community care project in line with community-based primary healthcare service, comprehensive management of chronic diseases, including health improvement and lifestyle modification, could be implemented. In particular, in Europe, where public health policies are in place, chronic diseases are effectively managed by strengthening the local clinic-centered services, such as the attending physician, to manage chronic diseases. For common goals such as chronic disease management, community care is implemented to ensure continuous health care. In view of this, chronic disease management through public health policy should be implemented prior to private medical insurance. Patients with private medical insurance have a lower risk of developing chronic diseases, but this can be seen as a problem of low insurance coverage for chronic diseases. This can be resolved through community care projects such as in Europe. Because of this, patient-centered chronic disease management will ultimately improve the health of chronic disease patients.

Author Contributions: Conceptualization, M.L.; methodology, S.P.; software, S.P.; validation, M.L. and K.-S.L.; formal analysis, M.L.; writing—original draft preparation, S.P.; writing—review and editing, M.L.; supervision, K.-S.L.; project administration, M.L. All authors have read and agreed to the published version of the manuscript.

References

1.   Janowski, K.; Kurpas, D.; Kusz, J.; Mroczek, B.; Jedynak, T. Health-related behavior, profile of health locus of control and acceptance of illness in patients suffering from chronic somatic diseases. *PLoS ONE* **2013**, *8*, e63920. [CrossRef] [PubMed]
2.   Mullen, P.D.; Hersey, J.C.; Iverson, D.C. Health behavior models compared. *Soc. Sci. Med.* **1987**, *24*, 973–981. [CrossRef]
3.   Berrigan, D.; Dodd, K.; Troiano, R.P.; Krebs-Smith, S.M.; Barbash, R.B. Patterns of health behavior in U.S. adults. *Prev. Med.* **2003**, *36*, 615–623. [CrossRef]
4.   McGinnis, J.M.; Williams-Russo, P.; Knickman, J.R. The case for more active policy attention to health promotion. *Health Aff.* **2002**, *21*, 78–93. [CrossRef]
5.   Jarvandi, S.; Yan, Y.; Schootman, M. Income disparity and risk of death: The importance of health behaviors and other mediating factors. *PLoS ONE* **2012**, *7*, e49929. [CrossRef]
6.   Nettle, D. Why are there social gradients in preventative health behavior? A perspective from behavioral ecology. *PLoS ONE* **2010**, *5*, e13371. [CrossRef]
7.   Paudel, S.; Owen, A.J.; Owusu-Addo, E.; Smith, B.J. Physical activity participation and the risk of chronic diseases among South Asian adults: A systematic review and meta-analysis. *Sci. Rep.* **2019**, *9*, 9771. [CrossRef]
8.   Strong, K.; Mathers, C.; Leeder, S.; Beaglehole, R. Preventing chronic diseases: How many lives can we save? *Lancet* **2005**, *366*, 1578–1582. [CrossRef]
9.   Yach, D.; Hawkes, C.; Gould, C.L.; Hofman, K.J. The Global Burden of Chronic DiseasesOvercoming Impediments to Prevention and Control. *JAMA* **2004**, *291*, 2616–2622. [CrossRef]

10. Bae, E.-J.; Park, N.-J.; Sohn, H.-S.; Kim, Y.-H. Handgrip strength and all-cause mortality in middle-aged and older Koreans. *Int. J. Environ. Res. Public Health* **2019**, *16*, 740. [CrossRef]

11. Gansevoort, R.T.; Correa-Rotter, R.; Hemmelgarn, B.R.; Jafar, T.H.; Heerspink, H.J.L.; Mann, J.F.; Matsushita, K.; Wen, C.P. Chronic kidney disease and cardiovascular risk: Epidemiology, mechanisms, and prevention. *Lancet* **2013**, *382*, 339–352. [CrossRef]

12. Halpin, H.A.; Morales-Suárez-Varela, M.M.; Martin-Moreno, J.M. Chronic Disease Prevention and the New Public Health. *Public Health Rev.* **2010**, *32*, 120–154. [CrossRef]

13. Sturm, R. The effects of obesity, smoking, and drinking on medical problems and costs. *Health Aff.* **2002**, *21*, 245–253. [CrossRef] [PubMed]

14. Strine, T.W.; Chapman, D.P.; Balluz, L.S.; Moriarty, D.G.; Mokdad, A.H. The associations between life satisfaction and health-related quality of life, chronic illness, and health behaviors among US community-dwelling adults. *J. Community Health* **2008**, *33*, 40–50. [CrossRef]

15. Harris, M. The role of primary health care in preventing the onset of chronic disease, with a particular focus on the lifestyle risk factors of obesity, tobacco and alcohol. *Canberra Natl. Prev. Health Taskforce* **2008**, *1*, 21.

16. Steyn, K.; Damasceno, A. Lifestyle and related risk factors for chronic diseases. *Dis. Mortal. Sub-Sahar. Afr.* **2006**, *2*, 247–265.

17. Reeves, M.J.; Rafferty, A.P. Healthy lifestyle characteristics among adults in the United States, 2000. *Arch. Intern. Med.* **2005**, *165*, 854–857. [CrossRef]

18. Kang, Y.J.; Kang, M.-Y. Chronic diseases, health behaviors, and demographic characteristics as predictors of ill health retirement: Findings from the Korea Health Panel Survey (2008–2012). *PLoS ONE* **2016**, *11*, e0166921. [CrossRef]

19. Winkleby, M.A.; Cubbin, C. Changing patterns in health behaviors and risk factors related to chronic diseases, 1990–2000. *Am. J. Health Promot.* **2004**, *19*, 19–27. [CrossRef]

20. Speake, D.L.; Cowart, M.E.; Pellet, K. Health perceptions and lifestyles of the elderly. *Res. Nurs. Health* **1989**, *12*, 93–100. [CrossRef]

21. Cho, Y.I.; Lee, S.-Y.D.; Arozullah, A.M.; Crittenden, K.S. Effects of health literacy on health status and health service utilization amongst the elderly. *Soc. Sci. Med.* **2008**, *66*, 1809–1816. [CrossRef] [PubMed]

22. Lee, T.W.; Ko, I.S.; Lee, K.J. Health promotion behaviors and quality of life among community-dwelling elderly in Korea: A cross-sectional survey. *Int. J. Nurs. Stud.* **2006**, *43*, 293–300. [CrossRef] [PubMed]

23. Winkleby, M.A.; Jatulis, D.E.; Frank, E.; Fortmann, S.P. Socioeconomic status and health: How education, income, and occupation contribute to risk factors for cardiovascular disease. *Am. J. Public Health* **1992**, *82*, 816–820. [CrossRef] [PubMed]

24. Innes, H.; McAuley, A.; Alavi, M.; Valerio, H.; Goldberg, D.; Hutchinson, S.J. The contribution of health risk behaviors to excess mortality in American adults with chronic hepatitis C: A population cohort-study. *Hepatology* **2018**, *67*, 97–107. [CrossRef] [PubMed]

25. Lim, J.; Kim, S.; Ke, S.; Cho, B. The Association Chronic Liver Diseases with Health Related Behaviors in South Korea. *Korean J. Fam. Med.* **2010**, *31*, 302–307. [CrossRef]

26. Caspersen, C.J.; Pereira, M.A.; Curran, K.M. Changes in physical activity patterns in the United States, by sex and cross-sectional age. *Med. Sci. Sports Exerc.* **2000**, *32*, 1601–1609. [CrossRef]

27. Chang, O.; Choi, E.-K.; Kim, I.-R.; Nam, S.-J.; Lee, J.E.; Lee, S.K.; Im, Y.-H.; Park, Y.H.; Cho, J. Association between socioeconomic status and altered appearance distress, body image, and quality of life among breast cancer patients. *Asian Pac. J. Cancer Prev.* **2014**, *15*, 8607–8612. [CrossRef]

28. Fine, L.J.; Philogene, G.S.; Gramling, R.; Coups, E.J.; Sinha, S. Prevalence of multiple chronic disease risk factors: 2001 National Health Interview Survey. *Am. J. Prev. Med.* **2004**, *27*, 18–24. [CrossRef]

29. Lee, M.; Yoon, K. Catastrophic Health Expenditures and Its Inequality in Households with Cancer Patients: A Panel Study. *Processes* **2019**, *7*, 39. [CrossRef]

30. McCann, B.A.; Ewing, R. Measuring the Health Effects of Sprawl: A National Analysis of Physical Activity, Obesity and Chronic Disease. *Geography* **2003**. [CrossRef]

31. Katzmarzyk, P.; Lear, S. Physical activity for obese individuals: A systematic review of effects on chronic disease risk factors. *Obes. Rev.* **2012**, *13*, 95–105. [CrossRef] [PubMed]

32. Mukamal, K.J.; Ding, E.L.; Djoussé, L. Alcohol consumption, physical activity, and chronic disease risk factors: A population-based cross-sectional survey. *BMC Public Health* **2006**, *6*, 118. [CrossRef] [PubMed]

33. Cho, E.R.; Shin, A.; Kim, J.; Jee, S.H.; Sung, J. Leisure-time physical activity is associated with a reduced risk for metabolic syndrome. *Ann. Epidemiol.* **2009**, *19*, 784–792. [CrossRef] [PubMed]

34. Choban, P.; Flancbaum, L. Nourishing the obese patient. *Clin. Nutr.* **2000**, *19*, 305–311. [CrossRef]

35. Chan, M.; Lim, Y.; Ernest, A.; Tan, T. Nutritional assessment in an Asian nursing home and its association with mortality. *J. Nutr. Health Aging* **2010**, *14*, 23–28. [CrossRef]

36. Kim, Y.-H.; Kim, S.M.; Han, K.-D.; Jung, J.-H.; Lee, S.-S.; Oh, S.W.; Park, H.S.; Rhee, E.-J.; Lee, W.-Y.; Yoo, S.J. Waist Circumference and All-Cause Mortality Independent of Body Mass Index in Korean Population from the National Health Insurance Health Checkup 2009–2015. *J. Clin. Med.* **2019**, *8*, 72. [CrossRef]

37. Virtanen, M.; Oksanen, T.; Batty, G.D.; Ala-Mursula, L.; Salo, P.; Elovainio, M.; Pentti, J.; Lybäck, K.; Vahtera, J.; Kivimäki, M. Extending employment beyond the pensionable age: A cohort study of the influence of chronic diseases, health risk factors, and working conditions. *PLoS ONE* **2014**, *9*, e88695. [CrossRef]

38. Park, M.; Park, Y.; Kim, S.; Park, S.; Seol, H.; Woo, S.; Cho, S.; Lim, D.-S. Introduction and effectiveness of The Seoul Metabolic Syndrome Management. *Public Health Aff.* **2017**, *1*, 25–39. [CrossRef]

39. Zhao, C.; Wong, L.; Zhu, Q.; Yang, H. Prevalence and correlates of chronic diseases in an elderly population: A community-based survey in Haikou. *PLoS ONE* **2018**, *13*, e0199006. [CrossRef]

40. Cockerham, W.C.; Hamby, B.W.; Oates, G.R. The social determinants of chronic disease. *Am. J. Prev. Med.* **2017**, *52*, S5–S12. [CrossRef]

41. Martínez-García, M.; Salinas-Ortega, M.; Estrada-Arriaga, I.; Hernández-Lemus, E.; García-Herrera, R.; Vallejo, M. A systematic approach to analyze the social determinants of cardiovascular disease. *PLoS ONE* **2018**, *13*, e0190960. [CrossRef] [PubMed]

42. Taylor, L.A.; Tan, A.X.; Coyle, C.E.; Ndumele, C.; Rogan, E.; Canavan, M.; Curry, L.A.; Bradley, E.H. Leveraging the social determinants of health: What works? *PLoS ONE* **2016**, *11*, e0160217. [CrossRef] [PubMed]

43. Nicholas, S.B.; Kalantar-Zadeh, K.; Norris, K.C. Socioeconomic disparities in chronic kidney disease. *Adv. Chronic Kidney Dis.* **2015**, *22*, 6–15. [CrossRef] [PubMed]

44. Jeon, B.; Kwon, S. Effect of private health insurance on health care utilization in a universal public insurance system: A case of South Korea. *Health Policy* **2013**, *113*, 69–76. [CrossRef] [PubMed]

45. Lee, M.; Yoon, K.; Choi, M. Private health insurance and catastrophic health expenditures of households with cancer patients in South Korea. *Eur. J. Cancer Care* **2018**, *27*, e12867. [CrossRef]

46. Mulcahy, A.W.; Eibner, C.; Finegold, K. Gaining coverage through Medicaid or private insurance increased prescription use and lowered out-of-pocket spending. *Health Aff.* **2016**, *35*, 1725–1733. [CrossRef]

47. Culica, D.; Rohrer, J.; Ward, M.; Hilsenrath, P.; Pomrehn, P. Medical checkups: Who does not get them? *Am. J. Public Health* **2002**, *92*, 88–91. [CrossRef]

48. Liu, Y.; Croft, J.B.; Wheaton, A.G.; Kanny, D.; Cunningham, T.J.; Lu, H.; Onufrak, S.; Malarcher, A.M.; Greenlund, K.J.; Giles, W.H. Clustering of Five Health-Related Behaviors for Chronic Disease Prevention Among Adults, United States, 2013. *Prev. Chronic Dis.* **2016**, *13*, E70. [CrossRef]

49. Campbell, D.J.; Ronksley, P.E.; Manns, B.J.; Tonelli, M.; Sanmartin, C.; Weaver, R.G.; Hennessy, D.; King-Shier, K.; Campbell, T.; Hemmelgarn, B.R. The association of income with health behavior change and disease monitoring among patients with chronic disease. *PLoS ONE* **2014**, *9*, e94007. [CrossRef]

50. Thande, N.K.; Hurstak, E.E.; Sciacca, R.E.; Giardina, E.G.V. Management of obesity: A challenge for medical training and practice. *Obesity* **2009**, *17*, 107–113. [CrossRef]

51. Lee, M.; Yoon, K.; Lee, K.-S. Subjective health status of multimorbidity: Verifying the mediating effects of medical and assistive devices. *Int. J. Equity Health* **2018**, *17*, 164. [CrossRef] [PubMed]

52. Zhu, X.; Cahan, A. Wearable technologies and telehealth in Care Management for Chronic Illness. In *Healthcare Information Management Systems*; Springer: Cham, Switzerland, 2016; pp. 375–398.

53. Kang, S.Y. The ICT Technology for Geriatric Diseases Healthcare. In *Information Science and Applications (ICISA) 2016*; Springer: Singapore, 2016; pp. 1495–1500.

54. Bodenheimer, T.; Lorig, K.; Holman, H.; Grumbach, K. Patient self-management of chronic disease in primary care. *JAMA* **2002**, *288*, 2469–2475. [CrossRef] [PubMed]

55. Chiauzzi, E.; Rodarte, C.; DasMahapatra, P. Patient-centered activity monitoring in the self-management of chronic health conditions. *BMC Med.* **2015**, *13*, 77. [CrossRef] [PubMed]

7

Factors Associated with Health-Related Quality of Life in Community-Dwelling Older Adults: A Multinomial Logistic Analysis

Encarnación Blanco-Reina [1,*], Jenifer Valdellós [2], Ricardo Ocaña-Riola [3,4], María Rosa García-Merino [5], Lorena Aguilar-Cano [6], Gabriel Ariza-Zafra [7] and Inmaculada Bellido-Estévez [1]

[1]   Pharmacology and Therapeutics Department, School of Medicine, Instituto de Investigación Biomédica de Málaga-IBIMA, University of Málaga, 29016 Málaga, Spain; ibellido@uma.es

[2]   Health District of Málaga-Guadalhorce, 29009 Málaga, Spain; jenny_dok7@hotmail.com

[3]   Escuela Andaluza de Salud Pública, 18011 Granada, Spain; ricardo.ocana.easp@juntadeandalucia.es

[4]   Instituto de Investigación Biosanitaria ibs.GRANADA, 18012 Granada, Spain

[5]   Health District of Córdoba Sur, 14940 Córdoba, Spain; rosaballet@yahoo.es

[6]   Physical Medicine and Rehabilitation Department, Hospital Regional Universitario, 29010 Málaga, Spain; loagca2011@hotmail.com

[7]   Geriatrics Department, Complejo Hospitalario Universitario, 02006 Albacete, Spain; gariza@sescam.jccm.es

*   Correspondence: eblanco@uma.es

Abstract: The main aim of this study was to determine the association of various clinical, functional and pharmacological factors with the physical (PCS) and mental (MCS) summary components of the health-related quality of life (HRQoL) of community-dwelling older adults. Design: Cross-sectional study. Patients and setting: Sample of 573 persons aged over 65 years, recruited at 12 primary healthcare centres in Málaga, Spain. Sociodemographic, clinical, functional, and comprehensive drug therapy data were collected. The main outcome was HRQoL assessed on the basis of the SF-12 questionnaire. A multinomial logistic regression model was constructed to study the relationship between independent variables and the HRQoL variable, divided into intervals. The average self-perceived HRQoL score was 43.2 (± 11.02) for the PCS and 48.5 (± 11.04) for the MCS. The factors associated with a poorer PCS were dependence for the instrumental activities of daily living (IADL), higher body mass index (BMI), number of medications, and presence of osteoarticular pathology. Female gender and the presence of a psychopathological disorder were associated with worse scores for the MCS. The condition that was most strongly associated with a poorer HRQoL (in both components, PCS and MCS) was that of frailty (odds ratio (OR) = 37.42, 95% confidence interval (CI) = 8.96–156.22, and OR = 20.95, 95% CI = 7.55–58.17, respectively). It is important to identify the determinant factors of a diminished HRQoL, especially if they are preventable or modifiable.

Keywords: health-related quality of life; older adults; frailty; medication; primary care

1. Introduction

The aging of the population is a global phenomenon that is producing dramatic sociodemographic transformations. In this respect, a recent study modelled life expectancy, all-cause mortality and cause of death forecasts for 250 causes of death from 2016 to 2040 in 195 countries and territories. For 2040, Japan, Singapore, Spain and Switzerland were forecast to have an average life expectancy exceeding 85 years for both genders, and another 59 countries, including China, were projected to surpass a life expectancy of 80 years. According to these forecasts, Spain will then have the greatest life expectancy in the world (85.8 years) [1]. This pattern of aging poses a major challenge to health and social assistance services, as older people present more chronic conditions and generate higher per capita healthcare costs. Multimorbidity is strongly associated with adverse health outcomes, such as disability, dependence, mortality, increased need for health and social services and polymedication, and diminished health-related quality of life (HRQoL) [2].

Increased longevity should not be achieved at the expense of quality of life. A poor HRQoL has been associated with reduced activities of daily living, a higher frequency of hospitalisation and increased mortality [3,4]. Therefore, enhancing HRQoL should be a major consideration in the design and implementation of health care for older persons [5]. In addition, assigning a greater importance to the quality of life, in preference to disease-based outcomes, is consistent with the opinions expressed by such persons themselves [6,7]. As a consequence of the interest being generated by this topic, patient-perceived quality of life is now widely used as a measure of health care in clinical research and in health economics assessments [8].

HRQoL has been defined as "the subjective perception influenced by the current health status of the ability to perform activities important for the person" [9,10]. In response to heightened interest in assessing HRQoL and in determining the effectiveness of health care interventions in older patients, a range of instruments—both generic and specific—have been developed for these purposes.

Many factors can influence the HRQoL of older adults, including health status, social engagement and cognitive function [11]. In this area, studies have been undertaken to analyse the association between factors (such as female sex, age, functional impairment and comorbidities) and HRQoL, and in recent years, the role of medication as a determinant of overall health outcomes has emerged as an area of great interest. Various aspects of treatment regimens call for special attention, because they may have a negative influence on the HRQoL of older persons, such as polymedication, and potentially inappropriate or harmful medication [12–17]. It is important to recall that the benefits of medication should always outweigh the potential harm, and therefore individual circumstances should be taken into account. In recent studies, frailty, too, has been highlighted as a possible determinant of worsened quality of life [18–22]. Frailty is defined as an abnormal health state characterised by the loss of biological reserves, related to the aging process [23]. Therefore, in providing care for persons with frailty, special emphasis should be placed on quality of life considerations.

Evaluation of HRQoL can help clinicians to determine the needs of older patients and thus optimise their decision making. Therefore, we believe it is important to explore factors influencing HRQoL in this population in order to identify suitable intervention strategies. In this respect, we note that many previous studies have not addressed all the factors that might have a significant impact on HRQoL, and in some cases the results presented are contradictory. For all of these reasons, we consider it interesting to investigate HRQoL in older adults, resident in one of the countries where life expectancy is highest, to assess clinical, functional and pharmacological aspects of the question. In this study, we hypothesise that there are multiple predictive factors of a poor HRQoL and that they may affect its physical and mental components in different ways and to different degrees. Accordingly, our aim was to determine levels of HRQoL among community-dwelling older people and to analyse the factors associated with a poor HRQoL.

2. Patients and Methods

2.1. Study Design, Setting and Participants

In this cross-sectional investigation, the study population was composed of 89,615 community-dwelling residents aged 65 years or more, living in Málaga, Spain. Assuming a standard deviation for HRQoL of 11.0 [24], an absolute precision of $\delta = 0.9$ and a level of confidence of $1-\alpha = 0.95$, we calculated that the minimum sample size needed to estimate the average physical and mental HRQoL was 570. Finally, the total sample was composed of 573 persons. These patients were recruited from twelve primary care centres, by stratified random sampling designed to obtain a representative sample of the population, allocating the population in proportion to the size of each healthcare centre.

Participants were selected randomly within each healthcare centre from a general list of healthcare cards issued by the Spanish National Health Service. The inclusion criteria were people 65 years of age or older, included in the database of healthcare cards, belonging to the outpatient setting (not institutionalized), and giving their informed consent to participate in the study (people who did not give consent were excluded).

2.2. Data Collection and Measures

To obtain the study data for analysis, patients were interviewed using a structured questionnaire. Further data were obtained from medication packaging and digital medical records. The questionnaire was used to obtain detailed information on the patients' regular drug use, together with clinical, functional and sociodemographic data. Clinical diagnoses were examined, and the number of chronic conditions presented by each participant was determined. Patients' independence in performing instrumental activities of daily living (IADL) was assessed using the Lawton scale [25]. In addition, the body mass index was determined for all patients, and frailty was assessed according to Fried's criteria (as robust, pre-frail or frail) [26].

Medication assessment. Data were obtained for the medication prescribed (indication, dosage and duration of treatments during the last three months or more). The presence of polymedication was considered, defining this as the regular use of five or more medications, as was that of potentially inappropriate medication (PIM), according to the STOPP v2 criteria (Screening Tool of Older Person's Potentially Inappropriate Prescriptions, version 2) [27]. The latter variable was operationalised as the percentage of patients receiving at least one PIM.

Quality of life assessment. The main study outcome was HRQoL assessed by the SF-12 questionnaire, a widely used generic instrument. The SF-12 is an abbreviated version of the Short Form-36 Health Survey (SF-36), in which a subset of 12 items/questions are used to derive summary scores for physical health (PCS score) and mental health (MCS score) [28]. The response options form Likert-type scales that assess the intensity and/or frequency of people's health status. The final score obtained can be between 0 and 100, where lower scores indicate worse, and higher scores better HRQoL. Using only one-third of the SF-36 items, the SF-12 reproduces the two summary scores originally developed for the SF-36 with remarkable accuracy, but more quickly and requiring less effort from the respondent [29]. The SF-12 has been validated for use in the USA, the UK, Spain and many other European countries [24].

2.3. Statistical Analysis

Exploratory data analysis and frequency tables were used to describe the study variables. Using the standardised scores of the SF-12 questionnaire for the Spanish population [24], the HRQoL score of each participant was assigned to one of the following intervals, taking into account the population reference group according to age and sex:

- Very low: QoL ≤ 20th percentile of the Spanish population corresponding to their age group and sex;
- Low: QoL > 20th percentile and ≤50th percentile of the Spanish population corresponding to their age group and sex;
- High: QoL > 50th percentile and ≤80th percentile of the Spanish population corresponding to their age group and sex;
- Very high: QoL > 80th percentile of the Spanish population corresponding to their age group and sex.

A multinomial logistic regression model was used to study the relationship between the independent variables and the HRQoL variable, grouped into the corresponding intervals [30]. A 5% significance level was assumed to indicate statistical significance. Statistical data analysis was performed using SPSS version 23.0 (IBM SPSS Statistics, Armonk, NY, USA).

2.4. Ethical Considerations

This study was conducted in accordance with the provisions of the 1975 Declaration of Helsinki, revised in 2013. The Málaga Clinical Research Ethics Committee approved the study (PI-0234-14), and informed consent was obtained from all patients prior to their inclusion.

3. Results

3.1. Characteristics of the Study Population

The study sample was composed of 573 patients, with a mean age of 73.1 years (standard deviation 5.5, range 65–104) and of whom 57.2% were female. Most lived with their partner (62.4%) or family (16.5%), but 21.1% lived alone. On average, each patient presented 7.8 chronic conditions (standard deviation 3.3, range 0–20). The most prevalent diagnoses were bone and joint disorders (mainly osteoarthritis of the knee, hip, hand and shoulder) (75.2%), hypertension (70.5%) and dyslipidaemia (51.6%). Most of the patients presented with overweight (40.9%) or obesity (45.7%) and their mean body mass index was 30.2 (standard deviation 5.1, range 17–54.5). Half were independently capable of performing IADL, and the mean score on the Lawton scale was 6.6 (standard deviation 1.8, range 0–8). Frailty was present in 137 patients (23.9%; 95% confidence interval (CI) = 20.5–27.5), according to Fried's criteria. The main characteristics of the study population are detailed in Table 1.

The prevalence of polymedication was 68% (95% CI = 64.1–71.7), and on average each patient consumed 6.8 drugs (standard deviation 4.0; range 0–23). The most widely prescribed drugs were omeprazole and acetaminophen, followed by aspirin, simvastatin, metformin, metamizole, enalapril and bromazepam. The use of potentially inappropriate medication, according to the STOPP v2 criteria, was identified in 66.8% of patients (95% CI = 62.9–70.6). The number of PIMs per patient ranged from 0–10 (mean 2.1, standard deviation 2.2). The most frequent PIMs detected were benzodiazepines (61% of all PIMs).

3.2. Assessment of HRQoL and Analysis of Related Factors

The patients' perceptions of their HRQoL produced an average score of 43.2 (standard deviation 11.02, range 16.2–65.4) for the physical component summary (PCS) and a somewhat higher one, 48.5 (standard deviation 11.04, range 14.1–66.6), for the mental component (MCS). Males obtained higher scores than females in both the PCS and the MCS, with average values of 45.91 vs. 41.27 and 51.95 vs. 45.91, respectively. Table 2 shows the distribution within the global sample among the categories of perceived HRQoL (very low, low, high and very high). A notable feature of this distribution is that a higher proportion of patients perceived their HRQoL as very high in the mental component than in the physical one.

To further examine the impact of the independent variables on the HRQoL categories, a multinomial logistic regression analysis was performed (Tables 3–5). The factors related to having high vs. very high HRQoL (P_{50}–P_{80} and $\geq P_{80}$, respectively) were the level of dependence for IADL in the PCS, and BMI, respiratory disease and frailty in the MCS (Table 3). The presence of a low HRQoL (P_{20}–P_{50}) with respect to a very high score for the PCS was associated with the level of dependence for IADL, with accompanied living, with the presence of osteoarticular pathology and with frailty (Table 4). The odds of these older persons having a low HRQoL decrease by 30% for each additional point of independence on the Lawton scale (odds ratio (OR) = 0.70, 95% CI = 0.55–0.88). However, they double for those who do not live alone (OR = 2.13, 95% CI = 1.07–4.27), are 2.5 times greater for those with osteoarticular pathology compared to those without it (OR = 2.57, 95% CI = 1.35–4.85) and are seven times greater for those who are frail (OR = 7.43, 95% CI = 2.13–25.82) compared to those who are robust. In the case of the MCS, the presence of frailty was associated with a three times greater perception of low HRQoL (OR = 3.2, 95% CI = 1.21–8.46).

Table 1. Characteristics of study population (n = 573).

Quantitative Variables	Mean	Standard Deviation
Age (years)	73.1	5.5
Lawton (IADL)	6.6	1.8
BMI (Kg/m^2)	30.2	5.1
Number of comorbidities	7.8	3.3
Number of drugs per patient	6.8	4.0
Number of PIMs per patient	2.1	2.2

Qualitative Variables	Subjects	Percentage
Gender		
Male	245	42.8
Female	328	57.2
Living Arrangements		
Living alone	121	21.1
Accompanied living	452	78.9
Frailty		
Robust	124	21.6
Pre-frail	312	54.5
Frail	137	23.9
Most Frequent Comorbidities		
Bone and joint disorders	431	75.2
Hypertension	404	70.5
Dyslipidaemia	292	51.0
Insomnia	254	44.3
Gastrointestinal disease	241	42.0
Peripheral vascular disease	227	39.6
Psychopathology	207	36.1
Diabetes mellitus	172	30.0
Heart disease	139	24.3
Respiratory Disease	123	21.5
Polymedication	390	68.0
PIM prevalence	383	66.8

IADL: Instrumental Activities of Daily Living; BMI: Body Mass Index; PIM: Potentially Inappropriate Medication (according to STOPP v2 criteria).

Table 2. HRQoL assessment according to SF-12 questionnaire.

HRQoL Component	HRQoL Categories, n (%)			
Summary Score	Very low ($\leq P_{20}$)	Low (P_{20}–P_{50})	High (P_{50}–P_{80})	Very high ($\geq P_{80}$)
PCS	137 (23.9%)	170 (29.7%)	150 (26.2%)	116 (20.2%)
MCS	143 (25.0%)	117 (20.4%)	125 (21.8%)	188 (32.8%)

PCS: Physical Component Summary; MCS: Mental Component Summary; P: Percentile.

A very low perception of HRQoL ($\leq P_{20}$) in the PCS was also related to the level of dependence for IADL (OR = 0.62, 95% CI = 0.48–0.79), with the presence of osteoarticular pathology (OR = 4.38, 95% CI = 1.98–9.70) and with the states of prefrailty (OR = 4.19, 95% CI = 1.61–10.86) and frailty (OR = 37.42, 95% CI = 8.96–156.22). In addition, the odds of a very low HRQoL increase by 15% for each additional drug in the treatment regimen (OR = 1.15, 95% CI = 1.02–1.30) and by 8% for each unit increase in BMI (OR = 1.08, 95% CI = 1.01–1.15). However, age was inversely related to HRQoL. Thus, all other variables being equal, for each additional year of life, the odds of the patient perceiving a very low HRQoL decreased by 8% (Table 5). A similar pattern for the age effect was observed with respect to the mental component of HRQoL; thus, each additional year of life decreased the odds of a very low HRQoL by 7%. In the MCS, too, the states of prefrailty and frailty were associated with a very low

HRQoL. In this mental component, and with all other variables being equal, the female patients were 88% more likely than the males to have a very low HRQoL. Finally, the presence of a psychopathology (usually anxiety and/or depression) was related to a poorer HRQoL; the presence of any such disorder quadrupled the odds of the patient perceiving a very low HRQoL (OR = 4.69, 95% CI = 2.60–8.47).

Table 3. Factors related to HRQoL. Multinomial logistic regression for High HRQoL (with respect to Very High HRQoL) for physical and mental health components (PCS-MCS).

Independent Variable	PCS OR (95% CI)	MCS OR (95% CI)
Age	1.02 (0.96–1.07)	1.01 (0.95–1.05)
No. of comorbidities	1.06 (0.93–1.20)	1.02 (0.91–1.14)
BMI	0.99 (0.94–1.05)	0.94 (0.89–0.99) *
Independence (IADL)	0.74 (0.58–0.94) *	1.17 (0.98–1.39)
No. of medications	1.07 (0.96–1.19)	1.00 (0.91–1.10)
No. of PIMs	1.10 (0.85–1.43)	1.08 (0.87–1.34)
Female gender (ref. male)	0.72 (0.38–1.34)	1.45 (0.81–2.59)
Living accompanied (ref. alone)	1.26 (0.67–2.38)	1.14 (0.61–2.14)
Bone and joint disease	1.40 (0.79–2.49)	0.94 (0.53–1.66)
Heart disease	1.35 (0.62–2.92)	0.81 (0.42–1.54)
Respiratory disease	0.71 (0.33–1.53)	2.05 (1.10–3.84) *
Hypertension	1.20 (0.67–2.15)	1.20 (0.67–2.14)
Diabetes mellitus	1.22 (0.63–2.37)	0.76 (0.42–1.36)
Psychopathology	1.11 (0.58–2.12)	1.65 (0.91–2.98)
Insomnia	1.18 (0.64–2.16)	1.26 (0.73–2.16)
Pre–frail (ref. robust)	0.87 (0.48–1.57)	0.95 (0.53–1.69)
Frail (ref. robust)	0.46 (0.11–1.81)	3.39 (1.35–8.51) **

PIMs: Potentially Inappropriate Medications (according to STOPP v2 criteria). * $p < 0.05$; ** $p < 0.01$.

Table 4. Factors related to HRQoL. Multinomial Logistic Regression for Low HRQoL (with respect to Very High HRQoL) for physical and mental health components (PCS-MCS).

Independent Variable	PCS OR (95% CI)	MCS OR (95% CI)
Age	0.97 (0.92–1.03)	0.98 (0.93–1.03)
No. of comorbidities	1.08 (0.95–1.23)	1.11 (0.98–1.24)
BMI	1.04 (0.98–1.10)	0.95 (0.90–0.99) *
Independence (IADL)	0.70 (0.55–0.88) **	0.99 (0.84–1.18)
No. of medications	1.11 (0.99–1.24)	0.98 (0.89–1.08)
No. of PIMs	0.94 (0.72–1.22)	1.12 (0.89–1.39)
Female gender (ref. male)	1.01 (0.52–1.91)	1.67 (0.93–3.00)
Living accompanied (ref. alone)	2.13 (1.07–4.27) *	0.84 (0.45–1.57)
Bone and joint disease	2.57 (1.35–4.85) **	0.96 (0.53–1.72)
Heart disease	1.19 (0.54–2.62)	0.85 (0.45–1.62)
Respiratory disease	1.32 (0.64–2.71)	1.54 (0.81–2.92)
Hypertension	1.75 (0.94–3.27)	0.73 (0.41–1.31)
Diabetes mellitus	0.96 (0.48–1.92)	0.75 (0.42–1.36)
Psychopathology	1.20 (0.62–2.30)	1.36 (0.74–2.50)
Insomnia	1.33 (0.71–2.47)	1.01 (0.58–1.74)
Pre–frail (ref. robust)	1.48 (0.77–2.87)	1.50 (0.81–2.78)
Frail (ref. robust)	7.43 (2.13–25.82) **	3.20 (1.21–8.46) **

* $p < 0.05$; ** $p < 0.01$.

Table 5. Factors related to HRQoL. Multinomial Logistic Regression for Very Low HRQoL (with respect to Very High HRQoL) for physical and mental health components (PCS-MCS).

Independent Variable	PCS OR (95% CI)	MCS OR (95% CI)
Age	0.92 (0.86–0.98) *	0.93 (0.88–0.98) *
No. of comorbidities	1.11 (0.96–1.28)	0.98 (0.87–1.10)
BMI	1.08 (1.01–1.15) *	0.99 (0.95–1.05)
Independence (IADL)	0.62 (0.48–0.79) ***	0.94 (0.79–1.12)
No. of medications	1.15 (1.02–1.30) *	0.99 (0.90–1.10)
No. of PIMs	0.94 (0.70–1.24)	1.08 (0.87–1.35)
Female gender (ref. male)	1.58 (0.76–3.29)	1.88 (1.01–3.49) *
Living accompanied (ref. alone)	1.63 (0.76–3.50)	0.63 (0.33–1.17)
Bone and joint disease	4.38 (1.98–9.70) **	1.14 (0.60–2.18)
Heart disease	0.87 (0.36–2.08)	0.74 (0.37–1.49)
Respiratory disease	1.01 (0.45–2.22)	0.94 (0.47–1.89)
Hypertension	1.50 (0.73–3.05)	0.93 (0.51–1.72)
Diabetes mellitus	1.11 (0.52–2.36)	0.88 (0.47–1.63)
Psychopathology	1.53 (0.75–3.11)	4.69 (2.60–8.47) ***
Insomnia	1.24 (0.62–2.46)	1.66 (0.94–2.91)
Pre-frail (ref. robust)	4.19 (1.61–10.86) **	2.92 (1.36–6.26) **
Frail (ref. robust)	37.42 (8.96–156.22) ***	20.95 (7.55–58.17) ***

$* p < 0.05; ** p < 0.01; *** p < 0.001.$

4. Discussion

Overall, our results for perceived HRQoL among community-dwelling older patients in Malaga (southern Spain) are consistent with those reported in similar studies conducted in other regions of Spain [31,32] and elsewhere in Europe [33]. With respect to the components of physical and mental health, the average PCS score (43.2) is slightly higher than that obtained in previous research [31–34], while the MCS (48.5) is somewhat lower than the average value for six European countries (54.3), also obtained using the SF-12 [33]. This lower score in the MCS could be due to cultural differences, and/or the non-negligible prevalence of psychopathological disorders (mainly anxiety and/or depression) in our region (these pathologies affect 36% of the older population). Regarding the influence of age on HRQoL, previous studies have produced conflicting results [32–35]. Our investigation revealed an inverse relationship between advanced age and the odds of a very low HRQoL. Therefore, other questions such as comorbidities, frailty, dependence and other possible confounders being equal, as the patient ages there is a lower probability of him/her perceiving a very low HRQoL, and this is true for both the physical and the mental components. These findings might be explained in terms of a better psychological adaptation to aging and perhaps to the fact that with age comes not only wisdom, but also the attribution of greater meaning or value to life. As concerns the influence of gender, previous studies have reported a poorer HRQoL among women than among men [31–34,36,37], and our own results corroborate this difference. Thus, women obtained poorer scores in both components of HRQoL, although the association was only significant for the mental component of a very low quality of life. In the physical component, female gender is probably not a determinant factor of a poorer HRQoL due to the adjustment made for confounding variables such as frailty or osteoarticular pathology, both of which are more prevalent among women.

One of the most consistent predictors of a poor quality of life is the level of dependence for IADL. According to the multinomial logistic regression model, with a higher score on the Lawton scale, i.e., with greater independence, the possibility of a poorer HRQoL decreased significantly (in all the categories considered: high, low and very low, with respect to very high) always with respect to the physical component. It seems logical that the higher the degree of independence among older persons, in activities such as handling economic affairs, using the telephone or managing different forms of transport, the better the quality of life they will perceive. According to a recent study, functional dependence, together with the presence of depressive symptoms, would be an important factor mediating the well-known association between multimorbidity and a poor quality of life [38]. In this line, too, it has been shown that disability is one of the most significant conditions worsening the HRQoL [39]. Older adults who live in cohabitation are twice as likely to have a low physical HRQoL than are those living alone. This finding may be related to the level of functional dependence presented, but further study is needed to confirm this possibility.

Regarding medication, the number of drugs prescribed was positively associated with a very low HRQoL in the PCS. This finding is consistent with previous research, in which polymedication has been identified as a determinant factor of a poorer quality of life [12–14,40]. In our opinion, this association may be related to the side effects produced by the joint presence of several drugs within the patient. On the other hand, we found no evidence of any association between having at least one PIM and the perception of a poorer HRQoL. We speculate that such a relationship might not have been demonstrated because the STOPP v2 criteria contain a large number of items, of varying clinical significance, and therefore the impact produced on HRQoL by a single PIM might be slight. In other words, the sensitivity of this means of measuring the risk might be insufficient. Other authors, too, have failed to observe any significant association between the presence of a PIM and HRQoL, whether using the Beers [16] or the STOPP v2 criteria [41]. On the other hand, other previous studies do suggest that the prescription of drugs with a high anticholinergic load may be associated with a diminished quality of life [15–17,42].

Among this population, the most prevalent pathologies observed were osteoarthritis and hypertension. This is a common profile and similar to that reported in previous research in this field [39]. Our assessment of the impact on HRQoL of different conditions shows that physical disorders mostly affected the "physical" HRQoL while mental disorders mainly affected the "mental" aspect—as is only logical. The presence of bone and joint disease was significantly associated with a low or very low HRQoL, which corroborates previous findings in which this diagnosis was associated both with disability and with a diminished HRQoL [39]. We believe this relationship may be explained by the chronic pain which often accompanies these diseases, as well as a degree of physical limitation that is usually provoked. This association contrasts with its absence for other diagnoses, perhaps with a worse prognosis but of a more 'silent' nature, such as hypertension and diabetes mellitus. On the other hand, the presence of a psychopathology in an older person raises the possibility of his/her perceiving a very low HRQoL, in the mental component, by 400%, as has also been indicated in previous studies [12,31,32,43,44]. It would seem that the distress generated by these diseases has a negative impact on emotional regulation, motivation and other components of subjective perceptions of health and well-being. According to other researchers, and taking into account the significant impact on the patient's quality of life, we believe more screening for depression and anxiety among older populations should be performed, because these conditions tend to be under-diagnosed and also because a more active approach to this question would promote healthy aging [31]. In our sample, the BMI values observed presented two interesting aspects: on the one hand, at the mental level, a higher BMI was associated with a better HRQoL, but for the physical component it was significantly associated with a very low quality of life. It seems clear that overweight and obese patients perceive a poorer physical health [40,45–47]. This is corroborated by the fact that interventions aimed at achieving weight loss have been shown to improve the physical quality of life [48].

It is interesting to note that the factor most strongly associated with a diminished HRQoL was that of frailty, which severely affected both the MCS and the PCS, but especially the latter. The odds of a very low physical quality of life were 37 times greater among frail older persons than among those who were robust, while the MCS reflected 20 times greater odds of their presenting a poor mental quality of life. Previous studies, too, have reported this association [18–21,49], which was reinforced in a recent systematic review and meta-analysis that described it as clear and often substantial [22]. Although the growing numbers of frail older people pose a real challenge to health systems around the world, this state of pre-discapacity can in fact be prevented and treated. Furthermore, in our study sample, the pre-frail persons also perceived a poorer quality of life than those who were relatively robust. Accordingly, we believe it necessary to design and incorporate care programmes specifically adapted to this emerging population of frail and pre-frail patients, to help them age with a better quality of life.

In our opinion, the type of study described in this paper is useful for identifying the characteristics and clinical conditions that are associated with a poorer HRQoL, with particular attention to those factors that may be preventable or treatable. As improving the quality of life and well-being of older persons is a priority objective, it is of major importance to extend our knowledge of these questions.

The strengths of our study lie in the analysis made of a representative sample of healthcare centres, the global approach taken, and the great variety of clinical, functional and treatment data compiled. We acknowledge that selecting a sample population from a single region or country may result in a certain lack of external validity. Nevertheless, the sample examined in this study may be representative of the population of older adults in the ambulatory setting, which is where the largest number of such patients are to be found. Another limitation to our study is its cross-sectional design, which does not allow causal relationships to be established, although it can detect factors related to HRQoL.

With regard to the analysis performed, since HRQoL is a quantitative variable, a multivariate linear regression model might, in principle, be considered appropriate to identify the factors related to it. However, in the present case the linear model considered did not meet the conditions of homoscedasticity and normality of the residuals necessary for the correct estimation of the study parameters. Previous statistical research has reached similar conclusions, i.e., that HRQoL cannot be analysed using linear regression models [50]. Neither nonlinear modelling, nor generalised least squares nor other more complex statistical techniques overcame the problem of achieving an adequate fit, and therefore we adopted the solution of treating QoL as a qualitative variable and using a multinomial logistic regression model. This approach provided a good fit to the data considered.

5. Conclusions

In conclusion, many factors may be predictive of a poor HRQoL and they affect its physical and mental components in different ways. For the PCS, the associated factors were dependence for IADL, a higher BMI, the number of medications and the presence of osteoarticular pathology. The main factors associated with a lower MCS score were female gender and the presence of a psychopathological disorder. Some factors may be preventable or modifiable, and so recognising them and optimising the response made are crucial to the priority objective of enhancing the quality of life among older people. Clearly and consistently, the factor that was most strongly associated with a poorer overall HRQoL was the state of frailty (and also, albeit to a lesser extent, that of pre-frailty). Frailty is a dynamic syndrome, in which transitions are possible between the states of normality, pre-frailty and frailty. Accordingly, detecting frailty and addressing it in a suitable way are questions of major importance.

Author Contributions: Conceptualization, E.B.-R., R.O.-R., G.A.-Z.; Methodology, E.B.-R., R.O.-R.; Formal analysis, E.B.-R., R.O.-R.; Investigation, E.B.-R., R.O.-R., G.A.-Z., J.V., L.A.-C., M.R.G.-M., I.B.-E.; Resources, E.B.-R., I.B.-E.; Data curation: J.V., L.A.-C., M.R.G.-M.; Writing—original draft preparation, E.B.-R., R.O.-R., J.V.; Writing—review & editing, E.B.-R., R.O.-R., J.V., I.B.-E.; Visualization, E.B.-R., R.O.-R., I.B.-E.; Supervision, E.B.-R., I.B.-E.; Project administration, E.B.-R.; Funding acquisition: E.B.-R.

Acknowledgments: The authors wish to thank the Primary Care Management Team (Health District of Málaga) for providing access to the health centres and patient lists.

References

1. Foreman, K.J.; Márquez, N.; Dolgert, A.; Fukutaki, L.; Fullman, N.; McGaughey, M.; Pletcher, M.A.; Smith, A.E.; Tang, K.; Yuan, C.W.; et al. Forecasting life expectancy, years of life lost, and all-cause and cause-specific mortality for 250 causes of death: Reference and alternative scenarios for 2016-40 for 195 countries and territories. *Lancet* **2018**, *392*, 2052–2090. [CrossRef]

2. Marengoni, A.; Angleman, S.; Melis, R.; Mangialasche, F.; Karp, A.; Garmen, A.; Meinow, B.; Fratiglioni, L. Aging with multimorbidity: A systematic review of the literatura. *Ageing Res. Rev.* **2011**, *10*, 430–439. [CrossRef] [PubMed]

3. Lee, D.T.F.; Yu, D.S.F.; Kwong, A.N.L. Quality of life of older people in residential care home: A literature review. *J. Nurs. Healthc Chronic Illn.* **2009**, *1*, 116–125. [CrossRef]

4. Otero-Rodríguez, A.; León-Muñoz, L.M.; Balboa-Castillo, T.; Banegas, J.R.; Rodríguez-Artalejo, F.; Guallar-Castillón, P. Change in health-related quality of life as a predictor of mortality in the older adults. *Qual. Life Res.* **2010**, *19*, 15–23. [CrossRef] [PubMed]

5. World Health Organization. World Report on Ageing and Health. Geneva: World Health Organization. 2015. Available online: https://www.who.int/ageing/events/world-report-2015-launch/en/ (accessed on 29 July 2019).

6. Gabriel, Z.; Bowling, A. Quality of life from the perspectives of older people. *Ageing Soc.* **2004**, *24*, 675–691. [CrossRef]

7. National Voices, Age, U. K. & UCL Partners. I'm Still Me: A Narrative for Coordinated Support for Older People: National Voices. 2014. Available online: https://www.nationalvoices.org.uk/sites/default/files/public/publications/im_still_me.pdf (accessed on 29 July 2019).

8. Makai, P.; Brouwer, W.B.; Koopmanschap, M.A.; Stolk, E.A.; Nieboer, A.P. Quality of life instruments for economic evaluations in health and social care for older people: A systematic review. *Soc. Sci. Med* **2014**, *102*, 83–93. [CrossRef] [PubMed]

9. Group WHOQoL. Study protocol for the World Health Organization project to develop a Quality of Life assessment instrument (WHOQOL). *Qual. Life Res.* **1993**, *2*, 153–159. [CrossRef]

10. Shumaker, S.A.; Berzon, R.A. *The International Assessment of Health-Related Quality of Life: Theory, Translation, Measurement, and Analysis*; Rapid Communications of Oxford Ltd.: Oxford, UK, 1995.

11. Borowiak, E.; Kostka, T. Predictors of quality of life in older people living at home and in institutions. *Aging Clin. Exp. Res.* **2004**, *16*, 212–220. [CrossRef]

12. Montiel-Luque, A.; Núñez-Montenegro, A.J.; Martín-Aurioles, E.; Canca-Sánchez, J.C.; Toro-Toro, M.C.; González-Correa, J.A.; Polipresact Research Group. Medication-related factors associated with health-related quality of life in patients older than 65 years with polypharmacy. *PLoS ONE.* **2017**, *11*, e0171320. [CrossRef]

13. Schenker, Y.; Park, S.Y.; Jeong, K.; Pruskowski, J.; Kavalieratos, D.; Resick, J.; Abernethy, A.; Kutner, J.S. Associations Between Polypharmacy, Symptom Burden, and Quality of Life in Patients with Advanced, Life-Limiting Illness. *J. Gen. Intern. Med.* **2019**, *34*, 559–566. [CrossRef]

14. Tegegn, H.G.; Erku, D.A.; Sebsibe, G.; Gizaw, B.; Seifu, D.; Tigabe, M.; Belachew, S.A.; Ayele, A.A. Medication-related quality of life among Ethiopian elderly patients with polypharmacy: A cross-sectional study in an Ethiopia university hospital. *PLoS ONE.* **2019**, *14*, e0214191. [CrossRef] [PubMed]

15. Juola, A.L.; Pylkkanen, S.; Kautiainen, H.; Bell, J.S.; Bjorkman, M.P.; Finne-Soveri, H.; Soini, H.; Pitkälä, K.H. Burden of Potentially Harmful Medications and the Association with Quality of Life and Mortality Among Institutionalized Older People. *J. Am. Med. Dir. Assoc.* **2016**, *17*, e9–e14. [CrossRef] [PubMed]

16. Ie, K.; Chou, E.; Boyce, R.D.; Albert, S.M. Potentially Harmful Medication Use and Decline in Health-Related Quality of Life among Community-Dwelling Older Adults. *Drugs Real World Outcomes.* **2017**, *4*, 257–264. [CrossRef] [PubMed]

17. Harrison, S.L.; Kouladjian O'Donnell, L.; Bradley, C.E.; Milte, R.; Dyer, S.M.; Gnanamanickam, E.S.; Liu, E.; Hilmer, S.N.; Crotty, M. Associations between the Drug Burden Index, Potentially Inappropriate Medications and Quality of Life in Residential Aged Care. *Drugs Aging* **2018**, *35*, 83–91. [CrossRef]

18. Rivera-Almaraz, A.; Manrique-Espinoza, B.; Ávila-Funes, J.A.; Chatterji, S.; Naidoo, N.; Kowal, P.; Salinas-Rodríguez, A. Disability, quality of life and all-cause mortality in older Mexican adults: Association with multimorbidity and frailty. *BMC Geriatr.* **2018**, *18*, 236. [CrossRef]

19. Godin, J.; Armstrong, J.J.; Wallace, L.; Rockwood, K.; Andrew, M.K. The impact of frailty and cognitive impairment on quality of life: Employment and social context matter. *Int. Psychogeriatr.* **2018**, *13*, 1–9. [CrossRef]

20. Kirkhus, L.; Šaltytė Benth, J.; Grønberg, B.H.; Hjermstad, M.J.; Rostoft, S.; Harneshaug, M.; Selbæk, G.; Wyller, T.B.; Jordhøy, M.S. Frailty identified by geriatric assessment is associated with poor functioning, high symptom burden and increased risk of physical decline in older cancer patients: Prospective observational study. *Palliat. Med.* **2019**, *33*, 312–322. [CrossRef]

21. Siriwardhana, D.D.; Weerasinghe, M.C.; Rait, G.; Scholes, S.; Walters, K.R. The association between frailty and quality of life among rural community-dwelling older adults in Kegalle district of Sri Lanka: A cross-sectional study. *Qual. Life Res.* **2019**, *28*, 2057–2068. [CrossRef]

22. Crocker, T.F.; Brown, L.; Clegg, A.; Farley, K.; Franklin, M.; Simpkins, S.; Young, J. Quality of life is substantially worse for community-dwelling older people living with frailty: Systematic review and meta-analysis. *Qual. Life Res.* **2019**, *28*, 2041–2056. [CrossRef]

23. Clegg, A.; Young, J.; Iliffe, S.; Rikkert, M.O.; Rockwood, K. Frailty in elderly people. *Lancet.* **2013**, *381*, 752–762. [CrossRef]

24. Vilagut, G.; Valderas, J.M.; Ferrer, M.; Garin, O.; López-García, E.; Alonso, J. Interpretation of SF-36 and SF-12 questionnaires in Spain: Physical and mental components. *Med. Clin.* **2008**, *130*, 726–735. [CrossRef] [PubMed]

25. Lawton, M.P.; Brody, E.M. Assessment of older people: Self-maintaining and instrumental activities of daily living. *Gerontologist* **1969**, *9*, 179–186. [CrossRef]

26. Fried, L.P.; Tangen, C.M.; Walston, J.; Newman, A.B.; Hirsch, C.; Gottdiener, J.; Seeman, T.; Tracy, R.; Kop, W.J.; Burke, G.; et al. Frailty in Older Adults: Evidence for a Phenotype. *J. Gerontol. A Biol. Sci. Med. Sci.* **2001**, *56*, M146–M156. [CrossRef] [PubMed]

27. O'Mahony, D.; O'Sullivan, D.; Byrne, S.; O'Connor, M.N.; Ryan, C.; Gallagher, P. STOPP/START criteria for potentially inappropriate prescribing in older people: Version 2. *Age Ageing* **2015**, *44*, 213–218.

28. Ware, J., Jr.; Kosinski, M.; Keller, S.D. A 12-Item Short-Form Health Survey: Construction of scales and preliminary tests of reliability and validity. *Med. Care* **1996**, *34*, 220–233. [CrossRef]

29. Jenkinson, C.; Layte, R.; Jenkinson, D.; Lawrence, K.; Petersen, S.; Paice, C.; Stradling, J. A shorter form health survey: Can the SF-12 replicate the results from the SF-36 in longitudinal studies? *J. Public. Health. Med.* **1997**, *19*, 179–186. [CrossRef]

30. Hosmer, D.W.; Lemeshow, S.; Sturdivant, R.X. *Applied Logistic Regression*, 3rd ed.; John Wiley & Sons: Hoboken, NJ, USA, 2013.

31. Baladón, L.; Rubio-Valera, M.; Serrano-Blanco, A.; Palao, D.J.; Fernández, A. Gender differences in the impact of mental disorders and chronic physical conditions on health-related quality of life among non-demented primary care elderly patients. *Qual. Life Res.* **2016**, *25*, 1461–1474. [CrossRef]

32. Naveiro-Rilo, J.C.; Diez-Juárez, M.D.; Flores-Zurutuza, L.; Javierre Pérez, P.; Alberte Pérez, C.; Molina Mazo, R. Quality of life in the elderly on polymedication and with multiple morbidities. *Rev. Esp. Geriatr. Gerontol.* **2014**, *49*, 158–164. [CrossRef]

33. König, H.H.; Heider, D.; Lehnert, T.; Riedel-Heller, S.G.; Angermeyer, M.C.; Matschinger, H.; Vilagut, G.; Bruffaerts, R.; Haro, J.M.; de Girolamo, G.; et al. Health status of the advanced elderly in six European countries: Results from a representative survey using EQ-5D and SF-12. *Health Qual. Life Outcomes.* **2010**, *29*, 143.

34. Juste, M.P.; Barbosa, F.B.; Carreiro, J.P. Calidad de vida en personas mayores. Apuntes para un programa de educación para la salud. *Revista de Investigación en Educación.* **2009**, *6*, 70–78. (In Spanish)

35. Van der Vorst, A.; Zijlstra, G.A.R.; De Witte, N.; Vogel, R.G.M.; Schols, J.M.G.A.; Kempen, G.I.J.M.; D-SCOPE Consortium. Explaining discrepancies in self-reported quality of life in frail older people: A mixed-methods study. *BMC Geriatr.* **2017**, *17*, 251. [CrossRef] [PubMed]

36. Orfila, F.; Ferrer, M.; Lamarca, R.; Tebe, C.; Domingo-Salvany, A.; Alonso, J. Gender differences in health-related quality of life among the elderly: The role of objective functional capacity and chronic conditions. *Soc. Sci. Med.* **2006**, *63*, 2367–2380. [CrossRef] [PubMed]

37. Padua, L.; Pasqualetti, P.; Coraci, D.; Imbimbo, I.; Giordani, A.; Loreti, C.; Marra, C.; Molino-Lova, R.; Pasquini, G.; Simonelli, I.; et al. Gender effect on well-being of the oldest old: A survey of nonagenarians living in Tuscany: The Mugello study. *Neurol. Sci.* **2018**, *39*, 509–517. [CrossRef]

38. She, R.; Yan, Z.; Jiang, H.; Vetrano, D.L.; Lau, J.T.F.; Qiu, C. Multimorbidity and Health-Related Quality of Life in Old Age: Role of Functional Dependence and Depressive Symptoms. *J. Am. Med. Dir. Assoc.* **2019**, *20*, 1143–1149. [CrossRef] [PubMed]

39. Forjaz, M.J.; Rodríguez-Blazquez, C.; Ayala, A.; Rodríguez-Rodríguez, V.; de Pedro-Cuesta, J.; García-Gutiérrez, S.; Prados-Torres, A. Chronic conditions, disability, and quality of life in older adults with multimorbidity in Spain. *Eur. J. Intern. Med.* **2015**, *26*, 176–181. [CrossRef]

40. Acar Tek, N.; Karaçil-Ermumcu, M.S. Determinants of Health Related Quality of Life in Home Dwelling Elderly Population: Appetite and Nutritional Status. *J. Nutr. Health Aging* **2018**, *22*, 996–1002. [CrossRef]

41. Akkawi, M.E.; Nik Mohamed, M.H.; Md Aris, M.A. Does inappropriate prescribing affect elderly patients' quality of life? A study from a Malaysian tertiary hospital. *Qual. Life Res.* **2019**, *28*, 1913–1920. [CrossRef]

42. Cossette, B.; Bagna, M.; Sene, M.; Sirois, C.; Lefebvre, G.P.; Germain, O.; Morais, J.A.; Gaudreau, P.; Payette, H. Association Between Anticholinergic Drug Use and Health-Related Quality of Life in Community-Dwelling Older Adults. *Drugs Aging* **2017**, *34*, 785–792. [CrossRef]

43. Sivertsen, H.; Bjørkløf, G.H.; Engedal, K.; Selbæk, G.; Helvik, A.S. Depression and Quality of Life in Older Persons: A Review. *Dement. Geriatr. Cogn. Disord.* **2015**, *40*, 311–339. [CrossRef]

44. Chang, Y.C.; Yao, G.; Hu, S.C.; Wang, J.D. Depression Affects the Scores of All Facets of the WHOQOL-BREF and May Mediate the Effects of Physical Disability among Community-Dwelling Older Adults. *PLoS ONE.* **2015**, *10*, e0128356. [CrossRef]

45. De Almeida Roediger, M.; de Fátima Nunes Marucci, M.; Duim, E.L.; Santo, J.L.F.; de Oliveira Duarte, Y.A.; de Oliveira, C. Inflammation and quality of life in later life: Findings from the health, well-being and aging study (SABE). *Health Qual. Life Outcomes.* **2019**, *17*, 26. [CrossRef] [PubMed]

46. Banegas, J.R.; López-García, E.; Graciani, A.; Guallar-Castillón, P.; Gutierrez-Fisac, J.L.; Alonso, J.; Rodríguez-Artalejo, F. Relationship between obesity, hypertension and diabetes, and health-related quality of life among the elderly. *Eur. J. Cardiovasc. Prev. Rehabil.* **2007**, *14*, 456–462. [CrossRef] [PubMed]

47. Giovannini, S.; Macchi, C.; Liperoti, R.; Laudisio, A.; Coraci, D.; Loreti, C.; Vannetti, F.; Onder, G.; Padua, L.; Mugello Study Working Group. Association of Body Fat with Health-Related Quality of Life and Depression in Nonagenarians: The Mugello Study. *J. Am. Med. Dir. Assoc* **2019**, *20*, 564–568. [CrossRef] [PubMed]

48. Payne, M.E.; Porter Starr, K.N.; Orenduff, M.; Mulder, H.S.; McDonald, S.R.; Spira, A.P.; Pieper, C.F.; Bales, C.W. Quality of Life and Mental Health in Older Adults with Obesity and Frailty: Associations with a Weight Loss Intervention. *J. Nutr. Health Aging* **2018**, *22*, 1259–1265. [CrossRef]

49. Masel, M.C.; Graham, J.E.; Reistetter, T.A.; Markides, K.S.; Ottenbacher, K.J. Frailty and health related quality of life in older Mexican Americans. *Health Qual. Life Outcomes.* **2009**, *7*. [CrossRef]

50. Madariaga, I.A.; Antón, V.A.N. Aspectos estadísticos del cuestionario de calidad de vida relacionada con salud Short Form-36 (SF-36). *Estadística Española.* **2008**, *50*, 147–192. (In Spanish)

Epidemiology and Burden of Diabetic Foot Ulcer and Peripheral Arterial Disease in Korea

Dong-il Chun [1,†]**, Sangyoung Kim** [2,†]**, Jahyung Kim** [1]**, Hyeon-Jong Yang** [3]**, Jae Heon Kim** [4]**,
Jae-ho Cho** [5]**, Young Yi** [6]**, Woo Jong Kim** [7] **and Sung Hun Won** [1,*]

[1] Department of Orthopaedic Surgery, Soonchunhyang University Hospital Seoul, 59, Daesagwan-ro, Yongsan-gu, Seoul 04401, Korea; orthochun@gmail.com (D.-i.C.); hpsyndrome@naver.com (J.K.)
[2] SCH Biomedical Informatics Research Unit, Soonchunhyang University Seoul Hospital, Seoul 04401, Korea; kkimsy@naver.com
[3] Department of Pediatrics, Soonchunhyang University Hospital Seoul, 59, Daesagwan-ro, Yongsan-gu, Seoul 04401, Korea; pedyang@schmc.ac.kr
[4] Department of Urology, Soonchunhyang University Hospital Seoul, 59, Daesagwan-ro, Yongsan-gu, Seoul 04401, Korea; piacekjh@hanmail.net
[5] Department of Orthopaedic Surgery, Chuncheon Sacred Heart Hospital, Hallym University, 77, Sakju-ro, Chuncheon-si 24253, Korea; hohotoy@nate.com
[6] Department of Orthopaedic Surgery, Seoul Foot and Ankle Center, Inje University, 85, 2-ga, Jeo-dong, Jung-gu, Seoul 04551, Korea; 20vvin@naver.com
[7] Department of Orthopaedic Surgery, Soonchunhyang University Hospital Cheonan, 31, Soonchunhyang 6-gil, Dongnam-gu, Cheonan 31151, Korea; kwj9383@hanmail.net
* Correspondence: orthowon@gmail.com; Tel.:
† Dong-il Chun and Sangyoung Kim contributed equally to this work and should be considered co-first authors.

Abstract: Information about the epidemiology of diabetic foot ulcer (DFU) with peripheral arterial disease (PAD) is likely to be crucial for predicting future disease progression and establishing a health care budget. We investigated the incidence and prevalence of DFU and PAD in Korea. In addition, we examined costs of treatments for DFU and PAD. This study was conducted using data from Health Insurance Review and Assessment Service from 1 January 2011 to 31 December 2016. The incidence of DFU with PAD was 0.58% in 2012 and 0.49% in 2016. The prevalence of DFU with PAD was 1.7% in 2011 to 1.8% in 2016. The annual amputation rate of DFU with PAD was 0.95% in 2012 and 1.10% in 2016. Major amputation was decreased, while minor amputation was increased. The direct cost of each group was increased, especially the limb saving group. which was increased from 296 million dollars in 2011 to 441 million dollars in 2016. The overall incidence of DFU with PAD was about 0.5% of total population in Korea, from 2012 to 2016. Furthermore, costs for treatments of diabetic foot ulcer are increasing, especially those for the limb saving group.

Keywords: diabetic foot ulcer; peripheral arterial disease; incidence; prevalence; cost; National Health Insurance Service data

1. Introduction

The prevalence of diabetes mellitus is expected to increase and the number of diabetic patients worldwide is on the rise. The global prevalence of diabetic foot varies from 3% in Oceania to 13% in North America, with a global average of 6.4% [1]. The annual incidence of diabetic foot ulcer (DFU) or necrosis in diabetic patients is known to be about 2% to 5% and the lifetime risk ranges from 15% to 20% [2–4]. Peripheral arterial disease (PAD), like cardiovascular disease, is a major arterial disease caused by atherosclerosis [5]. Diabetes is one of the high risk factors of PAD [5], and Olinic et al. [6]

reported that the prevalence of PAD in Europe is increasing, parallel with increasing age and other risk factors for cardiovascular disease. PAD is associated with a 20-fold higher prevalence in patients with diabetes. It is known to be a risk factor for the highest severity of single factors in diabetic patients [7–9]. In addition, the probability of amputation within one year after the first ulcer or gangrene is 34.1% and the mortality rate has been reported to be 5.5% [8]. Information about the epidemiology of peripheral arterial disease associated with DFU is likely to be crucial for predicting future disease progression and establishing a health care budget.

About 20% to 33% of costs related to diabetes mellitus are used for treatments of diabetic foot [3,10]. The incidence of diabetes represented by chronic diseases is increasing. The cost of medical care for diabetic foot is increasing. Korea has recently entered an aging society. The increase in the number of diabetic patients has become an important issue in the decision of the health and welfare budget in Korea. In addition, the increase in complications due to diabetes is a burden, not only for patients, but also for the nation. Furthermore, such information is important for public health policy makers to advocate for implementation of prevention and treatment recommendations. However, there are no recent studies on the incidence, prevalence, or costs of treatments of DFU and PAD in Korea.

Thus, the primary objective of this study was to investigate the incidence and prevalence of DFU and PAD in Korea. The secondary objective was to analyze the costs of treatments for DFU and PAD using National Health Insurance Service data provided by the Health Insurance Review and Assessment Service (HIRA).

2. Materials and Methods

This study was approved by the Institutional Review Board of Soonchunhyang University Hospital Seoul (Institutional Review Board number: SCHUH 2018-01-007). The use of codes directly signifying DFU began on 1 January 2011, when the sixth edition of the Korean statistical classification of disease and related health problems-6 system (KCD-6) was applied. Until the year 2010, the disease code indicating the gangrene and ulcer was used separately from the diabetes code. If the disease code of the foot wound was not actively recorded, even if there was a DFU, DFU patients were inevitably missing. Therefore, we judged that it was not accurate to investigate data before 2010. Finally, data after 2011 were examined in this study. This study was conducted using data from HIRA from 1 January 2011 to 31 December 2016.

The annual incidence and prevalence of diabetes foot ulcer and PAD among the total population of Korea (estimated population) reported by the National Statistical Office were calculated. We considered the wash-out period as one year to determine the annual incidence of DFU and PAD. Therefore, the annual incidence of newly diagnosed DFU and PAD patients was calculated from 2012.

The amputation rates in diabetic foot ulcer and PAD patients were also calculated according to amputation level (minor vs. major (above ankle)). Diabetic foot ulcer and PAD codes and behavior codes (such as amputation, debridement, etc.) included in this study are summarized in Table 1.

Table 1. Diabetic foot ulcer (DFU) and peripheral arterial disease (PAD) codes and behavior codes included in this study.

Diabetic Foot
E105: E1050, E1051, E1058
E107: E1070, E1071, E1072, E1078
E115: E1150, E1151, E1158
E117: E1170, E1171, E1172, E1178
E125: E1250, E1251, E1258
E127: E1270, E1271, E1272, E1278
E135: E1350, E1351, E1358
E137: E1370, E1371, E1372, E1378

Table 1. *Cont.*

E145: E1450, E1451, E1458
E147: E1470, E1471, E1472, E1478

Peripheral Arterial Disease
I7022, I7023, I7024, I7025, I7029

Behavior
SC021, SC022, SC023, SC024, SC025, SC026, SC027
M0111, M0115, M0121, M0122, M0123, M0125, M0135, M0137
N0571, N0572, N0573, N0574, N0575, N0579

The direct cost for each amputation was calculated. We also analyzed the direct costs of DFU and PAD care in three groups. Group I was a limb-saving group. Group II was for those who had one amputation. Group III was for patients who had repeated amputation. The cost was based on the direct cost of patient contributions plus insurance claims. The direct cost was adjusted by taking into account the medical price index presented by the Korean Statistical Information Service (KOSIS, Daejeon, Korea). The data of this study were analyzed using SAS Enterprise Guide, ver. 6.1 M1 (SAS Institute Inc., Cary, NC, USA).

3. Results

Regarding the overall annual incidence of DFU from 2012 to 2016, 0.43% of total populations were diagnosed with DFU in 2012 whereas 0.34% were diagnosed in 2016, showing a remarkable incidence plateau with a mild decrease over five years. The annual incidence of PAD was 0.19% in 2012 and 0.20% in 2016, showing an incidence plateau with a mild increase over five years. The annual incidence of DFU with PAD was 0.58% in 2012 and 0.49% in 2016 (Figure 1). The overall prevalence of DFU in the study period was 1.4% in 2011 and 1.3% in 2016. The prevalence of PAD was 0.4% in 2011 and 0.5% in 2016. The prevalence of DFU with PAD showed a mild increase from 1.7% in 2011 to 1.8% in 2016 (Figure 1).

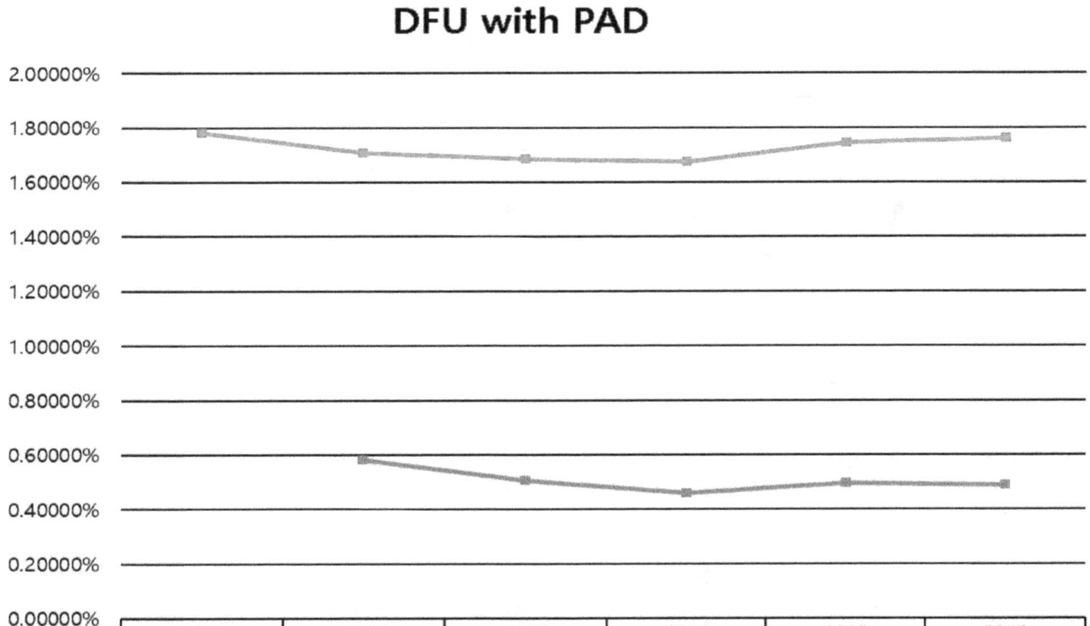

DFU with PAD

	2011	2012	2013	2014	2015	2016
Prevalence	1.78035%	1.70875%	1.68292%	1.67338%	1.74344%	1.76196%
Incidence		0.58268%	0.50460%	0.45971%	0.49460%	0.48764%

Figure 1. Annual the incidence and prevalence of diabetic foot ulcer with PAD.

The annual amputation rate of DFU with PAD was increased from 0.95% in 2012 to 1.10% in 2016. Of these, the major amputation rate was decreased from 0.28% in 2012 to 0.27% in 2016, while the minor amputation rate was increased from 0.66% in 2012 to 0.82% in 2016 (Figure 2).

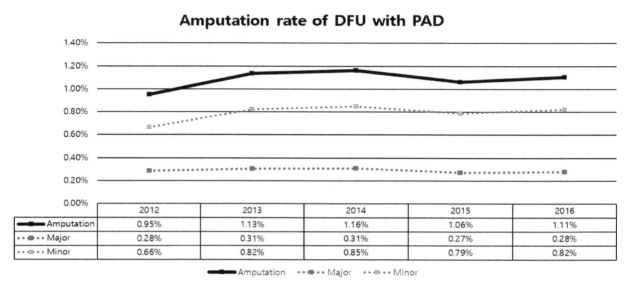

	2012	2013	2014	2015	2016
Amputation	0.95%	1.13%	1.16%	1.06%	1.11%
Major	0.28%	0.31%	0.31%	0.27%	0.28%
Minor	0.66%	0.82%	0.85%	0.79%	0.82%

Figure 2. Annual amputation rate of diabetic foot ulcer with PAD.

The direct cost of amputation was increased from 17 million dollars in 2011 to 25 million dollars in 2016. Especially, the sum of direct costs of minor amputation increased from 11 million dollars in 2011 to 17 million dollars in 2016 (Figure 3). The average cost of amputation per person was also increased from 6100 dollars in 2011 to 7300 dollars in 2016 (Figure 4). The direct cost of each group was increased from 2011 to 2016. Direct costs for group 1 increased from 296 million dollars in 2011 to 441 million dollars in 2016. These costs for group 2 increased from 7.1 million dollars in 2011 to 9.3 million dollars in 2016, while those for group 3 increased from 10 million dollars in 2011 to 15 million dollars in 2016 (Figure 5).

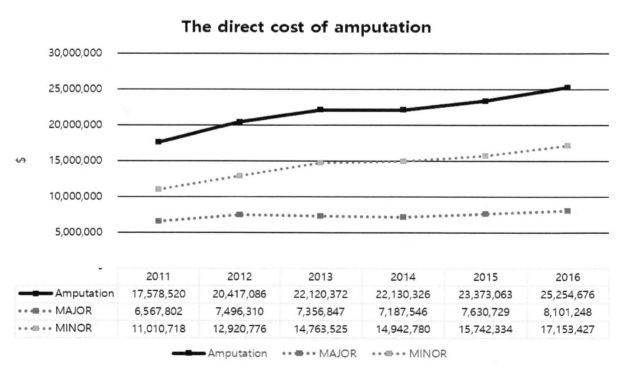

	2011	2012	2013	2014	2015	2016
Amputation	17,578,520	20,417,086	22,120,372	22,130,326	23,373,063	25,254,676
MAJOR	6,567,802	7,496,310	7,356,847	7,187,546	7,630,729	8,101,248
MINOR	11,010,718	12,920,776	14,763,525	14,942,780	15,742,334	17,153,427

Figure 3. The direct cost of amputation of diabetic foot ulcer with PAD.

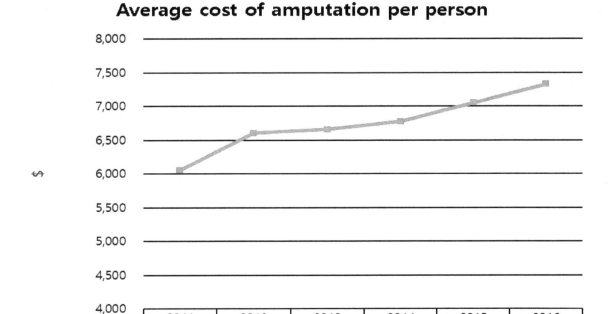

Figure 4. The average cost of amputation, per person, of diabetic foot ulcer with PAD.

	2011	2012	2013	2014	2015	2016
Average cost	6,055	6,603	6,659	6,776	7,051	7,329

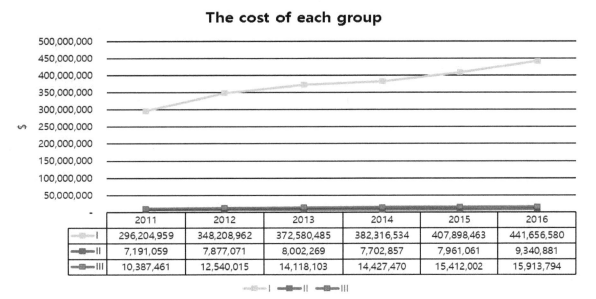

	2011	2012	2013	2014	2015	2016
I	296,204,959	348,208,962	372,580,485	382,316,534	407,898,463	441,656,580
II	7,191,059	7,877,071	8,002,269	7,702,857	7,961,061	9,340,881
III	10,387,461	12,540,015	14,118,103	14,427,470	15,412,002	15,913,794

Figure 5. The direct cost of each group for diabetic foot ulcer with PAD.

4. Discussion

Overall incidence and prevalence of DFU with PAD in Korea from 2012 to 2016 were about 0.5% and 1.7% of the total population, respectively. The amputation rate was increased, especially the minor amputation rate, which increased from 0.66% in 2011 to 0.82% in 2016. Furthermore, direct costs for diabetes treatment were increased, especially the expense for the limb saving group.

We investigated the annual incidence and prevalence of DFU and PAD among the total population in Korea. The incidence and prevalence of DFU are also important for determining the number of diabetic patients. We requested HIRA to provide the total data for diabetic patients. However, the organization explained to us that these data were too large to release. Therefore, we could not obtain information for the total number of diabetic patients during the study period. Thus, we calculated the incidence and prevalence of DFU patients in the total population. However, the Korean diabetic association reported that the prevalence of diabetes increased from 12.4% in 2012 to 14.4% in 2016 through a diabetic fact sheet in 2018. Thus, we could investigate the prevalence of diabetic foot ulcer among the diabetic patients indirectly, showing 10% in 2012 and 9% in 2016. Recently, Zhang et al. [1] reported that the global prevalence of diabetic foot ulceration is 6.3% and the prevalence is 13.0% in North America and 5.5% in Asia. However, in their systematic review and meta-analysis study, the definitions for diabetic foot and diabetic foot ulceration were ambiguous. Furthermore, two epidemiologic studies using only Korean data focused on the epidemiology of diabetic peripheral neuropathy [11,12]. However, our study investigated not only DFU, but also PAD. Thus, we believe that our study has a more accurate prevalence of DFU in Korea.

Concerning amputation, our results showed that annual amputation rate of DFU with PAD increased from 0.95% in 2012 to 1.10% in 2016. Of these, the major amputation rate decreased from 0.28% in 2012 to 0.27% in 2016, while the minor amputation rate was increased from 0.66% in 2012 to 0.82% in 2016. The overall amputation rate was increased. This might be due to the increased minor amputation rate, rather than the decrease of the major amputation rate. Goodney et al. reported that lower extremity amputation decreased by 45% from 1996 to 2011 (above the knee amputation decreased by 48% and below the knee amputation decreased by 39%) [13]. Although, in our study, we did not show a clear causal relationship about the reason for this situation, two reasons might be important. The first one is the increased awareness of the risk of diabetic foot in diabetic patients. Previous studies have reported that education about foot care to diabetic patients is important because it is associated with a significant reduction in lower extremity amputation. In addition, monthly foot checks are associated with the reduction of major lower limb amputations in diabetic incident hemodialysis patients [14,15]. Future studies are needed to examine awareness of risk of DFU in diabetic patients. The second reason is the improvement of vascular conditions due to increase of revascularization. This is also important for the reduction of major amputation. Peripheral vascular disease is known to be the most significant risk factor for diabetic foot amputation [8]. A previous study also reported that it is evident that the increasing use of vascular and preventive care, especially among patients with diabetes, is temporally associated with lower rates of major amputation [16]. Future studies focusing on understanding this relationship are needed.

The increase in the cost of medical care, due to the increased number of diabetic patients, has been reported all over the world. It is a useful indicator for planning and enforcing health care policies and budgets [17–19]. To the best of our knowledge, our research is the first to investigate the cost of medical care for diabetic foot ulcer in Korea. Our study showed that, although the cost of amputation was increased a lot, the expense for the limb saving group increased exponentially. Such a cost increase might be due to the development of medications and dressing materials. This could increase the burden on the patient. Understanding the cost of DFU should support future decisions on investment in diabetic foot care.

Some limitations of the study need to be addressed. First, DFU and PAD codes are diverse, unclear, and sometimes missing. There was no defined disease code for DFU until 2010. Thus, data on DFU from 2007 to 2010 could not be used. This is considered the limit for using National Health Insurance Service data provided by HIRA. It is necessary to agree on codes of diabetic foot and PAD more clearly and uniformly in the future. Second, diabetic neuropathy was not included in this study, because the disease code and operational definition for diabetic neuropathy were not established in the Big Data. Furthermore, extracted data using the provided diabetic neuropathy code revealed that too many patients were included, so the extracted data could not be trusted. Therefore, in this study, diabetic neuropathy was excluded in order to improve the quality of the study, but it is thought that studies to include neuropathy in the diabetic foot should be done through the operational definition defined later. Third, when calculating the incidence of chronic diseases, such as diabetes and PAD, a wash-out period of at least 2 years should be used. However, we used wash-out period of one year to calculate incidence of DFU and PAD. This was an inevitable choice due to too much missing data. If data for a longer period of time can be used, the wash-out period of 2 years can be used. Such study is needed in the future.

5. Conclusions

In conclusion, over 5 years, we found that the overall incidence and prevalence of DFU with PAD in Korea were about 0.5% and 1.7% of the total population, respectively. The amputation rate was increased, especially the minor amputation rate. Furthermore, the direct costs for DFU treatment were increased, especially the expense for the limb saving group. Our results suggest that we should pay attention to effective implementation of the budget when we make future health policies for diabetic foot. Further studies warrant the importance of productive and cost-effective methods for saving limbs in the healthcare system.

Author Contributions: Conceptualization, J.-h.C. and S.H.W.; Data curation, J.K.; Formal analysis, D.-i.C. and S.K.; Investigation, H.-J.Y., Y.Y., and W.J.K.; Methodology, J.H.K.

Acknowledgments: We thank Mi-soon Lim, Dong won Shin for contributing to collect the full text articles.

References

1. Zhang, P.; Lu, J.; Jing, Y.; Tang, S.; Zhu, D.; Bi, Y. Global epidemiology of diabetic foot ulceration: A systematic review and meta-analysis (dagger). *Ann. Med.* **2017**, *49*, 106–116. [CrossRef] [PubMed]
2. Schaper, N.C.; Apelqvist, J.; Bakker, K. The international consensus and practical guidelines on the management and prevention of the diabetic foot. *Curr. Diabetes Rep.* **2003**, *3*, 475–479. [CrossRef] [PubMed]
3. Mayfield, J.A.; Reiber, G.E.; Sanders, L.J.; Janisse, D.; Pogach, L.M.; American Diabetes, A. Preventive foot care in diabetes. *Diabetes Care* **2004**, *27* (Suppl. 1), S63–S64.
4. Jeffcoate, W.J.; Harding, K.G. Diabetic foot ulcers. *Lancet* **2003**, *361*, 1545–1551. [CrossRef]
5. Katsilambros, N.L.; Tsapogas, P.C.; Arvanitis, M.P.; Tritos, N.A.; Alexiou, Z.P.; Rigas, K.L. Risk factors for lower extremity arterial disease in non-insulin-dependent diabetic persons. *Diabet. Med.* **1996**, *13*, 243–246. [CrossRef]
6. Olinic, D.M.; Spinu, M.; Olinic, M.; Homorodean, C.; Tataru, D.A.; Liew, A.; Schernthaner, G.H.; Stanek, A.; Fowkes, G.; Catalano, M. Epidemiology of peripheral artery disease in Europe: VAS Educational Paper. *Int. Angiol.* **2018**, *37*, 327–334. [CrossRef] [PubMed]
7. Hirsch, A.T.; Criqui, M.H.; Treat-Jacobson, D.; Regensteiner, J.G.; Creager, M.A.; Olin, J.W.; Krook, S.H.; Hunninghake, D.B.; Comerota, A.J.; Walsh, M.E.; et al. Peripheral arterial disease detection, awareness, and treatment in primary care. *JAMA* **2001**, *286*, 1317–1324. [CrossRef] [PubMed]
8. Won, S.H.; Chung, C.Y.; Park, M.S.; Lee, T.; Sung, K.H.; Lee, S.Y.; Kim, T.G.; Lee, K.M. Risk factors associated with amputation-free survival in patient with diabetic foot ulcers. *Yonsei Med. J.* **2014**, *55*, 1373–1378. [CrossRef] [PubMed]
9. Behrendt, C.A.; Sigvant, B.; Szeberin, Z.; Beiles, B.; Eldrup, N.; Thomson, I.A.; Venermo, M.; Altreuther, M.; Menyhei, G.; Nordanstig, J.; et al. International Variations in Amputation Practice: A VASCUNET Report. *Eur. J. Vasc. Endovasc. Surg.* **2018**, *56*, 391–399. [CrossRef] [PubMed]
10. Driver, V.R.; Fabbi, M.; Lavery, L.A.; Gibbons, G. The costs of diabetic foot: The economic case for the limb salvage team. *J. Vasc. Surg.* **2010**, *52*, 17S–22S. [CrossRef] [PubMed]
11. Kim, S.S.; Won, J.C.; Kwon, H.S.; Kim, C.H.; Lee, J.H.; Park, T.S.; Ko, K.S.; Cha, B.Y. Prevalence and clinical implications of painful diabetic peripheral neuropathy in type 2 diabetes: Results from a nationwide hospital-based study of diabetic neuropathy in Korea. *Diabetes Res. Clin. Pract.* **2014**, *103*, 522–529. [CrossRef] [PubMed]
12. Won, J.C.; Kwon, H.S.; Kim, C.H.; Lee, J.H.; Park, T.S.; Ko, K.S.; Cha, B.Y. Prevalence and clinical characteristics of diabetic peripheral neuropathy in hospital patients with Type 2 diabetes in Korea. *Diabet. Med.* **2012**, *29*, e290–e296. [CrossRef] [PubMed]

13. Goodney, P.P.; Tarulli, M.; Faerber, A.E.; Schanzer, A.; Zwolak, R.M. Fifteen-year trends in lower limb amputation, revascularization, and preventive measures among medicare patients. *JAMA Surg.* **2015**, *150*, 84–86. [CrossRef] [PubMed]

14. Dargis, V.; Pantelejeva, O.; Jonushaite, A.; Vileikyte, L.; Boulton, A.J. Benefits of a multidisciplinary approach in the management of recurrent diabetic foot ulceration in Lithuania: A prospective study. *Diabetes Care* **1999**, *22*, 1428–1431. [CrossRef] [PubMed]

15. Marn Pernat, A.; Persic, V.; Usvyat, L.; Saunders, L.; Rogus, J.; Maddux, F.W.; Lacson, E., Jr.; Kotanko, P. Implementation of routine foot check in patients with diabetes on hemodialysis: Associations with outcomes. *BMJ Open Diabetes Res. Care* **2016**, *4*, e000158. [CrossRef] [PubMed]

16. Goodney, P.P.; Holman, K.; Henke, P.K.; Travis, L.L.; Dimick, J.B.; Stukel, T.A.; Fisher, E.S.; Birkmeyer, J.D. Regional intensity of vascular care and lower extremity amputation rates. *J. Vasc. Surg.* **2013**, *57*, 1471–1480. [CrossRef] [PubMed]

17. Toscano, C.; Sugita, T.; Rosa, M.; Pedrosa, H.; Rosa, R.; Bahia, L. Annual Direct Medical Costs of Diabetic Foot Disease in Brazil: A Cost of Illness Study. *Int. J. Environ. Res. Public Health* **2018**, *15*, 89. [CrossRef] [PubMed]

18. Hicks, C.W.; Selvarajah, S.; Mathioudakis, N.; Sherman, R.E.; Hines, K.F.; Black III, J.H.; Abularrage, C.J. Burden of Infected Diabetic Foot Ulcers on Hospital Admissions and Costs. *Ann. Vasc. Surg.* **2016**, *33*, 149–158. [CrossRef] [PubMed]

19. Kerr, M.; Rayman, G.; Jeffcoate, W.J. Cost of diabetic foot disease to the National Health Service in England. *Diabet. Med.* **2014**, *31*, 1498–1504. [CrossRef] [PubMed]

The Optimal Range of Serum Uric Acid for Cardiometabolic Diseases: A 5-Year Japanese Cohort Study

Masanari Kuwabara [1,2,*], Ichiro Hisatome [3], Koichiro Niwa [2], Petter Bjornstad [4,5],
Carlos A. Roncal-Jimenez [4], Ana Andres-Hernando [4], Mehmet Kanbay [6], Richard J. Johnson [4]
and Miguel A. Lanaspa [4]

[1] Intensive Care Unit and Department of Cardiology, Toranomon Hospital, Tokyo 105-8470, Japan
[2] Cardiovascular Center, St. Luke's International Hospital, Tokyo 104-8560, Japan; kniwa@aol.com
[3] Division of Regenerative Medicine and Therapeutics, Tottori University Graduate School of Medical
     Sciences, Tottori 683-8503, Japan; hisatome@med.tottori-u.ac.jp
[4] Division of Renal Diseases and Hypertension, School of Medicine, University of Colorado Denver, Aurora,
     CO 80045, USA; Petter.bjornstad@childrenscolorado.org (P.B.), Carlos.Roncal@ucdenver.edu (C.A.R.-J.);
     Ana.AndresHernando@ucdenver.edu (A.A.-H.); Richard.Johnson@ucdenver.edu (R.J.J.);
     Miguel.LanaspaGarcia@ucdenver.edu (M.A.L.)
[5] Children's Hospital Colorado and Barbara Davis Center for Childhood Diabetes, Aurora, CO 80045, USA
[6] Division of Nephrology, Department of Medicine, Koc University School of Medicine, Istanbul 34450,
     Turkey; mkanbay@ku.edu.tr
*   Correspondence: kuwamasa728@gmail.com
†   Optimal uric acid for cardiometabolic diseases.

Abstract: The optimal range of serum uric acid (urate) associated with the lowest risk for developing cardiometabolic diseases is unknown in a generally healthy population. This 5-year cohort study is designed to identify the optimal range of serum urate. The data were collected from 13,070 Japanese between ages 30 and 85 at the baseline (2004) from the Center for Preventive Medicine, St. Luke's International Hospital, Tokyo. We evaluated the number of subjects (and prevalence) of those free of the following conditions: hypertension, diabetes, dyslipidemia, and chronic kidney disease (CKD) over 5 years for each 1 mg/dL of serum urate stratified by sex. Furthermore, the odds ratios (ORs) for remaining free of these conditions were calculated with multiple adjustments. Except for truly hypouricemic subjects, having lower serum urate was an independent factor for predicting the absence of hypertension, dyslipidemia, and CKD, but not diabetes. The OR of each 1 mg/dL serum urate decrease as a protective factor for hypertension, dyslipidemia, and CKD was 1.153 (95% confidence interval, 1.068–1.245), 1.164 (1.077–1.258), and 1.226 (1.152–1.306) in men; 1.306 (1.169–1.459), 1.121 (1.022–1.230), and 1.424 (1.311–1.547) in women, respectively. Moreover, comparing serum urate of 3–5 mg/dL in men and 2–4 mg/dL in women, hypouricemia could be a higher risk for developing hypertension (OR: 4.532; 0.943–21.78) and CKD (OR: 4.052; 1.181–13.90) in women, but not in men. The optimal serum urate range associated with the lowest development of cardiometabolic diseases was less than 5 mg/dL for men and 2–4 mg/dL for women, respectively.

Keywords: uric acid; risk factor; epidemiology; cardiometabolic diseases; hypertension

---

1. Introduction

Both epidemiologically and in animal models, hyperuricemia is strongly associated with the development and progression of cardiovascular disease [1,2]. In this regard, a recent meta-analysis report estimated a 12% increase in coronary heart disease per 1 mg/dL elevation in serum uric acid (urate) levels. However, it is important to note that other studies could not support serum urate as a truly independent risk factor for cardiovascular diseases [3–5]. Furthermore, some studies have shown a J-shaped relationship between serum urate and cardiovascular disease supporting the idea that both low and high urate are associated with greater risk of developing cardiovascular events. As an example, according to the PIUMA study, serum urate levels lower than 4.5 mg/dL in men and 3.2 mg/dL in women with essential hypertension but also higher than 5.2 mg/dL in men and 3.9 mg/dL in women are associated with increased rates of cardiovascular disease and cardiovascular disease-related deaths. The J-curve phenomenon relating serum urate to cardiovascular events was also reported in the Syst-Eur trial [6]. The variability in the findings from the cross-sectional studies and the evidence supporting a J-shaped cause-effect between urate and cardiovascular disease suggests the need to identify the proper level range for which urate could be relatively safe, or in contrast, could exert a substantial deleterious role in the pathogenesis of cardiovascular disease. In this regard, little information is known on the optimal serum urate range associated with the lowest risk of disease in a generally healthy population.

Therefore, we aimed to evaluate whether a J-shaped curve exists for serum urate with cardiometabolic diseases (hypertension, diabetes, dyslipidemia, and chronic kidney disease (CKD)) and to identify the optimal range of serum urate that is associated with the lowest risk for developing these conditions by a longitudinal design.

2. Materials and Methods

2.1. Study Design and Study Subjects

This study included a single-center, large-scale, cross-sectional study and a 5-year longitudinal cohort study in Japan. We reviewed and used the database of health records from the Center for Preventive Medicine, St. Luke's International Hospital, Tokyo, Japan between 2004 and 2009. The study subjects came to the center to have annual regular health check-up by themselves, and also provided a general history for comorbidities. Every subject and/or their companies paid for the examinations and each subject had identical physical and laboratory examinations including blood pressure. In general, the patients with any symptoms go to their hospital or clinic with Japanese government insurance, and therefore this study population was defined as a 'generally healthy population'. Some of the findings from this database have already been published [7–15]. There were 30,227 subjects (15,263 men) who underwent an annual health check-up at the center in 2004. In this study, we enrolled 13,201 subjects who underwent health checks both in 2004 and in 2009. The background demographics between all the subjects in 2004 and this cohort study subjects were similar as shown in our previous manuscript [8]. The prevalence of hyperuricemia between the two groups showed no significant differences, including in men and in women, respectively [8]. For this study, we included subjects between the ages 30 and 85 in 2004 whose data were available at both 2004 and 2009. Subjects younger than 30 years of age were excluded due to their very modest risk for hypertension and cardiovascular diseases, while subjects aged 85 years old and above were excluded due to the substantial risk of death during a five-year follow-up. Out of the 13,201 subjects, only 121 subjects were less than 30 years old and 10 subjects were 85 years old and above in 2004, and 13,070 subjects were enrolled (mean age: 51.1 ± 11.3 years). Of these, 6367 were men (52.4 ± 11.5 years) and 6733 women (49.9 ± 11.1 years). For our first analysis (a cross-sectional study), we checked the prevalence of cardiometabolic diseases, like hypertension, diabetes, dyslipidemia, and CKD in each 1 mg/dL of serum urate range in each sex at baseline (2004). Then, we excluded the subjects with each cardiometabolic condition at baseline, and we checked whether they remained free of these conditions over the following five years, as it related to each serum urate quartile separated by sex (a 5-year cohort study). We also calculated the odds ratios (ORs) of each 1 mg/dL increase of serum urate for each cardiometabolic diseases after multiple adjustments for well-known factors associated with cardiovascular diseases including age, body mass index (BMI), smoking and drinking habits, serum urate, and the presence of other cardiometabolic diseases as detailed in Figure 1. When we assessed the protective factors for the development of hypertension, diabetes, dyslipidemia, and CKD, we excluded 2599 subjects with hypertensions, 575 subjects with diabetes, 5118 subjects with dyslipidemia, and 492 subjects with CKD at the baseline in each analysis, respectively. Moreover, we compared the cumulative incidence of any of these cardiometabolic diseases between hypouricemic subjects (serum urate of less than 3 mg/dL in men and less than 2 mg/dL in women) and normouricemic subjects (serum urate of 3–5 mg/dL in men and 2–4 mg/dL in women) to detect whether hypouricemia is a risk for developing cardiometabolic diseases compared with normouricemia. We also calculated the ORs of hypouricemia for each cardiometabolic diseases compared with normouricemia after multiple adjustments.

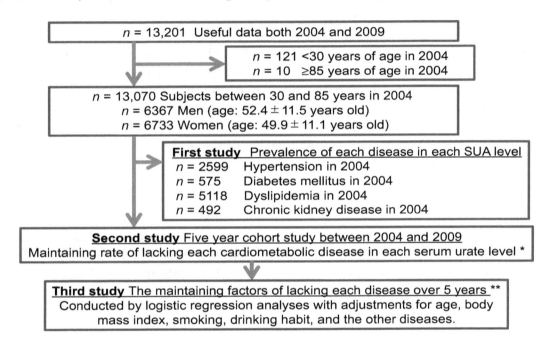

Figure 1. Flow diagram of study enrollment. All the analyses were stratified by sex. * Each cardiometabolic disease means hypertension, diabetes, dyslipidemia and chronic kidney disease. ** The number of subjects depends on the excluded subjects having the corresponding disorders at baseline.

2.2. Definition of Hypertension, Diabetes, Dyslipidemia, CKD, and Hypouricemia

Hypertension is defined as a condition when subjects are on current antihypertensive medication and/or systolic blood pressure of more than or equal to 140 mmHg and/or diastolic blood pressure of more than or equal to 90 mmHg [16,17]. Blood pressure readings were obtained using an automatic brachial sphygmomanometer (OMRON Corporation, Kyoto, Japan), which was upper arm blood pressure measuring and had passed validation. Two blood pressure examinations were taken after the participants were seated and rested quietly for more than five minutes with their feet on the ground and their back supported. The mean systolic and diastolic blood pressure of each of the subjects were calculated from the recorded measurements. Diabetes is defined as current diabetes mellitus on medication use and/or HbA1c (National Glycohemoglobin Standardization Program) more than or equal to 6.5%, according to International Expert Committee. Dyslipidemia is defined as current medication use for dyslipidemia and/or low-density lipoprotein cholesterol more than or equal to 140 mg/dL, high-density lipoprotein cholesterol less than 40 mg/dL, and/or triglyceride more than or equal to 150 mg/dL, according to Japan Atherosclerosis Society guidelines [18]. CKD is defined as estimated glomerular filtration rate (eGFR) is less than 60 mL/min/1.73m^2. We calculated eGFR using the Japanese GFR equation: eGFR (mL/min/1.73m^2) = 194 × serum creatinine $^{-1.094}$ × age $^{-0.287}$ (×0.739 if woman) [19]. Hypouricemia is defined as serum urate level lower than 3.0 mg/dL in men and 2.0 mg/dL in women in this study [20]

2.3. Statistical Analysis

All the statistical analyses were performed using the SPSS Statistics software (IBM SPSS Statistics version 22 for Windows; IBM, New York, NY, USA). The statistically significant level was set at probability $p < 0.05$ (two-tailed). Data are expressed as mean ± standard deviation or as percent frequency unless otherwise specified. Comparisons between two groups were performed with student t-tests for normally distributed variables, and χ^2 analyses for categorical data. The maintaining factors for lacking hypertension, diabetes, dyslipidemia, and CKD in the period of over five years were evaluated both by crude models and by multivariable logistic regression models with adjustments of the age, BMI, smoking and drinking habits, serum urate, and the other cardiometabolic diseases. We also calculated odds ratios (ORs) in each group. When we analyzed logistic regression analyses in the longitudinal study, we excluded hypouricemic subjects because there was not a linear association between serum urate levels and the maintaining rate of lacking prevalence of these cardiometabolic diseases only in hypouricemic subjects. Moreover, we compared cumulative incidence of each cardiometabolic disease between hypouricemia and normouricemia to clarify whether J. curve phenomenon exists or not. In this analysis, we used propensity score matching to combine the other factors (age, BMI, smoking and drinking habits, and cardiometabolic feathers; hypertension, diabetes, dyslipidemia, and CKD) into one parameter because the number of hypouricemic subjects were small (45 hypouricemic subjects).

2.4. Ethical Considerations

We adhered to the principles of the Declaration of Helsinki. All data were collected and compiled in a protected computer database. Individual data were anonymous without identifiable personal information. Informed consent was obtained from all subjects by a comprehensive agreement method provided by St. Luke's International Hospital. St. Luke's International Hospital Ethics Committee approved the protocol for this study (approval number: 16-R025).

3. Results

3.1. Demographics of this Study's Subjects

Table 1 shows the demographics of this study for men and women. In general, women were significantly older, and had lower BMI, lower blood pressure, less smoking and drinking habits, lower prevalence of hypertension, diabetes, dyslipidemia, and CKD, and lower serum urate compared to men.

Table 1. Demographics of study subjects at baseline (2004).

	Women	Men	p
Number of Subjects	**6733**	**6337**	
Age	49.9 ± 11.1	42.4 ± 11.5	<0.001
Body mass index (kg/m^2)	21.3 ± 3.0	23.8 ± 2.9	<0.001
Systolic blood pressure (mmHg)	114.5 ± 17.5	124.2 ± 17.2	<0.001
Diastolic blood pressure (mmHg)	70.8 ± 10.9	77.9 ± 10.9	<0.001
Pulse rate (bpm)	75.2 ± 10.8	71.6 ± 10.5	<0.001
Smoking	16.3%	63.0%	<0.001
Drinking habits	26.0%	61.5%	<0.001
Hypertension	13.4%	26.8%	<0.001
Diabetes mellitus	2.1%	6.8%	<0.001
Dyslipidemia	29.6%	49.3%	<0.001
Hypouricemia	0.22%	0.47%	0.016
Chronic kidney disease	2.3%	5.3%	<0.001
eGFR (mL/min/1.73m^2)	88.2 ± 15.7	82.6 ± 15.5	<0.001
Serum uric acid (mg/dL)	4.49 ± 0.95	6.24 ± 1.23	<0.001

bpm, beats per minute; p, probability. Data are presented as mean ± standard deviation.

3.2. Prevalence of Cardiometabolic Disease in Each Serum Urate Level (A Cross-Sectional Study)

Figure 2 shows the prevalence of hypertension, diabetes, dyslipidemia, and CKD for each 1mg/dL of serum urate range at baseline (2004). As shown in the figure, serum urate lower than 4 mg/dL were associated with the lowest prevalence of hypertension, dyslipidemia, and CKD in women while the range of serum urate between 2 and 4 mg/dL corresponded with the lowest prevalence of diabetes. In men, the range of serum urate associated with the lowest prevalence of these conditions was more variable. Interestingly, the prevalence of diabetes in men decreased with increasing serum urate, which may be due to the effect of glycosuria to cause uricosuria and decrease serum urate levels. As a result, serum urate levels in men ranging from 2 to 6 mg/dL corresponded with the lowest prevalence of dyslipidemia and CKD while levels ranging from 3 to 6 mg/dL were associated with the lowest prevalence of hypertension, respectively. However, it is important to note that this cross-sectional analysis at baseline did not account for medication for each disease, raising the possibility of a potential medication bias. Therefore, we conducted a 5-year cohort study to evaluate the odds for remaining free of these disease conditions over time.

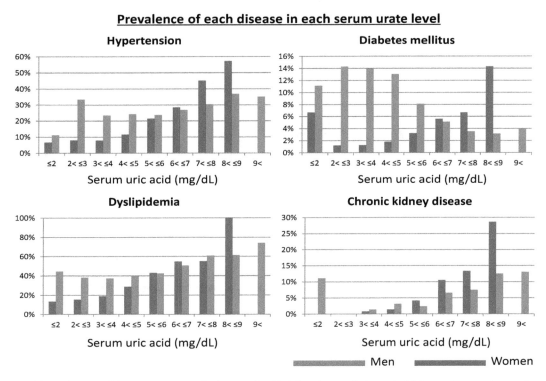

Figure 2. Prevalence of hypertension, diabetes, dyslipidemia, and chronic kidney disease in each serum urate at baseline (2004). Blue bars showed men and red bars showed women.

3.3. Rate of Being Free of Various Cardiometabolic Conditions According to Serum Urate Levels over Five Years (A Longitudinal Study)

The number of subjects with the new development of hypertension, diabetes, dyslipidemia, and CKD over 5 years was 1108/10,471 (10.6%), 318/12,495 (2.5%), 1454/7952 (18.3%), and 1961/12,578 (15.6%), respectively. Figure 3 shows the relative risk for being free of cardiometabolic disease (hypertension, diabetes, dyslipidemia, and CKD) for each serum urate group over a five-year period. There is a linear association between serum urate levels and the rate of being free of cardiometabolic disease except for subjects with hyporuricemia. and we excluded hypouricemic subjects. The multivariable analyses showed that serum urate levels were protective for developing hypertension, diabetes, dyslipidemia, and CKD irrespective of sex, except for hypouricemic subjects. Even when accounting for a J-curve phenomenon with hypouricemic subjects, hyperuricemic subjects had lower maintaining rates with respect to lacking hypertension, diabetes, dyslipidemia, and CKD than hypouricemic subjects.

We conducted additional analyses using four categories of serum urate levels; 2 or less (hypouricemia), from 2 to 4 mg/dL, from 4 to 6 mg/dL, and more than 6 mg/dL (hyperuricemia). We compared the relative risk for being free of cardiometabolic disease (hypertension, diabetes, dyslipidemia, and CKD) among these four serum urate categories over a five-year period. Figure 4 shows that the group with serum urate from 2 to 4 mg/dL exhibited maintaining rates of lacking hypertension or CKD compared to the other urate categories. The group with serum urate of 2 mg/dL or less had the highest maintaining rate with respect to lacking diabetes or dyslipidemia.

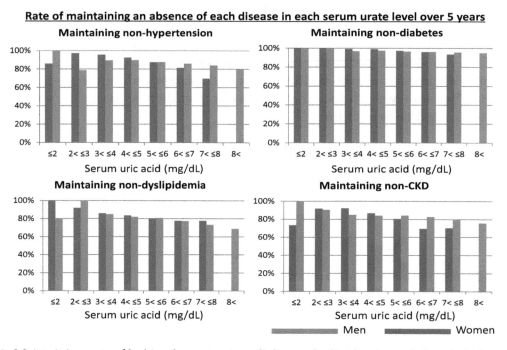

Figure 3. Maintaining rate of lacking hypertension, diabetes, dyslipidemia, and chronic kidney disease in each serum urate over five years. CKD, chronic kidney disease. Blue bars showed men and red bars showed women.

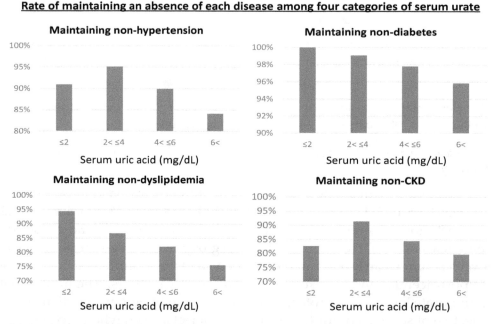

Figure 4. Maintaining rate of lacking hypertension, diabetes, dyslipidemia, and chronic kidney disease among four serum urate categories over five years. CKD, chronic kidney disease.

3.4. Optimal Serum Urate Range Associated with the Lowest Risk of Cardiometabolic Diseases

To determine the optimal range of serum urate to prevent the development of cardiometabolic disease, we conducted a multivariable logistic regression analysis and calculated ORs for maintaining conditions without hypertension, diabetes, dyslipidemia, and CKD after excluding 45 hypouricemic subjects (30 men and 15 women) since we intended to exclude the effects of *J.* curve phenomenon.

To evaluate factors that predict continued normotension, we analyzed 10,471 subjects after excluding 2599 subjects with hypertensions at baseline. After multivariable adjustments for age, BMI, smoking and drinking habits, diabetes, dyslipidemia, and CKD, lower serum urate was an independent factor that protects against the development of hypertension both in men (OR per 1 mg/dL decrease: 1.153; 95% CI, 1.068–1.245) and women (OR: 1.306; 95% CI, 1.169–1.459) (Table 2, Hypertension).

When we assessed the factors that protected against the development of diabetes, we analyzed 12,495 subjects after excluding 575 subjects with diabetes at the baseline. After multiple adjustments age, BMI, smoking and drinking habits, hypertension, dyslipidemia, and CKD, lower serum urate showed a tendency as a protective factor for the development of diabetes in women (OR per 1 mg/dL decrease: 1.206; 95% CI, 0.969–1.500), but it did not reach the significant ($p = 0.093$). In contrast, lower serum urate was not an independent protective factor for the development of diabetes in men ($p = 0.24$) (Table 2, Diabetes).

When we assessed the protective factor for the development of dyslipidemia, we analyzed 7952 subjects after excluding 5118 subjects with dyslipidemia at baseline. After multiple adjustments age, BMI, smoking and drinking habits, hypertension, diabetes, and CKD, lower serum urate was an independent protective factor for the development of dyslipidemia both in men (OR per 1 mg/dL decrease: 1.164; 95% CI, 1.077–1.258) and women (OR per 1 mg/dL decrease: 1.121; 95% CI, 1.022–1.230) (Table 2, Dyslipidemia).

When we assessed the factors that protected against the development of CKD, we analyzed 12,578 subjects after excluding 492 subjects with CKD at the baseline. After multiple adjustments age, BMI, smoking and drinking habits, hypertension, diabetes, and dyslipidemia, lower serum urate was an independent protective factor for the development of CKD both in men (OR per 1 mg/dL decrease: 1.226; 95% CI, 1.152–1.306) and women (OR per 1 mg/dL decrease: 1.424; 95% CI, 1.311–1.547) (Table 2, Chronic kidney disease).

We also compared the ORs for hypertension, diabetes, dyslipidemia, and CKD among four categories of serum urate levels. We referenced the group with serum urate from 2 to 4 mg/dL as shown in Table 3. Belonging to the group with serum urate from 2 to 4 mg/dL conferred protection from developing hypertension, dyslipidemia, and CKD when compared with the group with serum urate more than 4 mg/dL, but not diabetes (Table 3).

3.5. Hypouricemia as a Risk of Cardiometabolic Diseases Compared with Normouricemia

We compared the cumulative incidence of cardiometabolic diseases between hypouricemic subjects (30 men and 15 women) and normouricemic subjects (3–5 mg/dL for 958 men and 2–4 mg/dL for 2192 women). The number of hypouricemic subjects were small, and we could not analyze ORs of diabetes both in men and women and dyslipidemia in women. After multiple adjustments age, BMI, smoking and drinking habits, diabetes, dyslipidemia, and CKD, hypouricemia tends to be higher risk for the development of CKD in women (OR: 4.532; 95% CI, 0.943–21.78), but not reach significance ($p = 0.059$) (Table 4, Hypertension). After multiple adjustments that included age, BMI, smoking and drinking habits, hypertension, diabetes, and CKD, hypouricemia continued to show a higher risk for the development of CKD in women (OR: 4.052; 95% CI, 1.181–13.90), but not in men. (Table 4, Chronic kidney disease). The cumulative incidence of hypertension, dyslipidemia, and CKD in men was not significantly different between hypouricemic and normouricemic groups.

Table 2. Lower serum urate as a protective factor for the development of hypertension, diabetes, dyslipidemia and chronic kidney disease over 5 years.

	Crude			Adjusted		
Maintaining without Hypertension	OR	95% CI	p	Adjusted * OR	95% CI	p
Women						
Serum uric acid　per 1 mg/dL decreased	1.755	1.587–1.941	<0.001	1.306	1.169–1.459	<0.001
Men						
Serum uric acid　per 1 mg/dL decreased	1.180	1.099–1.266	<0.001	1.153	1.068–1.245	<0.001
Maintaining without diabetes mellitus	OR	95% CI	p	Adjusted † OR	95% CI	p
Women						
Serum uric acid　per 1 mg/dL decreased	1.822	1.507–2.202	<0.001	1.206	0.969–1.500	0.093
Men						
Serum uric acid　per 1 mg/dL decreased	1.160	1.037–1.298	0.010	1.074	0.953–1.210	0.24
Maintaining without dyslipidemia	OR	95% CI	p	Adjusted ‡ OR	95% CI	p
Women						
Serum uric acid　per 1 mg/dL decreased	1.311	1.202–1.429	<0.001	1.121	1.022–1.230	0.015
Men						
Serum uric acid　per 1 mg/dL decreased	1.205	1.120–1.296	<0.001	1.164	1.077–1.258	<0.001
Maintaining without chronic kidney disease	OR	95% CI	p	Adjusted ¶ OR	95% CI	p
Women						
Serum uric acid　per 1 mg/dL decreased	1.655	1.545–1.795	<0.001	1.424	1.311–1.547	<0.001
Men						
Serum uric acid　per 1 mg/dL decreased	1.144	1.082–1.210	<0.001	1.226	1.152–1.306	<0.001

OR, odds ratio; CI, confidence interval; p, probability. * Data adjusted for age, body mass index, smoking and drinking habits, diabetes mellitus, dyslipidemia, chronic kidney disease, and serum uric acid. † Data adjusted for age, body mass index, smoking and drinking habits, hypertension, dyslipidemia, chronic kidney disease, and serum uric acid. ‡ Data adjusted for age, body mass index, smoking and drinking habits, hypertension, diabetes mellitus, chronic kidney disease, and serum uric acid. ¶ Data adjusted for age, body mass index, smoking and drinking habits, hypertension, diabetes mellitus, dyslipidemia, and serum uric acid.

Table 3. Lower serum urate as a protective factor for the development of hypertension, diabetes, dyslipidemia and chronic kidney.

	Crude			Adjusted		
Maintaining without hypertension	OR	95% CI	P	OR *	95% CI	p
Serum uric acid						
2 mg/dL to 4 mg/dL	Reference			Reference		
2 mg/dL and less	1.922	0.444–8.328	0.38	1.705	0.385–7.564	0.48
4 mg/dL to 6 mg/dL	2.170	1.756–2.682	<0.001	1.543	1.237–1.926	<0.001
more than 6 mg/dL	3.630	2.920–4.512	<0.001	2.031	1.570–2.628	<0.001
Maintaining without diabetes mellitus	OR	95% CI	P	OR †	95% CI	p
Serum uric acid						
2 mg/dL to 4 mg/dL	Reference			Reference		
2 mg/dL and less	–	–	–	–	–	–
4 mg/dL to 6 mg/dL	2.404	1.530–3.779	<0.001	1.405	0.881–2.238	0.153
more than 6 mg/dL	4.634	2.957–7.262	<0.001	1.571	0.947–2.606	0.080
Maintaining without dyslipidemia	OR	95% CI	P	OR ‡	95% CI	p
Serum uric acid						
2 mg/dL to 4 mg/dL	Reference			Reference		
2 mg/dL and less	0.384	0.051–2.896	0.35	0.346	0.046–2.622	0.30
4 mg/dL to 6 mg/dL	1.437	1.233–1.674	<0.001	1.259	1.073–1.478	0.005
more than 6 mg/dL	2.116	1.784–2.508	<0.001	1.568	1.267–1.940	<0.001
Maintaining without chronic kidney disease	OR	95% CI	P	OR ¶	95% CI	p
Serum uric acid						
2 mg/dL to 4 mg/dL	Reference			Reference		
2 mg/dL and less	2.236	0.754–6.634	0.15	2.368	0.752–7.459	0.14
4 mg/dL to 6 mg/dL	1.949	1.665–2.281	<0.001	1.579	1.337–1.864	<0.001
more than 6 mg/dL	2.716	2.307–3.199	<0.001	2.345	1.927–2.854	<0.001

OR, odds ratio; CI, confidence interval; p, probability. * Data adjusted for age, body mass index, smoking and drinking habits, diabetes mellitus, dyslipidemia, chronic kidney disease, and serum uric acid. † Data adjusted for age, body mass index, smoking and drinking habits, hypertension, dyslipidemia, chronic kidney disease, and serum uric acid. ‡ Data adjusted for age, body mass index, smoking and drinking habits, hypertension, diabetes mellitus, chronic kidney disease, and serum uric acid. ¶ Data adjusted for age, body mass index, smoking and drinking habits, hypertension, diabetes mellitus, dyslipidemia, and serum uric acid.

Table 4. Hypouricemia (serum urate less than 3 mg/dL in men and less than 2 mg/dL in women) as a risk factor for the development of hypertension, diabetes, dyslipidemia and chronic kidney disease over 5 years compared with normouricemia (serum urate of 3–5 mg/dL in men and 2–4 mg/dL in women).

	Crude			Adjusted		
	OR	95% CI	p	OR	95% CI	p
Hypertension				(Adjusted *)		
Women						
Reference	Normouricemia (n = 2020)					
Hypouricemia (n = 14)	3.659	0.807–16.599	0.093	4.532	0.943–21.78	0.059
Men						
Reference	Normouricemia (n = 728)					
Hypouricemia (n = 22)	1.355	0.392–4.684	0.545	1.141	0.319–4.075	0.84
Diabetes				(Adjusted)		
Women						
Reference	normouricemia (n = 2165)					
Hypouricemia (n = 14)	–			–		
Men						
Reference	normouricemia (n = 831)					
Hypouricemia (n = 26)	–			–		
Dyslipidemia				(Adjusted †)		
Women						
Reference	normouricemia (n = 1789)					
Hypouricemia (n = 13)	–			–		
Men						
Reference	normouricemia (n = 582)					
Hypouricemia (n = 18)	0.28	0.037–2.129	0.219	0.238	0.031–1.847	0.17
Chronic kidney disease				(Adjusted ‡)		
Women						
Reference	normouricemia (n = 1795)					
Hypouricemia (n = 15)	4.212	1.327–13.37	0.015	4.052	1.181–13.90	0.026
Men						
Reference	normouricemia (n = 932)					
Hypouricemia (n = 29)	0.396	0.093–1.681	0.209	0.303	0.068–1.351	0.117

OR, odds ratio; CI, confidence interval; p, probability; N/A, not available for analysis. * Data adjusted for age, body mass index, smoking and drinking habits, diabetes mellitus, dyslipidemia, chronic kidney disease, and serum uric acid. † Data adjusted for age, body mass index, smoking and drinking habits, hypertension, diabetes mellitus, chronic kidney disease, and serum uric acid. ‡ Data adjusted for age, body mass index, smoking and drinking habits, hypertension, diabetes mellitus, dyslipidemia, and serum uric acid.

4. Discussion

The primary goal of our study was to identify the range of serum urate associated with the lowest risk for developing cardiometabolic diseases in a healthy Japanese population. Except for truly hypouricemic subjects (defined as ≤3 mg/dL in men and ≤2 mg/dL in women), our study indicates that lower serum urate level is an independent protective factor for the development of cardiometabolic disease. We show that in heathy subjects, for each 1 mg/dL decrease of serum urate in men, there was an 18% increment in the protection from developing hypertension, a 16% increment against dyslipidemia, and a 23% increment against CKD. Compared to men, lower serum urate in women conferred greater odds for preventing the appearance of cardiometabolic diseases. Specifically, for each 1 mg/dL decrease of serum urate in women, there was a 31% increment in the protection from developing hypertension, a 12% increment against dyslipidemia, and a 42% increment against CKD.

We also compared the cumulative incidence of cardiometabolic diseases over 5 years between hypouricemic subjects and normouricemic subjects (3–5 mg/dL for men and 2–4 mg/dL for women). The number of hypouricemic subjects was small (30 men and 15 women), and it might be difficult to apply the results to every population because of less power to analyze. However, our results suggest that hypouricemia could be a risk for development of hypertension and CKD in women, but not in men. Accounting for these results, we could see the *J.* curve phenomenon only in women, and the optimal serum urate range associated with the less development of cardiometabolic diseases could be less than 5 mg/dL for men and 2–4 mg/dL for women in a generally healthy population.

Other studies have also showed an inverse correlation between serum urate and the incidence of cardiovascular diseases in subjects with serum urate levels lower than 4.5 mg/dL in men and 3.2 mg/dL in women [6,21,22]. This phenomenon is observed primarily in those subjects with low serum urate levels. Of note, the study subjects in these previous reports often were hypertensive, diabetic or receiving medication against these conditions [6,21,22]. In our study, we can see the similar J-curve phenomenon in hypertension and CKD in women, but the serum urate levels required for this J-shape phenomenon were much lower compared to those reported in previous studies [6,21,22]

Our study also showed that hypouricemic subjects demonstrated greater risk for developing hypertension and CKD than normouricemic subjects in women. We postulate that the higher cumulative incidence of cardiometabolic diseases in hypouricemic women could well relate to the relatively frequent genetic loss of the urate transporter (URAT) in the Japanese population. Potential mechanisms for why this increases the risk for these conditions might relate to the marked uricosuria that may increase the risk for kidney disease, or potentially the possibility that a low serum urate may reduce antioxidant activity in the patients [23,24]. Importantly, there are no studies to determine whether lowering serum urate levels to very low levels with xanthine oxidase inhibitors increases cardiovascular risk compared to untreated controls.

Our study points out the necessity of addressing the risk of hypouricemia in addition to hyperuricemia in the pathogenesis of cardiovascular disease. Our published data demonstrated that hypouricemia is associated with endothelium dysfunction [23]. Consistently, a large-scale cross-sectional study showed that hypouricemic men had higher rates of kidney disease compared to non-hypouricemic subjects. However, the rates of other diseases including diabetes and urinary stones were not significantly different between hypouricemic and non-hypouricemic subjects [20]. In this regard, our longitudinal study showed that hypouricemia did not carry the lowest risk for developing cardiometabolic diseases. Since excess serum urate not only has an adverse effect, but also acts preferably as a reducing substance, this dual nature needs to be considered clinically.

This study showed a positive association between serum urate and cardiometabolic diseases, but most Mendelian randomization studies or meta-analyses suggested that elevated serum urate was only associated with gout [25–29]. However, Mendelian studies are often limited by not considering other influencing conditions, such as life habits including food, alcohol, and fructose intake. Most hyperuricemia is mainly acquired by life habits except for some genetic diseases [30], and it is therefore difficult to apply the results from Mendelian studies to most acquired hyperuricemic subjects. The gap of results between clinical studies and genetic studies suggest that acquired hyperuricemia may cause more cardiometabolic diseases than genetic hyperuricemia.

Our study has several limitations. First, this study is a retrospective single center study, which may have introduced selection bias. However, single center studies had some advantages of the similarity of the methodology. Second, we could not check the additional and withdrawal medication or gouty attacks over the periods. Some hyperuricemic subjects with gouty attacks might have medication especially non-steroidal anti-inflammatory drugs (NSAIDs), which might cause CKD or hypertension. However, our definition of each disease included medication use. Moreover, we did not exclude the subjects on medication for hyperuricemia or gout intentionally, because the serum urate levels on medication could be useful to evaluate the effects of serum urate on cardiometabolic diseases. However, there is a possibility of the influence of urate-lowering medications on the development (or prevention) of other cardiometabolic diseases, which thus may bias the present results. We additionally conducted the sensitivity analyses that excluded 373 (2.9%) subjects with urate-lowering medications (Supplementary Table S1). The results showed the same results, thus supporting our main results more robustly. However, this study was not able to show whether urate-lowering medications could prevent cardiometabolic diseases or not because this study was an observational study. We had to adjust the patient backgrounds between the medication group and the control group to show the efficacy of urate-lowering medications for hyperuricemia to prevent cardiometabolic diseases. Third, this longitudinal study lacks time-to-event data, which precluded survival analysis. Fourth, we measured serum urate only once, and blood pressure only at the center. Serum urate can fluctuate for natural or iatrogenic causes. Moreover, some hypertensive subjects might have white-coat hypertension and some non-hypertensive subjects might have masked hypertension. Measuring serum urate many times and ambulatory blood pressure monitoring are the best to evaluate serum urate and blood pressure precisely, but it is difficult in practice in the setting of an annual medical examination. Fifth, the number of hypouricemic subjects was small, and it might be less power to analyze the significant difference. Therefore, it is difficult to discuss the J-curve phenomenon precisely. Finally, causality cannot be inferred, because this is an observational study. Interventional studies are needed to further clarify whether the treatments for hyperuricemia are useful for preventing the development of cardiometabolic diseases.

5. Conclusions

Even in the normal range, having higher serum urate could be a risk for hypertension, dyslipidemia, and CKD. The optimal serum urate range, which conferred the lowest risk for developing cardiometabolic diseases, could be less than 5 mg/dL for men and 2–4 mg/dL for women in a generally healthy population. These findings suggest that routine screening of serum urate is useful as a predictor for cardiometabolic diseases in primary care settings.

Author Contributions: Conceptualization, M.K., I.H., R.J.J., and M.A.L.; Data Curation, M.K. and K.N.; Formal Analysis, M.K.; Investigation, M.K. and K.N.; Methodology, M.K., I.H., R.J.J. and M.A.L.; Software, M.K.; Validation, M.K. and K.N.; Visualization, M.K.; Writing—Original Draft M.K. and P.B.; Preparation, M.K.; Writing—Review and Editing, M.K., I.H., K.N., P.B., C.A.R.-J., A.A.-H., M.K., R.J.J., and M.A.L.; Supervision, M.K., I.H., K.N., P.B., C.A.R.-J, A.A.-H., M.K., R.J.J., and M.A.L. All authors have read and agreed to the published version of the manuscript.

Acknowledgments: All the authors of this paper fulfill the criteria of authorship. The authors thank the study subjects and all staff in Center for Preventive Medicine, St. Luke's International Hospital, for assistance with data collection.

References

1. Freedman, D.S.; Williamson, D.F.; Gunter, E.W.; Byers, T. Relation of serum uric acid to mortality and ischemic heart disease. The NHANES I Epidemiologic Follow-up Study. *Am. J. Epidemiol.* **1995**, *141*, 637–644. [CrossRef] [PubMed]

2. Ioachimescu, A.G.; Brennan, D.M.; Hoar, B.M.; Hazen, S.L.; Hoogwerf, B.J. Serum uric acid is an independent predictor of all-cause mortality in patients at high risk of cardiovascular disease: A preventive cardiology information system (PreCIS) database cohort study. *Arthritis Rheumatol.* **2008**, *58*, 623–630. [CrossRef] [PubMed]

3. Culleton, B.F.; Larson, M.G.; Kannel, W.B.; Levy, D. Serum uric acid and risk for cardiovascular disease and death: The Framingham Heart Study. *Ann. Intern. Med.* **1999**, *131*, 7–13. [CrossRef] [PubMed]

4. Moriarity, J.T.; Folsom, A.R.; Iribarren, C.; Nieto, F.J.; Rosamond, W.D. Serum uric acid and risk of coronary heart disease: Atherosclerosis Risk in Communities (ARIC) Study. *Ann. Epidemiol.* **2000**, *10*, 136–143. [CrossRef]

5. Sakata, K.; Hashimoto, T.; Ueshima, H.; Okayama, A.; Group, N.D.R. Absence of an association between serum uric acid and mortality from cardiovascular disease: NIPPON DATA 80, 1980-1994. National Integrated Projects for Prospective Observation of Non-communicable Diseases and its Trend in the Aged. *Eur. J. Epidemiol.* **2001**, *17*, 461–468. [CrossRef] [PubMed]

6. De Leeuw, P.W.; Thijs, L.; Birkenhager, W.H.; Voyaki, S.M.; Efstratopoulos, A.D.; Fagard, R.H.; Leonetti, G.; Nachev, C.; Petrie, J.C.; Rodicio, J.L.; et al. Prognostic significance of renal function in elderly patients with isolated systolic hypertension: Results from the Syst-Eur trial. *J. Am. Soc. Nephrol.* **2002**, *13*, 2213–2222. [CrossRef]

7. Kuwabara, M.; Hisatome, I.; Niwa, K.; Hara, S.; Roncal-Jimenez, C.A.; Bjornstad, P.; Nakagawa, T.; Andres-Hernando, A.; Sato, Y.; Jensen, T.; et al. Uric Acid Is a Strong Risk Marker for Developing Hypertension From Prehypertension: A 5-Year Japanese Cohort Study. *Hypertension* **2018**, *71*, 78–86. [CrossRef]

8. Kuwabara, M.; Niwa, K.; Hisatome, I.; Nakagawa, T.; Roncal-Jimenez, C.A.; Andres-Hernando, A.; Bjornstad, P.; Jensen, T.; Sato, Y.; Milagres, T.; et al. Asymptomatic Hyperuricemia Without Comorbidities Predicts Cardiometabolic Diseases: Five-Year Japanese Cohort Study. *Hypertension* **2017**, *69*, 1036–1044. [CrossRef]

9. Kuwabara, M.; Kuwabara, R.; Hisatome, I.; Niwa, K.; Roncal-Jimenez, C.A.; Bjornstad, P.; Andres-Hernando, A.; Sato, Y.; Jensen, T.; Garcia, G.; et al. "Metabolically Healthy" Obesity and Hyperuricemia Increase Risk for Hypertension and Diabetes: 5-year Japanese Cohort Study. *Obesity (Silver Spring)* **2017**, *25*, 1997–2008. [CrossRef]

10. Kuwabara, M.; Hisatome, I.; Roncal-Jimenez, C.A.; Niwa, K.; Andres-Hernando, A.; Jensen, T.; Bjornstad, P.; Milagres, T.; Cicerchi, C.; Song, Z.; et al. Increased Serum Sodium and Serum Osmolarity Are Independent Risk Factors for Developing Chronic Kidney Disease; 5 Year Cohort Study. *PLoS ONE* **2017**, *12*, e0169137. [CrossRef]

11. Kuwabara, M.; Bjornstad, P.; Hisatome, I.; Niwa, K.; Roncal-Jimenez, C.A.; Andres-Hernando, A.; Jensen, T.; Milagres, T.; Sato, Y.; Garcia, G.; et al. Elevated Serum Uric Acid Level Predicts Rapid Decline in Kidney Function. *Am. J. Nephrol.* **2017**, *45*, 330–337. [CrossRef] [PubMed]

12. Kuwabara, M.; Niwa, K.; Nishihara, S.; Nishi, Y.; Takahashi, O.; Kario, K.; Yamamoto, K.; Yamashita, T.; Hisatome, I. Hyperuricemia is an independent competing risk factor for atrial fibrillation. *Int. J. Cardiol.* **2017**, *231*, 137–142. [CrossRef] [PubMed]

13. Kuwabara, M.; Niwa, K.; Nishi, Y.; Mizuno, A.; Asano, T.; Masuda, K.; Komatsu, I.; Yamazoe, M.; Takahashi, O.; Hisatome, I. Relationship between serum uric acid levels and hypertension among Japanese individuals not treated for hyperuricemia and hypertension. *Hypertens. Res.* **2014**, *37*, 785–789. [CrossRef] [PubMed]

14. Kuwabara, M.; Motoki, Y.; Sato, H.; Fujii, M.; Ichiura, K.; Kuwabara, K.; Nakamura, Y. Low frequency of toothbrushing practices is an independent risk factor for diabetes mellitus in male and dyslipidemia in female: A large-scale, 5-year cohort study in Japan. *J. Cardiol.* **2017**, *70*, 107–112. [CrossRef] [PubMed]

15. Kuwabara, M.; Motoki, Y.; Ichiura, K.; Fujii, M.; Inomata, C.; Sato, H.; Morisawa, T.; Morita, Y.; Kuwabara, K.; Nakamura, Y. Association between toothbrushing and risk factors for cardiovascular disease: A large-scale, cross-sectional Japanese study. *BMJ Open* **2016**, *6*, e009870. [CrossRef] [PubMed]

16. Shimamoto, K.; Ando, K.; Fujita, T.; Hasebe, N.; Higaki, J.; Horiuchi, M.; Imai, Y.; Imaizumi, T.; Ishimitsu, T.; Ito, M.; et al. The Japanese Society of Hypertension Guidelines for the Management of Hypertension (JSH 2014). *Hypertens. Res.* **2014**, *37*, 253–390. [CrossRef]

17. Black, H.R.; Sica, D.; Ferdinand, K.; White, W.B. Eligibility and Disqualification Recommendations for Competitive Athletes With Cardiovascular Abnormalities: Task Force 6: Hypertension: A Scientific Statement from the American Heart Association and the American College of Cardiology. *J. Am. Coll. cardiol.* **2015**, *66*, 2393–2397. [CrossRef]

18. Teramoto, T.; Sasaki, J.; Ishibashi, S.; Birou, S.; Daida, H.; Dohi, S.; Egusa, G.; Hiro, T.; Hirobe, K.; Iida, M.; et al. Executive summary of the Japan Atherosclerosis Society (JAS) guidelines for the diagnosis and prevention of atherosclerotic cardiovascular diseases in Japan-2012 version. *J. Atheroscler. Thromb.* **2013**, *20*, 517–523. [CrossRef]

19. Matsuo, S.; Imai, E.; Horio, M.; Yasuda, Y.; Tomita, K.; Nitta, K.; Yamagata, K.; Tomino, Y.; Yokoyama, H.; Hishida, A.; et al. Revised equations for estimated GFR from serum creatinine in Japan. *Am. J. Kidney Dis.* **2009**, *53*, 982–992. [CrossRef]

20. Kuwabara, M.; Niwa, K.; Ohtahara, A.; Hamada, T.; Miyazaki, S.; Mizuta, E.; Ogino, K.; Hisatome, I. Prevalence and complications of hypouricemia in a general population: A large-scale cross-sectional study in Japan. *PLoS ONE* **2017**, *12*, e0176055. [CrossRef]

21. Verdecchia, P.; Schillaci, G.; Reboldi, G.; Santeusanio, F.; Porcellati, C.; Brunetti, P. Relation between serum uric acid and risk of cardiovascular disease in essential hypertension. The PIUMA study. *Hypertension* **2000**, *36*, 1072–1078. [CrossRef] [PubMed]

22. Mazza, A.; Zamboni, S.; Rizzato, E.; Pessina, A.C.; Tikhonoff, V.; Schiavon, L.; Casiglia, E. Serum uric acid shows a J-shaped trend with coronary mortality in non-insulin-dependent diabetic elderly people. The CArdiovascular STudy in the ELderly (CASTEL). *Acta Diabetol.* **2007**, *44*, 99–105. [CrossRef] [PubMed]

23. Sugihara, S.; Hisatome, I.; Kuwabara, M.; Niwa, K.; Maharani, N.; Kato, M.; Ogino, K.; Hamada, T.; Ninomiya, H.; Higashi, Y.; et al. Depletion of Uric Acid Due to SLC22A12 (URAT1) Loss-of-Function Mutation Causes Endothelial Dysfunction in Hypouricemia. *Circ. J.* **2015**, *79*, 1125–1132. [CrossRef] [PubMed]

24. Waring, W.S.; McKnight, J.A.; Webb, D.J.; Maxwell, S.R. Uric acid restores endothelial function in patients with type 1 diabetes and regular smokers. *Diabetes* **2006**, *55*, 3127–3132. [CrossRef]

25. Li, X.; Meng, X.; Timofeeva, M.; Tzoulaki, I.; Tsilidis, K.K.; Ioannidis, J.P.; Campbell, H.; Theodoratou, E. Serum uric acid levels and multiple health outcomes: Umbrella review of evidence from observational studies, randomised controlled trials, and Mendelian randomisation studies. *BMJ* **2017**, *357*, j2376. [CrossRef] [PubMed]

26. Jordan, D.M.; Choi, H.K.; Verbanck, M.; Topless, R.; Won, H.H.; Nadkarni, G.; Merriman, T.R.; Do, R. No causal effects of serum urate levels on the risk of chronic kidney disease: A Mendelian randomization study. *PLoS Med.* **2019**, *16*, e1002725. [CrossRef]

27. Rasheed, H.; Hughes, K.; Flynn, T.J.; Merriman, T.R. Mendelian randomization provides no evidence for a causal role of serum urate in increasing serum triglyceride levels. *Circ. Cardiovasc. Genet.* **2014**, *7*, 830–837. [CrossRef]

28. Kottgen, A.; Albrecht, E.; Teumer, A.; Vitart, V.; Krumsiek, J.; Hundertmark, C.; Pistis, G.; Ruggiero, D.; O'Seaghdha, C.M.; Haller, T.; et al. Genome-wide association analyses identify 18 new loci associated with serum urate concentrations. *Nat. Genet.* **2013**, *45*, 145–154. [CrossRef]

29. Yang, Q.; Kottgen, A.; Dehghan, A.; Smith, A.V.; Glazer, N.L.; Chen, M.H.; Chasman, D.I.; Aspelund, T.; Eiriksdottir, G.; Harris, T.B.; et al. Multiple genetic loci influence serum urate levels and their relationship with gout and cardiovascular disease risk factors. *Circ. Cardiovasc. Genet.* **2010**, *3*, 523–530. [CrossRef]

30. Johnson, R.J.; Segal, M.S.; Sautin, Y.; Nakagawa, T.; Feig, D.I.; Kang, D.H.; Gersch, M.S.; Benner, S.; Sanchez-Lozada, L.G. Potential role of sugar (fructose) in the epidemic of hypertension, obesity and the metabolic syndrome, diabetes, kidney disease, and cardiovascular disease. *Am. J. Clin. Nutr.* **2007**, *86*, 899–906. [CrossRef]

Re-Evaluating the Protective Effect of Hemodialysis Catheter Locking Solutions in Hemodialysis Patients

Chang-Hua Chen [1,2,3,4,*], Yu-Min Chen [5], Yu Yang [6], Yu-Jun Chang [7], Li-Jhen Lin [2] and Hua-Cheng Yen [8]

1   Division of Infectious Disease, Department of Internal Medicine, Changhua Christian Hospital, Changhua 500, Taiwan
2   Center for Infection Prevention and Control, Changhua Christian Hospital, Changhua 500, Taiwan; 3344@cch.org.tw
3   Program in Translational Medicine, National Chung Hsing University, Taichung County 402, Taiwan
4   Rong Hsing Research Center for Translational Medicine, National Chung Hsing University, Taichung County 402, Taiwan
5   Department of Pharmacy, Changhua Christian Hospital, Changhua 500, Taiwan; 30855@cch.org.tw
6   Division of Nephrology, Department of Internal Medicine, Changhua Christian Hospital, Changhua 500, Taiwan; 2219@cch.org.tw
7   Epidemiology and Biostatistics Center, Changhua Christian Hospital, Changhua 500, Taiwan; 83686@cch.org.tw
8   Department of Neurosurgery, Changhua Christian Hospital, Changhua 500, Taiwan; 90211@cch.org.tw
*   Correspondence: chenchanghuachad@gmail.com

Abstract: Catheter-related bloodstream infections (CRBSIs) and exit-site infections (ESIs) are common complications associated with the use of central venous catheters for hemodialysis. The aim of this study was to analyze the impact of routine locking solutions on the incidence of CRBSI and ESI, in preserving catheter function, and on the rate of all-cause mortality in patients undergoing hemodialysis. We selected publications (from inception until July 2018) with studies comparing locking solutions for hemodialysis catheters used in patients undergoing hemodialysis. A total of 21 eligible studies were included, with a total of 4832 patients and 318,769 days of catheter use. The incidence of CRBSI and ESI was significantly lower in the treated group (citrate-based regimen) than in the controls (heparin-based regimen). No significant difference in preserving catheter function and all-cause mortality was found between the two groups. Our findings demonstrated that routine locking solutions for hemodialysis catheters effectively reduce the incidence of CRBSIs and ESIs, but our findings failed to show a benefit for preserving catheter function and mortality rates. Therefore, further studies are urgently needed to conclusively evaluate the impact of routine locking solutions on preserving catheter function and improving the rates of all-cause mortality.

Keywords: effect; protection; catheter; hemodialysis; meta-analysis; trial sequential analysis

1. Introduction

1.1. Variety of New Strategies for Locking Solutions to Avoid Catheter Infection and Catheter Malfunction in Hemodialysis Patients

Infections are widely prevalent in patients on chronic hemodialysis, and mortality from infection account for 10% of deaths observed in patients undergoing hemodialysis [1]. The use of central venous catheters in hemodialysis has been associated with catheter-related bloodstream infections (CRBSIs) and exit-site infections (ESIs) [2–4]. Although recent efforts have minimized the use of catheters, the proportion patients with end-stage renal disease undergoing dialysis using central venous catheters has not yet declined [5]. Protective strategies against CRBSI and catheter malfunction are necessary [6], and to this end, the use of heparin as a routine locking solution for central venous catheters has become an accepted clinical practice [4]. However, heparinized locking solutions might cause unintended complications, such as systemic anticoagulation effects, bleeding episodes, heparin-induced thrombocytopenia, and susceptibility to bacterial biofilm formation [7–9]. A variety of new locking solutions have been developed; this includes citrate, which has antimicrobial properties [10–12]. However, the disadvantages of citrate compared with heparin have been raised and included the ability of avoiding catheter malfunction, citrate toxicity, and induction of cardiac arrhythmia [13]. Weijmer et al. showed that a 30% citrate solution was superior to heparin in preventing CRBSI [14]. In contrast, other studies have reported that the use of citrate does not have an advantage over heparin in preventing CRBSI [4,12]. Currently, the findings of the studies comparing citrate with heparin locking solutions are inconclusive for protecting against CRBSI and ESI and preserving the catheter function. Clinicians question if locking solutions should be considered a modifiable risk factor for CRBSIs in patients undergoing hemodialysis. Furthermore, the recommended locking solution for the routine care of patients undergoing hemodialysis continue to remain questionable.

1.2. Rationale for Re-Evaluating the Protective Effect of Hemodialysis Catheter Locking Solutions in Hemodialysis Patients

Routine locking solutions for hemodialysis catheters are recommended with category II evidence according to the guideline by the Healthcare Infection Control Practices Advisory Committee in 2011 [15]; however, there are some limitations of the studies providing the current and update evidence. Mostly, conclusions of meta-analysis could be influenced by the heterogeneity between individual studies and insufficient information size. Quantification of the required information size [16] is important to ensure the reliability of the data. In addition, current meta-analyses lack information size calculation [17–24]. Additionally, the incidence of CRBSI is difficult to evaluate because of their subjectivity for case finding, lack of specificity, and high inter-observer variability. CRBSI is associated with high morbidity and mortality in patients undergoing hemodialysis [1], and the prevention of CRBSI and ESI is becoming increasingly essential. Given these limitations, we performed a meta-analysis and trial sequential analysis to assess the impact of routine locking solutions on the incidence of CRBSI and ESI, in preserving catheter function, and on the rate of all-cause mortality in patients undergoing hemodialysis. We grouped the eligible publications according to combination regimen, antimicrobial activity, and concentration of the locking solutions; thereafter, we grouped according to the study design to assess its potential effect on the reported outcomes.

2. Experimental Section

2.1. Search Strategy and Inclusion Criteria

The study was conducted in accordance with the Declaration of Helsinki, and the protocol was approved by the institutional review board of Changhua Christian Hospital (CCH IRB No. 180801). From the earliest record to July 2018, we searched PubMed, Scopus, Cochrane Central Register of Controlled Trials, Cochrane Database of Systematic Reviews, ClinicalTrials.gov, Embase, and Web of Science databases for studies on locking solutions for central venous catheters used in hemodialysis of patients. Full search strategies for each database are available in the Appendix A. The reference lists of the eligible publications were manually reviewed for relevant studies. Articles published in languages other than English or those with no available full text were excluded.

We included all trials and studies that provided data on one or more of our target outcomes for both the treated group and control group: CRBSIs and ESIs. Two investigators (CHC and YMC) independently reviewed potential trials and studies for inclusion. Disagreements were resolved by consensus. We also tried to contact the corresponding authors of selected papers to provide clarifications and missing data where needed.

2.2. Definition of Study Outcomes

Based on the original studies, the treated group comprised of patients undergoing hemodialysis using citrate as the locking solution for central venous catheters; for the control group heparin was used as the locking solution (Table 1). The outcomes of the original studies were included in this meta-analysis. The primary outcomes included (1) CRBSI, defined as bacteremia caused by an intravenous catheter, and (2) ESI, defined as the development of a purulent redness around the exit site that did not result from residual stitches. The secondary outcomes included (1), the need to remove the catheter due to catheter malfunction; and (2) the need for thrombolytic treatments due to catheter malfunction; and (3) all-cause mortality at any timeframe. Incidence was presented as the number of episodes per catheter or per patient depending on the available data.

2.3. Data Extraction and Quality Assessment

Two reviewers examined all retrieved articles and extracted data using a pre-determined form, recording the name of the first author, year of publication, country where the study was conducted, study design (RCT or observational studies), demographic and disease characteristics of participants, number of participants enrolled, and quality assessment of each study. Each reviewer independently evaluated the quality of the eligible studies, using Jadad scoring [25] for the RCTs and the Newcastle-Ottawa quality assessment scale [26] for the comparative experimental studies.

2.4. Data Synthesis and Analysis

The outcomes were measured by determining the odds ratios (ORs). A random effects model was used to pool individual ORs. Analyses were performed with the Comprehensive Meta-Analysis software version 3.0 (Biostat, Englewood, NJ, USA). Between-trial heterogeneity was determined using I^2 tests; values > 50% were regarded as considerable heterogeneity [27]. Funnel plots and Egger's test were used to examine potential publication bias [27]. Statistical significance was defined as $p < 0.05$, except for the determination of publication bias where $p < 0.10$ was considered significant. This study was conducted and reported in accordance with the Preferred Reporting Items for Systematic Reviews and Meta-Analyses (PRISMA) statement (Table S1) [28].

In trial sequential analyses, the inconsistency of heterogeneity (I^2) adjusted by determining the required information size. The required information size was calculated with an intervention effect of a 10% relative risk reduction, an overall 5% risk of a type I error, and a 20% risk of a type II error. All trial sequential analyses were performed using TSA version 0.9 Beta (www.ctu.dk/tsa/, Copenhagen Trial Unit, Copenhagen, Denmark).

Table 1. Summary of the retrieved trials investigating experimental group and control group.

Author, Year, Country, Reference	RCT	Total N	Treated (N)	Control (N)	QA
Buturovic et al., 1998, SI, [29]	No	30	4% CiT (20)	1666 U/mL HpR (10)	3 #
Dogra et al., 2002, AU, [30]	Yes	79	26.7 mg/mL GM + 1.04% CiT (42)	5000 U/mL HpR (37)	8 *
Betjes et al., 2004, NL, [31]	No	58	1.35% TRD +4% CiT (37)	5000 U/mL HpR (39)	3 #
Weijmer et al., 2005, NL, [14]	Yes	291	30% CiT (148)	5000 U/mL HpR (143)	8 *
Nori et al., 2006, USA, [32]	No	40	4 mg/mL GM + 3.13% CiT (41)	5000 U/mL HpR (21)	3 #
Lok et al., 2007, CA, [13]	No	250	4% CiT (129)	5000 U/mL HpR (121)	3 #
MacRae et al., 2008, CA, [12]	No	61	4% CiT (32)	5000 U/mL HpR (29)	3 #
Power et al., 2009, UK, [4]	Yes	232	46.7% CiT (132)	5000 U/mL HpR (100)	8 *
Solomon et al., 2010, UK, [33]	Yes	107	1.35% TRD + 4% CiT (53)	5000 U/mL HpR (54)	8 *
Filiopoulos et al., 2011, GR, [34]	Yes	117	1.35% TRD + 4% CiT (119)	5000 U/mL HpR (58)	8 *
Maki et al., 2011, USA, [6]	Yes	407	7.0% CiT + MMP (206)	5000 U/mL HpR (201)	8 *
Moran et al., 2012, USA, [8]	No	303	320 μg/mL GM + 4% CiT (155)	1000 U/mL HpR (148)	3 #
Chen et al., 2014, CH, [35]	Yes	72	10% NaCl (36)	3125 U/mL HpR (36)	8 *

Table 1. *Cont.*

Author, Year, Country, Reference	RCT	Total *N*	Treated (*N*)	Control (*N*)	QA
Souweine et al., 2015, FR, [19]	Yes	1460	60% *w/w* EtOH (730)	0.9% NaCl (730)	8 *
Moghaddas et al., 2015, IR, [18]	Yes	87	10 mg/mL TMP/SMX + 2500 U/mL HpR (46)	2500 U/mL HpR (41)	8 *
Kanaa et al., 2015, UK, [17]	Yes	115	4% EDTA (59)	5000 U/mL HpR (56)	8 *
Zwiech et al., 2016, PL, [21]	Yes	50	4% CiT (26)	5000 U/mL HpR (24)	8 *
Chu et al., 2016, AU, [20]	Yes	100	1000 U/mL HpR (52)	5000 U/mL HpR (48)	8 *
Correa Barcellos et al., 2017, BZ, [22]	Yes	464	30% CiT (231)	5000 U/mL HpR (233)	8 *
Sofroniadou et al., 2017, GR, [23]	Yes	103	70% *w/w* EtOH + UFH 2000 U/mL (52)	2000 U/mL HpR (51)	8 *
Winnicki et al., 2018, Au, [24]	No	406	1.35% TRD + 4% CiT + HpR (52)	4% CiT (54)	3 #

Abbreviations: AU, Australia; Au, Austria; BZ, Brazil; CA, Canada; CH, China; CiT, citrate; EDTA, tetra-sodium ethylenediaminetetraacetic acid; EtOH, ethanol; FR, France; GM, gentamicin; GR, Greece; HpR, heparin; IR, Iran; MMP, 0.15% methylene blue + 0.15% methylparaben + 0.015% propylparaben; NaCl, sodium chloride; N, number; NL, Netherlands; PL, Poland; QA, quality assessment; RCT, randomized controlled trial; SI, Slovenia; TMP/SMX, cotrimoxazole (=trimethoprim/sulfamethoxazole); TRD, taurolidine; UFH, unfractionated heparin; UK, United Kingdom; US, United States. #, the study was evaluated using Jadad scale. *, the study was assessed using the Newcastle-Ottawa scale.

3. Results

3.1. Eligible Studies

The literature search yielded 458 potentially eligible articles. By screening the abstracts, we removed 350 irrelevant articles. The remaining 100 articles were assessed further by full-text reading, of which 79 were excluded (Figure 1). Thus, 21 selected articles comparing citrate with heparin lockings for central venous catheters used in hemodialysis were included in this meta-analysis [4,6,8,12–14,17–24,29–35].

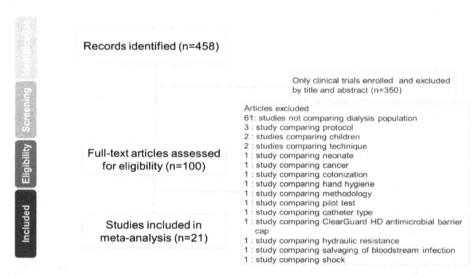

Figure 1. Preferred reporting items for systematic reviews and meta-analyses (PRISMA) flow diagram for the search and identification of the included studies.

The studies published in the selected articles were conducted from the earliest record to July 2018, with a total of 4832 patients and 318,769 total days of catheter use. Six studies compared citrate alone with heparin lockings; 14 studies tested regimens of citrate and other antimicrobials (gentamicin, taurolidine, methylparaben, methylene blue, and propylparaben) with heparin lockings; and two studies compared ethanol or combination solution (citrate, heparin and taurolidine) with non-heparin locking. Studies were conducted in North America (5 studies), South America (1), Europe (12), and Asia (3). A variety of end points were used in these studies. Most studies reported on CRBSI (17 studies [4,6,8,12–14,17,19,21–24,30–34]), followed by ESI (11 studies [4,8,12,14,17–19,24,30,31,33]), catheter removal for poor flow (9 studies [6,8,12,14,18,24,29,31,33]), thrombolytic treatment (8 studies [4,8,14,17,18,32,33]), and mortality (5 studies [6,14,19,32,33]). The characteristics of the studies fulfilling the inclusion criteria are listed in Table 1. Thirteen studies were identified as RCT, and 6 studies were not double-blinded (Table 1).

3.2. Pooled Odds for Primary Outcomes and Subgroup Analysis

3.2.1. Catheter-Related Bloodstream Infection (CRBSI)

Seventeen studies (1731 patients; 217,128 catheter days) reported on CRBSI. The incidence of CRBSI was significantly lower in the treated group compared with the control group (OR, 0.424; 95% CI, 0.267–0.673; $p < 0.001$) (Figure 2). CRBSI subgroup analysis showed that the OR appeared to have a tendency to favor the treatment groups with either the combined regimen (OR, 0.206; 95% CI, 0.058–0.730; $p = 0.027$), the single regimen (OR, 0.289; 95% CI, 0.083–0.365; $p = 0.037$), a regimen containing antibiotics (OR, 0.136; 95% CI, 0.051–0.365; $p = 0.002$), or a low concentration of a major regimen (OR, 0.421; 95% CI, 0.186–0.956; $p = 0.039$; Table 2).

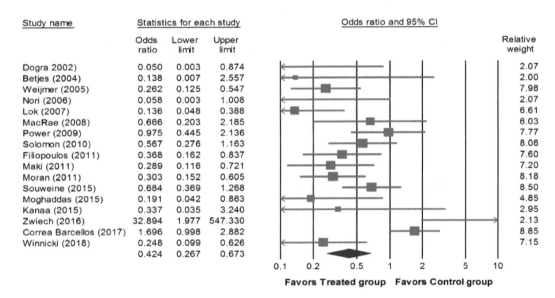

Figure 2. Forest plot of the overall odds ratios for catheter-related bloodstream infection in the treated group versus the control group. The random model of overall odds ratio showed a significant overall effect of interventions in reducing the risk for developing catheter-related bloodstream infections as compared with the control condition (OR, 0.424; 95% CI, 0.267–0.673; $p < 0.001$).

3.2.2. Exit-Site Infection (ESI)

A total of 11 RCTs (2,425 patients; 231,086 catheter days) described ESI. The incidence of ESI was significantly lower in the treated group compared with the control group (OR, 0.627; 95% CI, 0.441–0.893; $p = 0.001$; Figure 3). Further focusing at exit-site infection (Table 3), the subgroup analysis (combined regimen, regimen containing antibiotic, and concentration of regimen for exit-site infection) disclosed no significant differences between any groups except for combined regimen.

Table 2. Subgroup analysis of odds ratio based on study designs, combined regimen, regimen containing antibiotic, and concentration of regimen for CRBSI.

Subgroup	Odds Ratio	95% Confidence Interval
combined regimen		
RCT	0.606	0.298–1.230
Not RCT	0.206	0.058–0.730
Not combined regimen		
RCT	0.417	0.192–0.905
Not RCT	0.289	0.083–0.365
Regimen containing antibiotic		
RCT	0.191	0.023–1.564
Not RCT	0.136	0.051–0.365
Regimen Not containing antibiotic		
RCT	0.546	0.314–0.949
Not RCT	0.342	0.191–0.614
High Concentration of major regimen		
RCT	0.644	0.155–2.671
Low Concentration of major regimen		
RCT	0.421	0.186–0.956
Not RCT	0.260	0.135–0.497

Abbreviation: RCT, randomized controlled trial.

Table 3. Subgroup analysis of odds ratio based on study designs, combined regimen, regimen containing antibiotic, and concentration of regimen for exit site infection.

Subgroup	Odds Ratio	95% Confidence Interval
combined regimen		
RCT	0.849	0.358–2.011
Not RCT	0.706	0.307–1.62
Not combined regimen		
RCT	0.503	0.276–0.918
Not RCT	0.620	0.113–3.389
Regimen containing antibiotic		
RCT	0.571	0.189–1.725
Not RCT	0.735	0.284–1.905
Regimen Not containing antibiotic		
RCT	0.599	0.334–1.071
Not RCT	0.650	0.246–1.722
High Concentration of major regimen		
RCT	0.631	0.214–1.862
Low Concentration of major regimen		
RCT	0.805	0.282–2.297
Not RCT	0.692	0.35–1.368

Abbreviation: RCT, randomized controlled trial.

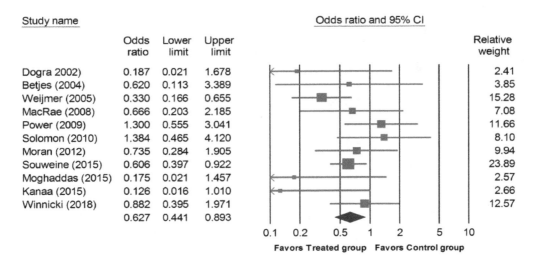

Figure 3. Forest plot of the overall odds ratios for exit-site infection in treated group versus the control group. The random model of overall odds ratio for exit-site infection showed a significant overall effect of interventions in reducing the risk for developing exit-site infection as compared with the control condition (OR, 0.627; 95% CI, 0.441–0.893; p = 0.001).

3.3. Pooled Odds for Secondary Outcomes and Subgroup Analysis

3.3.1. Catheter Withdrawal Due to Malfunction

Nine studies (1826 patients; 205,163 catheter days) reported catheters being removed for poor blood flow. As shown in Figure 4, no difference was identified between the two groups (OR, 0.696; 95% CI, 0.397–1.223; p = 0.208). Further subgroup analysis (combined regimen, regimen containing antibiotic, and concentration of regimen for catheter removal due to catheter malfunction) failed to reveal any differences between any groups (Table 4).

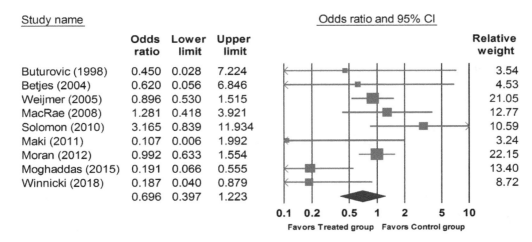

Figure 4. Forest plot of the overall odds ratios for catheter removal due to catheter malfunction in the treated group vs. the control group. The random model of overall odds ratio for the need to remove the catheter for malfunction showed a significant overall effect of the interventions in reducing the risk for catheter removal compared with the control condition (OR, 0.696; 95% CI, 0.397–1.223; p = 0.208).

Table 4. Subgroup analysis of odds ratio based on study designs, combined regimen, regimen containing antibiotic, and concentration of regimen for catheter removal due to catheter malfunction.

Subgroup	Odds Ratio	95% Confidence Interval
Combined regimen		
RCT	0.520	0.086–3.15
Not RCT	0.977	0.628–1.518
Not combined regimen		
RCT	0.434	0.068–2.786
Not RCT	1.106	0.392–3.124
Regimen containing antibiotic		
RCT	0.741	0.087–6.287
Not RCT	0.992	0.633–1.554
Regimen not containing antibiotic		
RCT	0.329	0.051–2.138
Not RCT	1.010	0.39–2.619
High concentration of major regimen		
RCT	0.896	0.029–27.554
Low concentration of major regimen		
RCT	0.479	0.051–4.537
Not RCT	0.995	0.663–1.494

Abbreviation: RCT, randomized controlled trial.

3.3.2. Thrombolytic Treatment Due to Catheter Malfunction

Overall, in eight RCTs (2092 patients; 220,460 catheter days) included in this meta-analysis the patients underwent thrombolytic treatment [4,8,14,17,18,32,33]. The incidence of thrombolytic treatment was not significantly lower in the treated group compared with the control group using the random-effects model (OR, 1.105; 95% CI, 0.655–1.573; $p = 0.946$; Figure 5). Thrombolytic treatment subgroup analysis showed no differences in the OR between the two groups (Table 5).

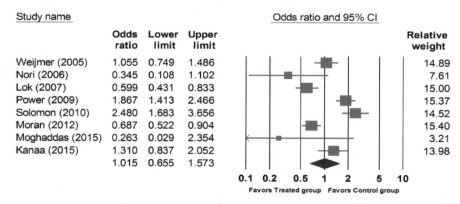

Figure 5. Forest plot of the overall odds ratios for thrombolytic treatments for catheter malfunction in the treated group versus the control group. The random model of overall odds ratio for the need to administer thrombolytic treatment for catheter malfunction showed a significant overall reduced risk for receiving thrombolytic treatments with interventions as compared with the control condition (OR, 1.105; 95% CI, 0.655–1.573; $p = 0.946$).

Table 5. Subgroup analysis of odds ratio based on study designs, combined regimen, regimen containing antibiotic, and concentration of regimen for the need of thrombolytic treatment for catheter malfunction.

Subgroup	Odds Ratio	95% Confidence Interval
Combined regimen		
RCT	2.480	1.214–5.066
Not RCT	0.620	0.382–1.004
Not combined regimen		
RCT	1.320	0.888–1.961
Not RCT	0.599	0.344–1.043
Regimen containing antibiotic		
RCT	1.969	0.944–4.107
Not RCT	0.620	0.382–1.004
Regimen not containing antibiotic		
RCT	1.385	0.893–2.149
Not RCT	0.345	0.108–1.102
High concentration of major regimen		
RCT	1.415	0.784–2.554
Low concentration of major regimen		
RCT	2.480	1.042–5.902
Not RCT	0.637	0.518–0.783

Abbreviation: RCT, randomized controlled trial.

3.3.3. All-Cause Mortality

The meta-analysis included five RCTs (2,327 patients) comparing all-cause mortality rate between the two groups; no significant difference was identified (OR, 0.909; 95% CI, 0.580–1.423; p = 0.676; Figure 6). The corresponding subgroup analysis (combined regimen, regimen containing antibiotic, and concentration of regimen for all-cause mortality) showed no apparent differences between the two groups (Table 6).

All-cause mortality

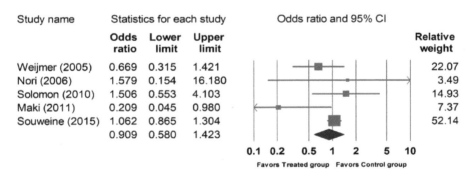

Figure 6. Forest plot of the overall odds ratios for all-cause mortality in the treated group versus the control group. The random model of overall odds ratio for all-cause mortality rate showed a significant overall effect of the interventions in reducing mortality rate as compared with the control condition (OR, 0.909; 95% CI, 0.580–1.423; p = 0.676).

Table 6. Subgroup analysis of odds ratio based on study designs, combined regimen, regimen containing antibiotic, and concentration of regimen for all-cause mortality.

Subgroup	Odds Ratio	95% Confidence Interval
Combined regimen		
RCT	0.725	0.237–2.211
Not RCT	1.579	0.154–16.18
Not combined regimen		
RCT	0.884	0.404–1.933
Regimen containing antibiotic		
RCT	1.506	0.388–5.838
Not RCT	1.579	0.154–16.18
Regimen not containing antibiotic		
RCT	0.723	0.367 – 1.425
High concentration of major regimen		
RCT	0.669	0.054–8.324
Low Concentration of major regimen		
RCT	0.615	0.09–4.22
Not RCT	1.579	0.154–16.18

Abbreviation: RCT, randomized controlled trial.

3.4. Pooled Odds for Outcomes in Trial Sequential Analysis

In trial sequential analysis between the treated and control groups, the overall OR of CRBSI was 0.439 (95% CI, 0.290–0.668; $p < 0.001$; Figure 7a), the OR of ESI was 0.644 (95% CI, 0.469–0.883; $p = 0.006$; Figure 7b), the OR of the need to remove the catheter for catheter malfunction was 0.746 (95% CI, 0.431–1.293; $p = 0.151$; Figure 7c), the OR of the need to receive thrombolytic treatment for catheter malfunction was 1.015 (95% CI, 0.655–1.573; $p = 0.461$; Figure 7d), and the OR of all-cause mortality was 0.976 (95% CI, 0.663–1.439; $p = 0.296$; Figure 7e).

(a) Trial sequential analysis of catheter-related bloodstream infection

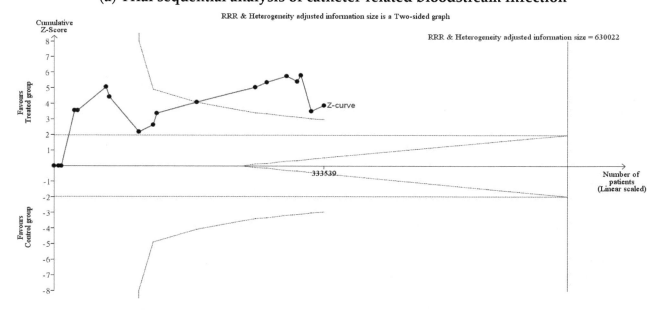

Figure 7. *Cont.*

(b) Trial sequential analysis of exit-site infection

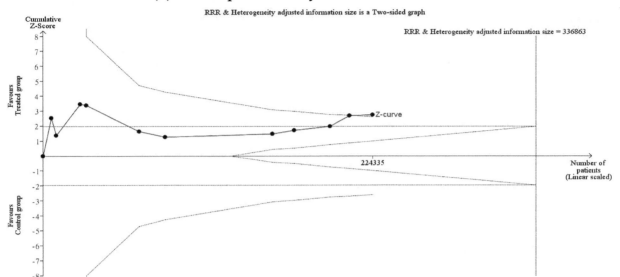

(c) Trial sequential analysis of catheter removal for catheter malfunction

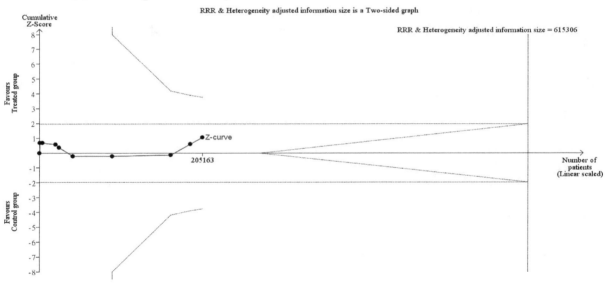

(d) Trial sequential analysis of thrombolytic treatments for catheter malfunction

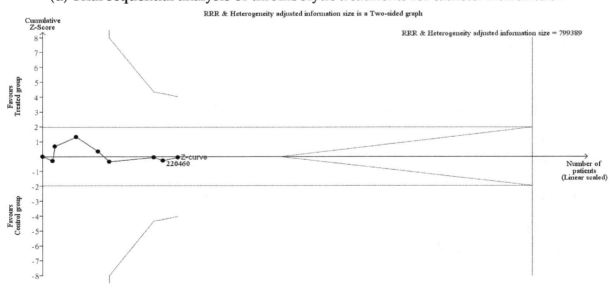

Figure 7. *Cont.*

(e) Trial sequential analysis of all-cause mortality

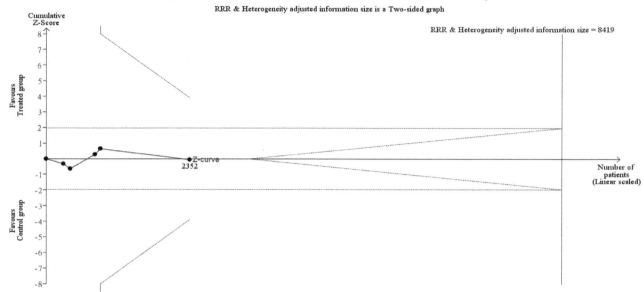

Figure 7. Trial sequential analysis of the odds ratio for evaluation event: (**a**) Trial sequential analysis of catheter-related bloodstream infection. Trial sequential analysis of 17 studies with a lower risk of bias in reporting catheter-related bloodstream infection, with a control event proportion of 17%, diversity of 45%, type I error of 5%, power of 80%, and relative risk reduction of 30%. The required information size of 630,022 was not reached and none of the boundaries for benefit, harm, or futility were crossed, leaving the meta-analysis inconclusive at a 30% relative risk reduction. The overall OR of CRBSI was 0.439 (95% CI, 0.290–1.668; $p < 0.001$); (**b**) trial sequential analysis of exit-site infection. Trial sequential analysis of eleven studies with low risk of bias reporting exit-site infection, with a control event proportion of 17%, diversity of 30%, type I error of 5%, power of 80%, and relative risk reduction of 30%. The required information size of 336,863 was not reached and none of the boundaries for benefit, harm, or futility were crossed, leaving the meta-analysis inconclusive at a 30% relative risk reduction. The OR of ESI was 0.644 (95% CI, 0.469–0.883; $p = 0.006$); (**c**) trial sequential analysis of nine studies with a lower risk of bias reporting the need to remove the catheter for catheter malfunction, with a control event proportion of 17%, diversity of 71%, type I error of 5%, power of 80%, and relative risk reduction of 30%. The required information size of 625,306 were not reached and none of the boundaries for benefit, harm, or futility were crossed, leaving the meta-analysis inconclusive at a 30% relative risk reduction. The OR of the need to remove the catheter for catheter malfunction was 0.746 (95% CI, 0.431–1.293; $p = 0.151$); (**d**) trial sequential analysis of thrombolytic treatments for catheter malfunction. Trial sequential analysis of nine studies with low risk of bias reporting the need to receive thrombolytic treatment for catheter malfunction, with a control event proportion of 17%, diversity of 91%, type I error of 5%, power of 80%, and relative risk reduction of 30%. The required information size of 615,306 were not reached and none of the boundaries for benefit, harm, or futility were crossed, leaving the meta-analysis inconclusive at a 30% relative risk reduction. The OR of the need to receive thrombolytic treatment for catheter malfunction was 1.015 (95% CI, 0.655–1.573; $p = 0.461$); (**e**) trial sequential analysis of all-cause mortality. Trial sequential analysis of five studies with a lower risk of bias reporting all-cause mortality, with a control event proportion of 17%, diversity of 78%, type I error of 5%, power of 80%, and relative risk reduction of 30%. The required information size of 8419were not reached and none of the boundaries for benefit, harm, or futility were crossed, leaving the meta-analysis inconclusive at a 30% relative risk reduction. The OR of all-cause mortality was 0.976 (95% CI, 0.663–1.439; $p = 0.296$). Notes: The solid blue line is the cumulative Z-curve. The vertical black dashed line is required information size. The green dashed lines represent the trial sequential monitoring boundaries and the futility boundaries.

3.5. Funnel Plot for the Overall OR of the Included Studies among Four Outcomes

We examined possible sources of underlying heterogeneity across studies. With regards to OR heterogeneity, the I^2 value was calculated in both the overall studies included. In the funnel plot of the OR for evaluation event, the I^2 value of CRBSI was 70.1% ($p = 0.303$, Figure 8a), ESI was 28.0% ($p = 0.010$; Figure 8b), the need to remove the catheter for catheter malfunction was 55.9% ($p = 0.208$; Figure 8c), the need to receive thrombolytic treatment for catheter malfunction was 88.69% ($p = 0.946$; Figure 8d), and all-cause mortality was 88.6% ($p = 0.804$; Figure 8e).

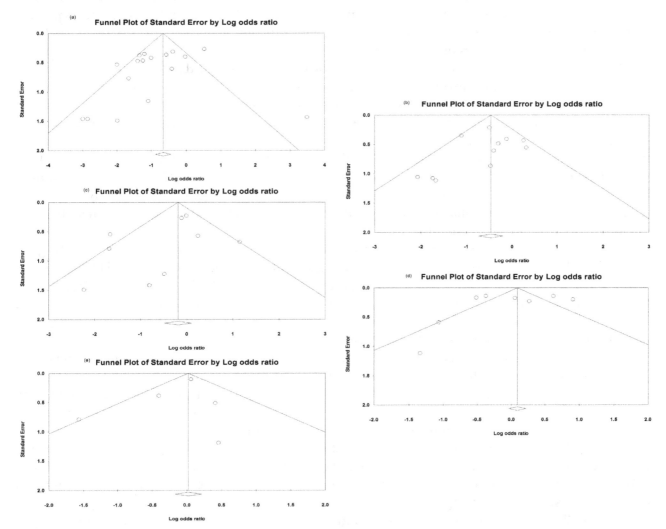

Figure 8. Funnel plot of the odds ratio for evaluation event: (**a**) Funnel plot of the odds ratio of catheter-related bloodstream infection. I^2 value, 70.1%; $p = 0.303$; (**b**) funnel plot of the odds ratio of exit-site infection. I^2 value, 28.0%; $p = 0.010$; (**c**) funnel plot of the odds ratio of catheter removal for catheter malfunction. I^2 value, 55.9%; $p = 0.208$; (**d**) funnel plot of the odds ratio of thrombolytic treatments for catheter malfunction. I^2 value, 88.69%; $p = 0.946$; (**e**) funnel plot of the odds ratio of all-cause mortality. I^2 value, 88.6%; $p = 0.804$. Regarding odds ratio heterogeneity, the I^2 value in both the overall studies included is indicated for each case. Egger's test revealed the existence of significant publication bias regarding the overall odds ratios, p-value is indicated for each case.

4. Discussion

Our meta-analysis and trial sequential analysis shows that routine locking solutions for hemodialysis catheters could effectively reduce the incidence of CRBSI and ESI. Our current meta-analysis, based on 21 selected studies with a total of 6118 participants, showed that the incidence of CRBSI and ESI significantly decreased in the treated group relative to the control group, that is less infections when using citrate or citrate mixtures versus heparin. Moreover, we found no significant difference in preserving catheter function, including in the need for catheter withdrawal or for thrombolytic treatment due to catheter malfunction, between the treated and control groups. We found no significant alteration in all-cause mortality between the two groups. The lack of statistical significance may not only be due to the heterogeneity and underlying variance in the outcomes of each regimen, but also due to inadequate required information sizes, as revealed by the trial sequential analysis. Regular locking care with citrate is standard practice for patients undergoing hemodialysis in many healthcare institutes, but not in some countries including Taiwan. Our updated review suggests that the role of routine locking solutions in preventing CRBSI and ESI in hemodialysis patients is robust. However, it does not show a benefit in preserving catheter function in hemodialysis patients, including in the need to remove catheters or in the need for thrombolytic treatment for catheter malfunction.

The current study shows that the incidence of CRBSI significantly decreased in the treated group relative to the control group, which is consistent with previous studies [36,37]. Subgroup analyses based on the type of locking solutions for hemodialysis catheters revealed that the usage of citrate-base regimens was associated with a lower incidence of CRBSI [4,14]. Our subgroup analysis for the concentration of citrate used showed that the incidence of CRBSI was similar in treated group, although the American Society of Diagnostic and Interventional Nephrology and the European Renal Best Practice recommend 4% citrate to be used as a catheter locking solution [38,39]. In some countries, including Taiwan, 4% citrate is still not routinely used in locking solutions for hemodialysis catheters. The current meta-analysis emphasizes that 4% citrate shows a benefit and could be routinely used as a locking solution for hemodialysis catheters.

Our current study shows that the incidence of ESI is significantly decreased in the treated group compared with the control group. Our result is in agreement with previous studies [14,19]. In some studies, patients received additional antibiotic ointments at the exit site during dressing changes, which could reduce the incidence of ESI [8,14,40]. After subgroup categorization, there is no significant difference between two groups except for combined regimen, which could result from the heterogeneity of the included studies and inadequate information size.

We found no significant difference in preserving catheter function between the treated and control groups, including the need to remove catheters or the need for thrombolytic treatment. However, Yahav et al. reported that citrate reduced catheter removals [41]. This incongruity may arise from the following: (1) Variation in enrollment criteria and definitions for the spectrum of catheter removal and (2) the number of cases is still limited because the meta-analysis information size does not meet the required information size. Concerning thrombolytic treatments and thrombosis episodes, our report is similar to previous studies [41,42]. Focusing on the need to remove catheters and to receive thrombolytic treatment for catheter malfunction, further large-scale RCTs are necessary to elucidate this issue for preserving catheter function.

The possible association between the two groups and all-cause mortality was not statistically significant in the current study (OR, 0.909; 95% CI, 0.580–1.423; $p = 0.676$). Subgroup analysis showed no difference in all-cause mortality. Mortality due to CRBSIs or ESIs account around one-tenth of all hemodialysis patient deaths [1–4]. Protective strategies with locking solutions to prevent CRBSIs and ESIs in hemodialysis patients still cannot decrease the mortality rate. Further large-scale RCTs are necessary to elucidate modifiable risk factor for decreasing morality in hemodialysis patients.

Guidelines for the Prevention of Intravascular Catheter-Related Infections has been published by the Center for Disease Control and Prevention [15], which recommends using prophylactic antimicrobial locking solution in patients undergoing hemodialysis who have a history of multiple CRBSI, despite optimal maximal adherence to aseptic techniques (Category II). This recommendation has been embraced by some dialysis centers due to the low execution rate of locking solutions in preventing CRBSI in hemodialysis patients. In fact, many challenges persist in managing daily care in dialysis centers, such as a lack of safety locking solutions for hemodialysis catheters, lack of a designated health-care workers to perform locking care, limited training on catheter care among health-care workers of dialysis centers, potential hemodialysis patients' noncompliance due to discomfort, as well as health-care workers being unable to maintain high adherence rates in conducting care procedures.

The current study has several limitations. Firstly, the enrolled trials and studies included in the primary analysis dealt with different indications for outcome measures by randomizing a variety of patient groups in different clinical settings. Thus, there is the risk of introducing potentially heterogeneity. Additionally, it is difficult to perform a subgroup analysis based on conditions, such as catheter type, heparin dosage, and other differences in individual unit practices. Secondly, differences in the study individuals, disease severity, setting, and type of infections between individual studies made the study population highly heterogeneous. The I^2 value for OR heterogeneity ranged from 25% to 50%, and this heterogeneity would impact the findings of this meta-analysis. Thus, the influence of measurement precision was considered when reporting treatment effectiveness using ORs. Due to the lack of adjusted data in our selected trials, we compiled the unadjusted ORs. We therefore suggest that future similar trials should record serial changes in catheter function and infection status to provide a more accurate indication of clinical effectiveness. Regardless of aforementioned limitations, we have minimized bias throughout the process by our methods of study identification, data selection, and statistical analysis, as well as in our control of publication bias. These steps should strengthen the stability and accuracy of the meta-analysis. Our findings of this meta-analysis are reliable to provide suggestions for improving clinical care.

5. Conclusions

In conclusion, our study demonstrated that routine locking solutions for hemodialysis catheters could effectively reduce the incidence of CRBSI and ESI. Our findings showed no benefit of routine locking solutions for hemodialysis catheters in decreasing all-cause mortality as well as preserving catheter function, including in the need to remove catheters and in the need to receive thrombolytic treatment, both due to catheter malfunction. The latter results lack statistical significance and the comparisons are limited due to the heterogeneity of the included trials and inadequate information size. Therefore, further well-conducted observational studies and randomized controlled trials are urgently needed to conclusively evaluate the impact of routine locking solutions on preserving catheter function and improving the rates of all-cause mortality.

Author Contributions: Conceptualization, C.-H.C., Y.-M.C., Y.Y., Y.-J.C., L.-J.Y. and H.-C.Y.; Methodology, C.-H.C., Y.-M.C. and Y.-J.C.; Software, C.-H.C., Y.-M.C. and Y.-J.C.; Validation, C.-H.C., Y.-M.C., Y.Y. and Y.-J.C.; Formal Analysis, C.-H.C., Y.-M.C. and Y.-J.C.; Investigation, X.X.; Data Curation, C.-H.C.; Writing—Original Draft Preparation, C.-H.C.; Writing—Review and Editing, C.-H.C., Y.-M.C., Y.Y. and Y.-J.C.; Writing—Approval, C.-H.C., Y.-M.C., Y.Y., Y.-J.C., L.-J.Y. and H.-C.Y.; Visualization, C.-H.C. and Y.-M.C.; Project Administration, C.-H.C.; Funding Acquisition, C.-H.C.

Acknowledgments: The authors thank Ping-Tao Tseng for technical analysis. The authors thank the staff at the Epidemiology and Biostatistics Center, the Department of Pharmacology, and the Department of Computer at Changhua Christian Hospital for the literature findings. This research project would not have been possible without the support of many people. The authors wish to express their gratitude to the staffs of the Department of Critical Care, Epidemiology and Biostatistics Center, the Division of Nephrology, the Division of Infectious Diseases, the Department of Pharmacology, the Department of Nursing, and the Department of Healthcare Quality at Changhua Christian Hospital who were extremely helpful and provided invaluable assistance and support.

Appendix A

Supplement Search strategy in PubMed

#1 lock

#2 filling solution

#3 #1 or #2

#4 End-Stage Kidney Disease or Disease, End-Stage Kidney, End Stage Kidney Disease, End-Stage Chronic Kidney Failure, End-Stage Renal Disease, End-Stage Renal Disease, Chronic Chronic Renal Failure, or ESRD

#5 Renal Dialyses, Renal Dialysis, Hemodialyses, Extracorporeal Dialysis or Renal replacement therapy

#6 Catheter Related Infections, Catheter-Related Infection

#7 #4 or #5 and #6

#8 #3 and #7

References

1. Liu, K.D.; Chertow, G.M. Dialysis in the Treatment of Renal Failure. In *Harrison's Principles of Internal Medicine, 20e*; Jameson, J.L., Fauci, A.S., Kasper, D.L., Hauser, S.L., Longo, D.L., Loscalzo, J., Eds.; McGraw-Hill Education: New York, NY, USA, 2018.

2. Schwab, S.J.; Beathard, G. The hemodialysis catheter conundrum: Hate living with them, but can't live without them. *Kidney Int.* **1999**, *56*, 1–17. [CrossRef] [PubMed]

3. Zhao, Y.; Li, Z.; Zhang, L.; Yang, J.; Yang, Y.; Tang, Y.; Fu, P. Citrate versus heparin locking for hemodialysis catheters: A systematic review and meta-analysis of randomized controlled trials. *Am. J. Kidney Dis.* **2014**, *63*, 479–490. [CrossRef] [PubMed]

4. Power, A.; Duncan, N.; Singh, S.K.; Brown, W.; Dalby, E.; Edwards, C.; Lynch, K.; Prout, V.; Cairns, T.; Griffith, M.; et al. Sodium citrate versus heparin catheter lockings for cuffed central venous catheters: A single-center randomized controlled trial. *Am. J. Kidney Dis.* **2009**, *53*, 1034–1041. [CrossRef] [PubMed]

5. Allon, M. Current management of vascular access. *Clin. J. Am. Soc. Nephrol.* **2007**, *2*, 786–800. [CrossRef]

6. Maki, D.G.; Ash, S.R.; Winger, R.K.; Lavin, P.; Investigators, A.T. A novel antimicrobial and antithrombotic locking solution for hemodialysis catheters: A multi-center, controlled, randomized trial. *Crit. Care Med.* **2011**, *39*, 613–620. [CrossRef] [PubMed]

7. Yevzlin, A.S.; Sanchez, R.J.; Hiatt, J.G.; Washington, M.H.; Wakeen, M.; Hofmann, R.M.; Becker, Y.T. Concentrated heparin locking is associated with major bleeding complications after tunneled hemodialysis catheter placement. In *Seminars in Dialysis*; Blackwell Publishing Ltd.: Oxford, UK, 2007; Volume 20, pp. 351–354.

8. Moran, J.; Sun, S.; Khababa, I.; Pedan, A.; Doss, S.; Schiller, B. A randomized trial comparing gentamicin/citrate and heparin lockings for central venous catheters in maintenance hemodialysis patients. *Am. J. Kidney Dis.* **2012**, *59*, 102–107. [CrossRef]

9. Shanks, R.M.; Donegan, N.P.; Graber, M.L.; Buckingham, S.E.; Zegans, M.E.; Cheung, A.L.; O'Toole, G.A. Heparin stimulates *Staphylococcus aureus* biofilm formation. *Infect. Immun.* **2005**, *73*, 4596–4606. [CrossRef]

10. Shanks, R.M.; Sargent, J.L.; Martinez, R.M.; Graber, M.L.; O'Toole, G.A. Catheter locking solutions influence staphylococcal biofilm formation on abiotic surfaces. *Nephrol. Dial. Transplant.* **2006**, *21*, 2247–2255. [CrossRef]

11. Ibberson, C.B.; Parlet, C.P.; Kwiecinski, J.; Crosby, H.A.; Meyerholz, D.K.; Horswill, A.R. Hyaluronan Modulation Impacts *Staphylococcus aureus* Biofilm Infection. *Infect. Immun.* **2016**, *84*, 1917–1929. [CrossRef] [PubMed]

12. Macrae, J.M.; Dojcinovic, I.; Djurdjev, O.; Jung, B.; Shalansky, S.; Levin, A.; Kiaii, M. Citrate 4% versus heparin and the reduction of thrombosis study (CHARTS). *Clin. J. Am. Soc. Nephrol.* **2008**, *3*, 369–374. [CrossRef]

13. Lok, C.E.; Appleton, D.; Bhola, C.; Khoo, B.; Richardson, R.M. Trisodium citrate 4%—An alternative to heparin capping of haemodialysis catheters. *Nephrol. Dial. Transplant.* **2007**, *22*, 477–483. [CrossRef] [PubMed]

14. Weijmer, M.C.; van den Dorpel, M.A.; Van de Ven, P.J.; ter Wee, P.M.; van Geelen, J.A.; Groeneveld, J.O.; van Jaarsveld, B.C.; Koopmans, M.G.; le Poole, C.Y.; Schrander-Van der Meer, A.M.; et al. Randomized, clinical trial comparison of trisodium citrate 30% and heparin as catheter-lockinging solution in hemodialysis patients. *J. Am. Soc. Nephrol.* **2005**, *16*, 2769–2777. [CrossRef]

15. O'grady, N.P.; Alexander, M.; Burns, L.A.; Dellinger, E.P.; Garland, J.; Heard, S.O.; Lipsett, P.A.; Masur, H.; Mermel, L.A.; Pearson, M.L. Guidelines for the prevention of intravascular catheter-related infections. *Clin. Infect. Dis.* **2011**, *52*, e162–e193. [CrossRef] [PubMed]

16. Thorlund, K.; Imberger, G.; Walsh, M.; Chu, R.; Gluud, C.; Wetterslev, J.; Guyatt, G.; Devereaux, P.J.; Thabane, L. The number of patients and events required to limit the risk of overestimation of intervention effects in meta-analysis—A simulation study. *PLoS ONE* **2011**, *6*, e25491. [CrossRef] [PubMed]

17. Kanaa, M.; Wright, M.J.; Akbani, H.; Laboi, P.; Bhandari, S.; Sandoe, J.A. Cathasept Line Locking and Microbial Colonization of Tunneled Hemodialysis Catheters: A Multicenter Randomized Controlled Trial. *Am. J. Kidney Dis.* **2015**, *66*, 1015–1023. [CrossRef] [PubMed]

18. Moghaddas, A.; Abbasi, M.R.; Gharekhani, A.; Dashti-Khavidaki, S.; Razeghi, E.; Jafari, A.; Khalili, H. Prevention of hemodialysis catheter-related blood stream infections using a cotrimoxazole-locking technique. *Future Microbiol.* **2015**, *10*, 169–178. [CrossRef]

19. Souweine, B.; Lautrette, A.; Gruson, D.; Canet, E.; Klouche, K.; Argaud, L.; Bohe, J.; Garrouste-Orgeas, M.; Mariat, C.; Vincent, F.; et al. Ethanol locking and risk of hemodialysis catheter infection in critically ill patients. A randomized controlled trial. *Am. J. Respir. Crit. Care Med.* **2015**, *191*, 1024–1032. [CrossRef]

20. Chu, G.; Fogarty, G.M.; Avis, L.F.; Bergin, S.; McElduff, P.; Gillies, A.H.; Choi, P. Low dose heparin locking (1000 U/mL) maintains tunnelled hemodialysis catheter patency when compared with high dose heparin (5000 U/mL): A randomised controlled trial. *Hemodial. Int.* **2016**, *20*, 385–391. [CrossRef]

21. Zwiech, R.; Adelt, M.; Chrul, S. A Taurolidine-Citrate-Heparin Locking Solution Effectively Eradicates Pathogens from the Catheter Biofilm in Hemodialysis Patients. *Am. J. Ther.* **2016**, *23*, e363–e368. [CrossRef]

22. Correa Barcellos, F.; Pereira Nunes, B.; Jorge Valle, L.; Lopes, T.; Orlando, B.; Scherer, C.; Nunes, M.; Araujo Duarte, G.; Bohlke, M. Comparative effectiveness of 30% trisodium citrate and heparin locking solution in preventing infection and dysfunction of hemodialysis catheters: A randomized controlled trial (CITRIM trial). *Infection* **2017**, *45*, 139–145. [CrossRef] [PubMed]

23. Sofroniadou, S.; Revela, I.; Kouloubinis, A.; Makriniotou, I.; Zerbala, S.; Smirloglou, D.; Kalocheretis, P.; Drouzas, A.; Samonis, G.; Iatrou, C. Ethanol combined with heparin as a lockinging solution for the prevention of catheter related blood stream infections in hemodialysis patients: A prospective randomized study. *Hemodial. Int.* **2017**, *21*, 498–506. [CrossRef] [PubMed]

24. Winnicki, W.; Herkner, H.; Lorenz, M.; Handisurya, A.; Kikic, Z.; Bielesz, B.; Schairer, B.; Reiter, T.; Eskandary, F.; Sunder-Plassmann, G.; et al. Taurolidine-based catheter locking regimen significantly reduces overall costs, infection, and dysfunction rates of tunneled hemodialysis catheters. *Kidney Int.* **2018**, *93*, 753–760. [CrossRef]

25. Jadad, A.R.; Moore, R.A.; Carroll, D.; Jenkinson, C.; Reynolds, D.J.M.; Gavaghan, D.J.; McQuay, H.J. Assessing the quality of reports of randomized clinical trials: Is blinding necessary? *Control. Clin. Trials* **1996**, *17*, 1–12. [CrossRef]

26. Wells, G.; Shea, B.; O'Connell, D.; Peterson, J.; Welch, V.; Losos, M. *Newcastle-Ottawa Quality Assessment Scale*; Ottawa Hospital Research Institute: Ottawa, ON, Canada, 2013.

27. Higgins, J.P.; Thompson, S.G. Quantifying heterogeneity in a meta-analysis. *Stat. Med.* **2002**, *21*, 1539–1558. [CrossRef]

28. Moher, D.; Liberati, A.; Tetzlaff, J.; Altman, D.G. Preferred reporting items for systematic reviews and meta-analyses: The PRISMA statement. *PLoS Med.* **2009**, *6*, e1000097. [CrossRef]

29. Buturovic, J.; Ponikvar, R.; Kandus, A.; Boh, M.; Klinkmann, J.; Ivanovich, P. Filling hemodialysis catheters in the interdialytic period: Heparin versus citrate versus polygeline: A prospective randomized study. *Artif. Organs* **1998**, *22*, 945–947. [CrossRef]

30. Dogra, G.K. Prevention of Tunneled Hemodialysis Catheter-Related Infections Using Catheter-Restricted Filling with Gentamicin and Citrate: A Randomized Controlled Study. *J. Am. Soc. Nephrol.* **2002**, *13*, 2133–2139. [CrossRef]

31. Betjes, M.G.; van Agteren, M. Prevention of dialysis catheter-related sepsis with a citrate-taurolidine-containing locking solution. *Nephrol. Dial. Transplant.* **2004**, *19*, 1546–1551. [CrossRef] [PubMed]

32. Nori, U.S.; Manoharan, A.; Yee, J.; Besarab, A. Comparison of low-dose gentamicin with minocycline as catheter locking solutions in the prevention of catheter-related bacteremia. *Am. J. Kidney Dis.* **2006**, *48*, 596–605. [CrossRef] [PubMed]

33. Solomon, L.R.; Cheesbrough, J.S.; Ebah, L.; Al-Sayed, T.; Heap, M.; Millband, N.; Waterhouse, D.; Mitra, S.; Curry, A.; Saxena, R.; et al. A randomized double-blind controlled trial of taurolidine-citrate catheter lockings for the prevention of bacteremia in patients treated with hemodialysis. *Am. J. Kidney Dis.* **2010**, *55*, 1060–1068. [CrossRef]

34. Filiopoulos, V.; Hadjiyannakos, D.; Koutis, I.; Trompouki, S.; Micha, T.; Lazarou, D.; Vlassopoulos, D. Approaches to prolong the use of uncuffed hemodialysis catheters: Results of a randomized trial. *Am. J. Nephrol.* **2011**, *33*, 260–268. [CrossRef]

35. Chen, F.K.; Li, J.J.; Song, Y.; Zhang, Y.Y.; Chen, P.; Zhao, C.Z.; Gong, H.Y.; Yao, D.F. Concentrated sodium chloride catheter locking solution—A new effective alternative method for hemodialysis patients with high bleeding risk. *Ren. Fail.* **2014**, *36*, 17–22. [CrossRef]

36. Jaffer, Y.; Selby, N.M.; Taal, M.W.; Fluck, R.J.; McIntyre, C.W. A meta-analysis of hemodialysis catheter lockinging solutions in the prevention of catheter-related infection. *Am. J. Kidney Dis.* **2008**, *51*, 233–241. [CrossRef]

37. Labriola, L.; Crott, R.; Jadoul, M. Preventing haemodialysis catheter-related bacteraemia with an antimicrobial locking solution: A meta-analysis of prospective randomized trials. *Nephrol. Dial. Transplant.* **2008**, *23*, 1666–1672. [CrossRef]

38. Moran, J.E.; Ash, S.R. Lockinging solutions for hemodialysis catheters; heparin and citrate—A position paper by ASDIN. *Semin. Dial.* **2008**, *21*, 490–492. [CrossRef] [PubMed]

39. Vanholder, R.; Canaud, B.; Fluck, R.; Jadoul, M.; Labriola, L.; Marti-Monros, A.; Tordoir, J.; Van Biesen, W. Catheter-related blood stream infections (CRBSI): A European view. *Nephrol. Dial. Transplant.* **2010**, *25*, 1753–1756. [CrossRef]

40. Jenks, M.; Craig, J.; Green, W.; Hewitt, N.; Arber, M.; Sims, A. Tegaderm CHG IV Securement Dressing for Central Venous and Arterial Catheter Insertion Sites: A NICE Medical Technology Guidance. *Appl. Health Econ. Health Policy* **2016**, *14*, 135–149. [CrossRef]

41. Yahav, D.; Rozen-Zvi, B.; Gafter-Gvili, A.; Leibovici, L.; Gafter, U.; Paul, M. Antimicrobial locking solutions for the prevention of infections associated with intravascular catheters in patients undergoing hemodialysis: Systematic review and meta-analysis of randomized, controlled trials. *Clin. Infect. Dis.* **2008**, *47*, 83–93. [CrossRef] [PubMed]

42. Yon, C.K.; Low, C.L. Sodium citrate 4% versus heparin as a locking solution in hemodialysis patients with central venous catheters. *Am. J. Health Syst. Pharm.* **2013**, *70*, 131–136. [CrossRef] [PubMed]

The Efficacy and Safety of Eravacycline in the Treatment of Complicated Intra-Abdominal Infections

Shao-Huan Lan [1], Shen-Peng Chang [2], Chih-Cheng Lai [3], Li-Chin Lu [4] and Chien-Ming Chao [3,*]

[1] School of Pharmaceutical Sciences and Medical Technology, Putian University, Putian 351100, Fujian, China; shawnlan0713@gmail.com

[2] Department of Pharmacy, Chi Mei Medical Center, Liouying 73657, Taiwan; httremoon@ms.szmc.edu.tw

[3] Department of Intensive Care Medicine, Chi Mei Medical Center, Liouying 73657, Taiwan; dtmed141@gmail.com

[4] School of Management, Putian University, Putian 351100, China; jane90467@gmail.com

* Correspondence: ccm870958@yahoo.com.tw

Abstract: This study aims to assess the clinical efficacy and safety of eravacycline for treating complicated intra-abdominal infection (cIAI) in adult patients. The PubMed, Web of Science, EBSCO, Cochrane databases, Ovid Medline, Embase, and ClinicalTrials.gov were searched up to May 2019. Only randomized controlled trials (RCTs) that evaluated eravacycline and other comparators for the treatment of cIAI were included. The primary outcome was the clinical cure rate at the test-of-cure visit based on modified intent-to-treat population, microbiological intent-to-treat population, clinically evaluable population, and microbiological evaluable population, and the secondary outcomes were clinical failure rate and the risk of adverse event. Three RCTs were included. Overall, eravacycline had a clinical cure rate (88.7%, 559/630) at test-of-cure in modified intent-to-treat population similar to comparators (90.1%, 492/546) in the treatment of cIAIs (risk ratio (RR), 0.99; 95% confidence interval (CI), 0.95–1.03; $I^2 = 0$%, Figure 3). In the microbiological intent-to-treat, clinically evaluable, and microbiological evaluable populations, no difference was found between eravacycline and comparators in terms of clinical cure rate at test-of-cure (microbiological intent-to-treat population, RR, 0.99; 95% CI, 0.95–1.04; $I^2 = 0$%, clinically evaluable population, RR, 1.00; 95% CI, 0.97–1.03; $I^2 = 0$%, microbiological evaluable population, RR, 0.98; 95% CI, 0.95–1.02; $I^2 = 0$%). In addition, eravacycline had clinical failure rate similar to comparators at test-of-cure in modified intent-to-treat population (RR, 1.01; 95% CI, 0.61–0.69; $I^2 = 0$%), microbiological intent-to-treat population (RR, 1.34; 95% CI, 0.77–2.31; $I^2 = 16$%), clinically evaluable population (RR, 1.03; 95% CI, 0.61–1.76; $I^2 = 0$%), and microbiological evaluable population (RR, 1.32; 95% CI, 0.75–2.32; $I^2 = 10$%). Although eravacycline was associated with higher risk of treatment-emergent adverse event than comparators (RR, 1.34; 95% CI, 1.13–1.58; $I^2 = 0$%), no significant differences were found between eravacycline and comparators for the risk of serious adverse event (RR, 1.04; 95% CI, 0.65–1.65; $I^2 = 0$%), discontinuation of study drug because of adverse event (RR, 0.68; 95% CI, 0.23–1.99; $I^2 = 13$%), and all-cause mortality (RR, 1.09; 95% CI, 0.41–2.9; $I^2 = 28$%). In conclusion, the clinical efficacy of eravacycline is as high as that of the comparator drugs in the treatment of cIAIs and this antibiotic is as well tolerated as the comparators.

Keywords: eravacycline; complicated intra-abdominal infection; efficacy; safety; mortality

1. Introduction

In contrast to uncomplicated abdominal infections, complicated intra-abdominal infections (cIAIs) can extend beyond the originally infected organ into peritoneal spaces, and can be associated with local or diffuse peritonitis [1,2]. *Enterobacteriaceae*, especially *Escherichia coli* and *Klebsiella pneumoniae*, are the most common pathogens causing cIAIs [3–5]. Emergence of multiple antibiotic resistances has become the major concern in this clinical entity and further limits the choice of optimal antibiotic treatment. *E. coli*, *Proteus* species, and *K. pneumoniae* are the most common pathogens; however, high resistance to broad-spectrum antibiotics, including extended-spectrum β-lactams and fluoroquinolones, among these pathogens, also emerges as a critical threat worldwide.

Eravacycline is a novel, synthetic fluorocycline antibacterial agent [6], and has excellent bactericidal activity against most antibiotic-resistant pathogens according to several in vitro studies [7–10]. Recently, the clinical efficacy of eravacycline in cIAI has been evaluated in several clinical studies [11–13]. However, an updated meta-analysis comparing the efficacy and safety of eravacycline and other comparators for the treatment of cIAI is lacking. Therefore, we conducted this meta-analysis to provide real-time evidence about the efficacy and safety of cIAI.

2. Methods

2.1. Study Search and Selection

All clinical studies were identified through a systematic review of the literature in PubMed, Web of Science, EBSCO, Cochrane databases, Ovid Medline, Embase, and ClinicalTrials.gov until May 2019 using the following search terms: "eravacycline", "Xerava™", "TP-434", and "abdom*" (Search strategy presented in Appendix A). Studies were considered eligible for inclusion if they directly compared the clinical efficacy and safety of eravacycline with other antimicrobial agents in the treatment of adult patients with cIAIs. Studies were excluded if they focused on in vitro activity, animal studies, or pharmacokinetic–pharmacodynamic assessment. Two authors (S.-P.C. and S.-H.L.) searched and examined publications independently. When they disagreed, the third author (C.-C.L.) resolved the issue. The following data including year of publication, study design, type of infections, patients' demographic features, antimicrobial regimens, clinical and microbiological outcomes, and adverse effects were extracted from every included study.

2.2. Outcome Measurement

The primary outcome of this meta-analysis was clinical response assessed at the test-of-cure visit, end-of-treatment, and follow-up visit based on modified intent-to-treat population, microbiological intent-to-treat population, clinically evaluable population, microbiological evaluable populations. The intent-to-treat population included all randomized patients, and the modified intent-to-treat population included all intent-to treat patients who received any amount of study drug. The microbiological intent-to-treat population included all modified intent-to-treat patients who met the minimal disease definition of cIAI and had a baseline pathogen identified. The clinically evaluable population included all modified intent-to-treat patients who met the minimal disease definition of cIAI and had a clinical response assessed at the test-of-cure visit. The microbiological evaluable population included all clinically evaluable patients who had a baseline pathogen identified and a microbiological response assessed. Clinical response was classified as cure, failure, or indeterminate based on clinical outcomes. Clinical cure was defined as resolution of all or most pretherapy signs or symptoms with no further requirement for antibiotics, radiological intervention, or surgery. The safety population included all patients who received any intravenous study therapy. Treatment-emergent adverse events were defined as adverse events that started during or after the first dose of study drug administration or increased in severity or relationship to the study drugs during the study. Serious adverse event is defined as an untoward medical occurrence or effect that at any dose results in death, is life-threatening, requires hospitalization or extension of existing hospitalization, or results in persistent or significant disability.

2.3. Data Analysis

The quality of enrolled RCTs and the risk of bias were assessed using Cochrane Risk of Bias Assessment tool [14]. Statistical analyses were conducted using the software Review Manager, version 5.3. The degree of heterogeneity was evaluated with the Q statistic generated from the χ^2 test. The proportion of statistical heterogeneity was assessed using the I^2 measure. Heterogeneity was considered significant when the p was less than 0.1 or I^2 was greater than 50%. The random-effects model was used when data were significantly heterogeneous and the fixed-effect model was used when data were homogeneous. Pooled risk ratios (RRs) and 95% confidence intervals (CIs) were calculated for outcome analyses.

3. Results

3.1. Study Selection and Characteristics

The search program yielded 147 references. After excluding 90 duplications, the remaining 57 abstracts were screened. Among them, we retrieved 11 articles for full-text review. Finally, three studies [11–13] fulfilling the inclusion criteria were included in this meta-analysis (Figure 1). All enrolled studies had the same principal investigator. All studies [11–13] were randomized, multicenter, and multinational studies designed to compare the clinical efficacy and safety of eravacycline with other comparators for adult patients with cIAI (Table 1). The inclusion criterion of these three studies was that adult patients had to have clinical evidence of cIAI requiring urgent surgical or percutaneous intervention within 48 hours of diagnosis. Two studies [11,13] compared eravacycline with ertapenem, and one [12] compared with meropenem. The test-of-cure evaluation was conducted 25 to 31 calendar days in two studies [11,12] and 10 to 14 days in one study [13] after the first dose of the study drug was administered for the patients with cIAI. The follow-up visit was performed 38 to 50 calendar days in one study [11] and 28 to 42 days in one study [13] after the first dose of study drug was administered. All of the domains in each study were classified as having a low risk of bias (Table 2).

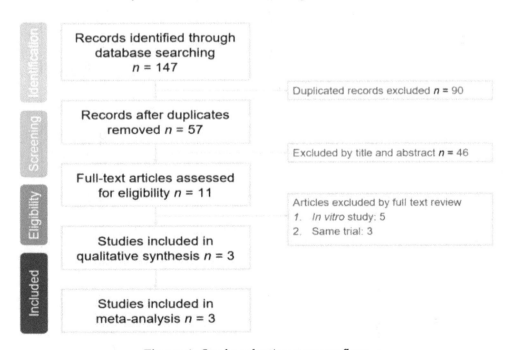

Figure 1. Study selection process flow.

Table 1. Characteristics of included studies.

Study, Published Year	Study Design	Study Site	Study Period	No. of Patients (ITT population)		Dose Regimen	
				Eravacycline	Comparator	Eravacycline	Comparator
Solomkin et al, 2014	Randomized, double-blind trial	19 sites in 6 countries	2011–2012	56 (1.5 mg/kg), 57 (1.0 mg/kg)	30	1.5 mg/kg or 1.0 mg/kg q24 h	Ertapenem 1 g q24 h
IGNITE1, 2017	Randomized, double-blind trial	66 sites in 11 countries	2013–2014	270	271	1.0 mg/kg q12 h	Ertapenem 1 g q24 h
IGNITE4, 2018	Randomized, double-blind trial	65 sites in 11 countries	2016–2017	250	250	1.0 mg/kg q12 h	Meropenem 1 g q8 h

ITT, intention to treat; q, every; h, hour; mg, milligram; g, gram.

Table 2. Risk of bias per study and domain.

Risk of Bias	Study		
	IGNITE1, 2017	IGNITE4, 2018	Solomkin et al, 2014
Random sequence generation	low	low	low
Allocation concealment	low	low	low
Blinding of participants and personnel	low	low	low
Blinding of outcome assessment	low	low	low
Incomplete outcome data	low	low	low
Selective reporting	low	low	low

3.2. Clinical Efficacy and Microbiologic Response

Overall, eravacycline had a clinical cure rate (88.7%, 559/630) at test-of-cure in modified intent-to-treat population similar to comparators (90.1%, 492/546) in the treatment of cIAIs (risk ratio (RR), 0.99; 95% CI, 0.95–1.03; I^2 = 0%, Figure 2). In the microbiological intent-to-treat, clinically evaluable, and microbiological evaluable populations, no difference was found between eravacycline and comparators in terms of clinical cure rate at test-of-cure (Figure 2). In addition, no significant difference was observed between eravacycline and comparator in terms of clinical failure rate at test-of-cure in modified intent-to-treat population, microbiological intent-to-treat population, clinically evaluable population, and microbiological evaluable population (Figure 3).

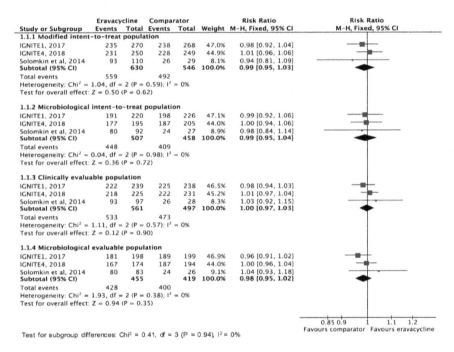

Figure 2. Overall clinical cure rates for eravacycline and comparators in the treatment of complicated intra-abdominal infections.

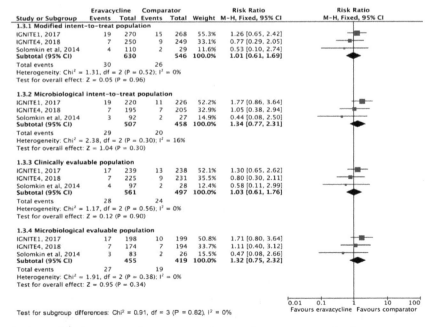

Figure 3. Overall clinical failure rates for eravacycline and comparators in the treatment of complicated intra-abdominal infections.

Only two studies [12,13] reported the outcome at end-of-treatment, and the pooled analysis showed no significant difference was observed between eravacycline and comparator in terms of clinical cure rate at end-of-treatment in modified intent-to-treat population (RR, 0.99; 95% CI, 0.95–1.03; I^2 = 1%), microbiological intent-to-treat population (RR, 0.98; 95% CI, 0.94–1.03; I^2 = 0%), clinically evaluable population (RR, 0.99; 95% CI, 0.96–1.01; I^2 = 0%), and microbiological evaluable population (RR, 0.98; 95% CI, 0.95–1.01; I^2 = 0%). In addition, these two studies[12,13] reported the outcome at follow-up, and the pooled analysis showed no significant difference was observed between eravacycline and comparator in terms of clinical cure rate at follow-up in modified intent-to-treat population (RR, 0.99; 95% CI, 0.93–1.04; I^2 = 0%), microbiological intent-to-treat population (RR, 0.98; 95% CI, 0.92–1.06; I^2 = 0%), clinically evaluable population (RR, 1.01; 95% CI, 0.97–1.06; I^2 = 0%), and microbiological evaluable population (RR, 1.02; 95% CI, 0.97–1.07; I^2 = 30%).

3.3. Adverse Events

In the pooled analysis of three studies reporting adverse events, we found that eravacycline was associated with a higher risk of treatment-emergent adverse events than comparators (Figure 4). However, no significant differences were found between eravacycline and comparators for the risk of serious adverse events, discontinuation of study drug because of adverse event, and all-cause mortality (Figure 4). The most common adverse event among the eravacycline group was nausea (6.5%, 41/629) and vomiting (3.8%, 24/629). Although the risks of nausea and vomiting in the eravacycline group were higher than those in the comparator group, these differences did not reach statistical significance (for nausea, RR, 4.79; 95% CI, 0.84–27.14;7 I^2 = 70%, for vomiting, RR, 1.46; 95% CI, 0.76–2.81;7 I^2 = 0%).

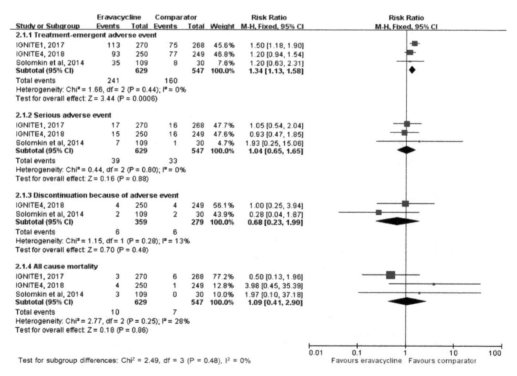

Figure 4. Adverse event risks with eravacycline and comparators in the treatment of complicated intra-abdominal infections.

4. Discussion

This first meta-analysis based on three RCTs [11–13] determined that the clinical efficacy of eravacycline is similar to that of other comparators in the treatment of adult patients with cIAIs. This significant finding is supported by the following analysis. First, the overall pooled clinical cure rate at test-of-cure of eravacycline in treating cIAIs was comparable to carbapenems in modified intent-to-treat, microbiological intent-to-treat, clinically evaluable, and microbiological evaluable populations. Second, pooled clinical failure rate at test-of-cure of eravacycline was as low as comparators in modified intent-to-treat, microbiological intent-to-treat, clinically evaluable, and microbiological evaluable populations. Third, this similarity in terms of clinical efficacy between eravacycline and comparators did not change with the timing of the outcome measure at end-of-treatment and follow-up. In summary, all of these findings indicated that eravacycline can be an effective therapeutic option in the treatment of adult patients with cIAIs.

The effectiveness of ceftaroline in the treatment of cIAIs in adult patients can be supported by in vitro studies [7,9,10,15,16]. In the surveillance of 2213 Gram-negative and 2423 Gram-positive pathogens in 13 Canadian hospitals, the minimum inhibitory concentration$_{90}$ (MIC$_{90}$) ranged from 0.5 to 2μg/mL for 9 species of *Enterobacteriaceae* tested ($n = 2067$) and extended-spectrum β-lactamase producing *E. coli* ($n = 141$) and *K. pneumoniae* ($n = 21$) did not affect the potency of eravacycline in this study [10]. In another survey of more than 4000 Gram-negative pathogens in New York hospitals [7], eravacycline demonstrated great in vitro activity against *Enterobacteriaceae*—*E. coli, K. pneumoniae, Enterobacter aerogenes,* and *Enterobacter cloacae* with minimum inhibitory concentration$_{50}$ (MIC$_{50}$)/MIC$_{90}$ of 0.12/0.5 μg/mL, 0.25/1 μg/mL, 0.25/1 μg/mL, and 0.5/1 μg/mL, respectively. Moreover, the potent activity was retained against multidrug-resistant (MDR) isolates, including carbapenem nonsusceptible strains [7,9]. In addition to aerobic bacteria, anaerobic bacteria play important roles in the cIAIs. Eravacycline showed good in vitro activity against *Bacteroides* spp., *Parabacteroides* spp., and *Clostridioides difficile* (formerly *Clostridium difficile*) and eravacycline remained potent against the strains with tetracycline-specific resistance determinants and MDR anaerobic pathogens [15,16]. Overall, the potent in vitro activity of eravacycline against commonly encountered pathogens causing cIAI largely explains the great in vivo clinical response in this meta-analysis.

In addition to clinical efficacy of eravacycline for the treatment of cIAIs, we should consider the risk of adverse event while prescribing eravacycline. Nausea and vomiting were the most common adverse events, and the overall incidence of these adverse events were higher than those of comparators. Moreover, the pooled risk of treatment-emergent adverse events was higher in the eravacycline group than in the control group. These findings are consistent with previous pooled analysis of IGNITE1 and IGNITE4, in which eravacycline recipients had higher incidence of nausea (6.5 vs. 0.6%) and vomiting (3.7 vs. 2.5%) [17]. In contrast, the incidence of serious adverse events, discontinuation of study drug because of adverse event, and all-cause mortality was similar between eravacycline and comparators. Therefore, the findings of this meta-analysis suggest that although eravacycline is associated with higher risk of mild adverse events than comparator, overall, eravacycline remains as safe as other comparators in the treatment of cIAI among adult patients.

This study has several limitations. First, only three RCTs were considered in this meta-analysis. Second, the usefulness of eravacycline in treating cIAIs was not assessed according to the disease severity. Third, we did not evaluate the correlation between in vitro activity and in vivo response of eravacycline against each specific pathogen, particularly antibiotic-resistant organisms, in this study.

5. Conclusions

In conclusion, eravacycline is as good as comparators in terms of efficacy and tolerance in the treatment of cIAI in adult patients.

Author Contributions: Conceptualization, S.-H.L., C.-C.L. and C.-M.C.; Data curation, S.-P.C., C.-C.L. and L.-C.L.; Formal analysis, S.-H.L., S.-P.C. and L.-C.L.; Writing—original draft, C.-C.L.; Writing—review & editing, C.-M.C.

Appendix A. Search Strategy

PubMed Search Strategy—Last Searched on 26 May 2019		Results
1	Eravacycline [Title/Abstract] OR TP-434 [Title/Abstract] OR Xerava [Title/Abstract]	74
2	abdom* [Title/Abstract]	330,674
3	1 AND 2	
4	Search (abdom* (Title/Abstract)) AND (((Eravacycline (Title/Abstract)) OR TP-434 (Title/Abstract)) OR Xerava (Title/Abstract))	22

Web of Science Search Strategy—Last Searched on 26 May 2019		Results
1	(Eravacycline) OR (Xerava) OR (TP-434)	71
2	(abdom*)	269,250
3	1 AND 2	
4	#1 AND #2	20

EBSCO Search Strategy—Last Searched on 26 May 2019		Results
1	AB Eravacycline OR AB Xerava OR AB TP-434	176
2	AB abdom*	495,125
3	1 AND 2	
4	S1 AND S2	40

Cochrane Library Search Strategy—Last Searched on 26 May 2019		Results
1	(Eravacycline):ti,ab,kw OR (TP-434):ti,ab,kw OR (Xerava):ti,ab,kw	12
2	(abdom*):ti,ab,kw	40,365
3	1 AND 2	
4	#1 AND #2	5

Ovid Medline Search Strategy—Last Searched on 26 May 2019		Results
1	(Eravacycline or Xerava or TP-434).ab.	82
2	abdom*.ab	373,974
3	1 AND 2	
4	1 and 2	24

Embase Search Strategy—Last Searched on 26 May 2019		Results
1	eravacycline:ti,ab,kw OR xerava:ti,ab,kw OR 'tp 434':ti,ab,kw	87
2	abdom*:ti,ab,kw	508,670
3	1 AND 2	
4	#1 AND #2	27

ClinicalTrials.gov Search Strategy—Last Searched on May 26, 2019		Results
1	Eravacycline (completed studies)	9

References

1. Solomkin, J.S.; Mazuski, J.E.; Baron, E.J.; Sawyer, R.G.; Nathens, A.B.; DiPiro, J.T.; Buchman, T.; Dellinger, E.P.; Jernigan, J.; Gorbach, S.; et al. Guidelines for the selection of anti-infective agents for complicated intra-abdominal infections. *Clin. Infect. Dis.* **2003**, *37*, 997–1005. [CrossRef] [PubMed]
2. Solomkin, J.S.; Mazuski, J.E.; Bradley, J.S.; Rodvold, K.A.; Goldstein, E.J.; Baron, E.J.; O'Neill, P.J.; Chow, A.W.; Dellinger, E.P.; Eachempati, S.R.; et al. Diagnosis and management of complicated intra-abdominal infection in adults and children: guidelines by the Surgical Infection Society and the Infectious Diseases Society of America. *Clin. Infect. Dis.* **2010**, *50*, 133–164. [CrossRef] [PubMed]

3.   Brink, A.J.; Botha, R.F.; Poswa, X.; Senekal, M.; Badal, R.E.; Grolman, D.C.; Richards, G.A.; Feldman, C.; Boffard, K.D.; Veller, M.; et al. Antimicrobial susceptibility of Gram-negative pathogens isolated from patients with complicated intra-abdominal infections in South African hospitals (SMART Study 2004–2009): Impact of the new carbapenem breakpoints. *Surg. Infect. (Larchmt)* **2012**, *13*, 43–49. [CrossRef] [PubMed]

4.   Lee, Y.L.; Chen, Y.S.; Toh, H.S.; Huang, C.C.; Liu, Y.M.; Ho, C.M.; Lu, P.L.; Ko, W.C.; Chen, Y.H.; Wang, J.H.; et al. Antimicrobial susceptibility of pathogens isolated from patients with complicated intra-abdominal infections at five medical centers in Taiwan that continuously participated in the Study for Monitoring Antimicrobial Resistance Trends (SMART) from 2006 to 2010. *Int. J. Antimicrob. Agents* **2012**, *40*, S29–S36. [PubMed]

5.   Sheng, W.H.; Badal, R.E.; Hsueh, P.R. Distribution of extended-spectrum beta-lactamases, AmpC beta-lactamases, and carbapenemases among *Enterobacteriaceae* isolates causing intra-abdominal infections in the Asia-Pacific region: Results of the study for Monitoring Antimicrobial Resistance Trends (SMART). *Antimicrob. Agents Chemother.* **2013**, *57*, 2981–2988. [PubMed]

6.   Zhanel, G.G.; Cheung, D.; Adam, H.; Zelenitsky, S.; Golden, A.; Schweizer, F.; Gorityala, B.; Lagacé-Wiens, P.R.; Walkty, A.; Gin, A.S.; et al. Review of Eravacycline, a Novel Fluorocycline Antibacterial Agent. *Drugs* **2016**, *76*, 567–588. [CrossRef] [PubMed]

7.   Abdallah, M.; Olafisoye, O.; Cortes, C.; Urban, C.; Landman, D.; Quale, J. Activity of eravacycline against *Enterobacteriaceae* and *Acinetobacter baumannii*, including multidrug-resistant isolates, from New York City. *Antimicrob. Agents Chemother.* **2015**, *59*, 1802–1805. [CrossRef] [PubMed]

8.   Livermore, D.M.; Mushtaq, S.; Warner, M.; Woodford, N. In vitro activity of eravacycline against Carbapenem-Resistant *Enterobacteriaceae* and *Acinetobacter baumannii*. *Antimicrob. Agents Chemother.* **2016**, *60*, 3840–3844. [CrossRef] [PubMed]

9.   Seifert, H.; Stefanik, D.; Sutcliffe, J.A.; Higgins, P.G. In-vitro activity of the novel fluorocycline eravacycline against carbapenem non-susceptible *Acinetobacter baumannii*. *Int. J. Antimicrob. Agents* **2018**, *51*, 62–64. [CrossRef] [PubMed]

10.   Zhanel, G.G.; Baxter, M.R.; Adam, H.J.; Sutcliffe, J.; Karlowsky, J.A. In vitro activity of eravacycline against 2213 Gram-negative and 2424 Gram-positive bacterial pathogens isolated in Canadian hospital laboratories: CANWARD surveillance study 2014–2015. *Diagn. Microbiol. Infect. Dis.* **2018**, *91*, 55–62. [CrossRef] [PubMed]

11.   Solomkin, J.; Evans, D.; Slepavicius, A.; Lee, P.; Marsh, A.; Tsai, L.; Sutcliffe, J.A.; Horn, P.A. Assessing the efficacy and safety of eravacycline vs ertapenem in complicated intra-abdominal infections in the Investigating Gram-Negative Infections Treated with Eravacycline (IGNITE 1) trial: A randomized clinical trial. *JAMA Surg.* **2017**, *152*, 224–232. [CrossRef] [PubMed]

12.   Solomkin, J.S.; Gardovskis, J.; Lawrence, K.; Montravers, P.; Sway, A.; Evans, D.; Tsai, L. IGNITE4: Results of a phase 3, randomized, multicenter, prospective trial of eravacycline vs. meropenem in the treatment of complicated intra-abdominal infections. *Clin. Infect. Dis.* **2018**. [CrossRef] [PubMed]

13.   Solomkin, J.S.; Ramesh, M.K.; Cesnauskas, G.; Novikovs, N.; Stefanova, P.; Sutcliffe, J.A.; Walpole, S.M.; Horn, P.T. Phase 2, randomized, double-blind study of the efficacy and safety of two dose regimens of eravacycline versus ertapenem for adult community-acquired complicated intra-abdominal infections. *Antimicrob. Agents Chemother.* **2014**, *58*, 1847–1854. [CrossRef]

14.   Higgins, J.P.; Altman, D.G.; Gotzsche, P.C.; Juni, P.; Moher, D.; Oxman, A.D.; Savovic, J.; Schulz, K.F.; Weeks, L.; Sterne, J.A. The Cochrane Collaboration's tool for assessing risk of bias in randomised trials. *BMJ* **2011**, *343*, d5928. [CrossRef]

15.   Goldstein, E.J.C.; Citron, D.M.; Tyrrell, K.L. In vitro activity of eravacycline and comparator antimicrobials against 143 recent strains of *Bacteroides* and *Parabacteroides* species. *Anaerobe* **2018**, *52*, 122–124. [CrossRef]

16.   Snydman, D.R.; McDermott, L.A.; Jacobus, N.V.; Kerstein, K.; Grossman, T.H.; Sutcliffe, J.A. Evaluation of the in vitro activity of eravacycline against a broad spectrum of recent clinical anaerobic isolates. *Antimicrob. Agents Chemother.* **2018**, *62*, e02206-17. [CrossRef]

17.   Tetraphase Pharmaceuticals Inc. Xerava (Eravacycline): US Prescribing Information. 2018. Available online: http://www.fda.gov (accessed on 23 May 2019).

Predictors of Discordance in the Assessment of Skeletal Muscle Mass between Computed Tomography and Bioimpedance Analysis

Min Ho Jo [1], Tae Seop Lim [1,2], Mi Young Jeon [1,2], Hye Won Lee [1,2], Beom Kyung Kim [1,2,3], Jun Yong Park [1,2,3], Do Young Kim [1,2,3], Sang Hoon Ahn [1,2,3], Kwang-Hyub Han [1,2,3] and Seung Up Kim [1,2,3,*]

[1] Department of Internal Medicine, Institute of Gastroenterology, Yonsei University College of Medicine, Seoul 03722, Korea; zns-1@hanmail.net (M.H.J.); TSLIM21@yuhs.ac (T.S.L.); HYUK4385@yuhs.ac (M.Y.J.); LORRY-LEE@yuhs.ac (H.W.L.); BEOMKKIM@yuhs.ac (B.K.K.); DRPJY@yuhs.ac (J.Y.P.); DYK1025@yuhs.ac (D.Y.K.); AHNSH@yuhs.ac (S.H.A.); GIHANKHYS@yuhs.ac (K.-H.H.)

[2] Yonsei Liver Center, Severance Hospital, Seoul 03722, Korea

[3] Institute of Gastroenterology, Severance Hospital Yonsei University College of Medicine, Seoul 03722, Korea

* Correspondence: KSUKOREA@yuhs.ac

Abstract: Computed tomography (CT) and bioimpedance analysis (BIA) can assess skeletal muscle mass (SMM). Our objective was to identify the predictors of discordance between CT and BIA in assessing SMM. Participants who received a comprehensive medical health check-up between 2010 and 2018 were recruited. The CT and BIA-based diagnostic criteria for low SMM are as follows: Defined CT cutoff values (lumbar skeletal muscle index (LSMI) <1 standard deviation (SD) and means of 46.12 cm^2/m^2 for men and 34.18 cm^2/m^2 for women) and defined BIA cutoff values (appendicular skeletal muscle/height^2 <7.0 kg/m^2 for men and <5.7 kg/m^2 for women). A total of 1163 subjects were selected. The crude and body mass index (BMI)-adjusted SMM assessed by CT were significantly associated with those assessed by BIA (correlation coefficient = 0.78 and 0.68, respectively; $p < 0.001$). The prevalence of low SMM was 15.1% by CT and 16.4% by BIA. Low SMM diagnosed by CT was significantly associated with advanced age, female gender, and lower serum albumin level, whereas low SMM diagnosed by BIA was significantly associated with advanced age, female gender, and lower BMI (all $p < 0.05$). Upon multivariate analysis, age >65 years, female and BMI <25 kg/m^2 had significantly higher risks of discordance than their counterparts (all $p < 0.05$). We found a significant association between SMM assessed by CT and BIA. SMM assessment using CT and BIA should be interpreted cautiously in older adults (>65 years of age), female and BMI <25 kg/m^2.

Keywords: sarcopenia; bioimpedance analysis; computed tomography; discordance

1. Introduction

Sarcopenia is a syndrome characterized by the loss of skeletal muscle mass, strength, and performance [1–3] that results in an increased risk of fracture, dysfunction, reduced quality of life, and increased mortality [4,5]. Due to the varying diagnostic cutoff values for muscle mass and the varying diagnostic tools used in previous studies, the reported prevalence of sarcopenia has been inconsistent [6,7]. Several studies of sarcopenia have been performed, and multiple guidelines have been proposed; these have enhanced our knowledge of the condition. Sarcopenia is now officially recognized as a disorder in some countries, with an ICD-10-MC diagnostic code [8].

The measurement of skeletal muscle mass (SMM) is of paramount importance to diagnose sarcopenia. Several imaging techniques that can assess SMM are currently available: Dual-energy X-ray absorptiometry (DXA), computed tomography (CT), magnetic resonance imaging (MRI), and bioimpedance analysis (BIA) [2]. DXA has several advantages over the other methods, such as safety, accuracy, and non-invasiveness, but it can overestimate muscle mass in cases of muscle edema or intramuscular fat deposition [9]. CT can accurately measure the quantity and quality of SMM, but it is costly and exposes the patient to radiation [2,10]. MRI has no radiation exposure for the patient and accurately measures SMM, but its clinical application is significantly limited due to its high cost [11]. BIA has been recognized as a rapid, inexpensive, portable, and safe methodology but, because BIA measures the resistance to a current that is applied through a body of water, the assessment of SMM may be inaccurate if the patients are dehydrated, overhydrated fluid status or obese [12]. BIA tends to overestimate SMM because it cannot discriminate among appendicular, non-appendicular fat, and non-fat mass [13].

To date, measurement of SMM by BIA has typically been performed using the Kyle, Jassen, Ergi, and Scafoglieri prediction models [14–17]. SMM can now be assessed directly using vertical, eight-point analyzers. Several studies have reported the accuracy and reproducibility of direct segmental multi-frequency BIA and the strong correlation between its results and SMM measured by DXA [18–23]. CT provides an accurate measurement of SMM, with a significant correlation to whole-body muscle mass [24,25]. Accordingly, CT has been considered to be the gold standard for measuring SMM [2,10]. Despite its drawbacks, BIA is more easily applied in clinical practice. Thus, investigating the prevalence of discordance in the assessment of SMM between CT and BIA and identifying predictors of this discordance is valuable. This investigation can ultimately help physicians select the optimal candidates for each modality to diagnose low SMM and interpret the results appropriately.

The primary aim of this study was to identify predictors of discordance between SMM measured by BIA and by CT. The secondary aims were to investigate the prevalence of low SMM by CT and BIA and the correlation between SMM measured by CT and BIA in apparently healthy subjects undergoing comprehensive medical health check-ups.

2. Methods

2.1. Study Subjects

A total of 1191 subjects who visited the health promotion center in Severance Hospital, a university-affiliated tertiary care hospital, for a comprehensive medical health check-up from June 2010 to April 2018 were included, see Figure 1. Severance Hospital is a 2000-bed academic referral hospital in Northwestern Seoul, Republic of Korea. Severance Hospital is supported by Yonsei University College of Medicine. Exclusion criteria were as follows: (1) no BIA data, (2) limited access to BIA data due to personal privacy, (3) poor CT quality, and (4) major operation in the lumbar area.

The study's protocol adhered to the tenets of the Declaration of Helsinki and was approved by the Institutional Review Board of Severance Hospital. Informed consents were waived due to the retrospective nature of the study.

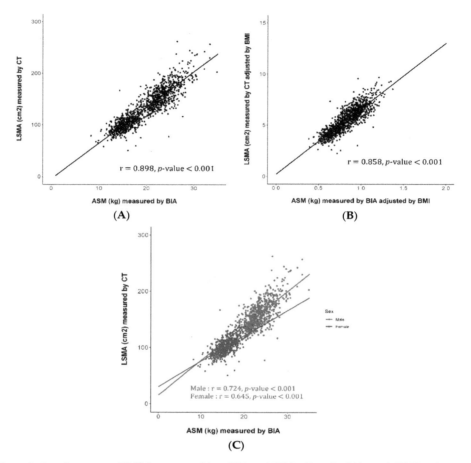

Figure 1. Correlation between SMM assessed by CT and BIA. Crude (**A**) and BMI-adjusted SMM (**B**) assessed by CT were significantly correlated with those by BIA (all $p < 0.001$, correlation coefficient = 0.898 and 0.858, respectively). The correlation between crude SMM assessed by CT and BIA was significant in men and women (**C**) (all $p < 0.001$, correlation coefficient = 0.724 in men and 0.645 in women, respectively). LSMA (cm^2) = −4.366 + 6.920 * ASM (kg), Standard error = 0.099 LSMI adjusted by BMI = 0.212 + 6.424 * (ASM adjusted by BMI), Standard error = 0.113. SMM, skeletal muscle mass; LSMA, lumbar skeletal mass area; AMS, appendicular skeletal mass; CT, computed tomography; BIA, bioimpedance analysis; BMI, body mass index; LMSI, lumbar skeletal muscle index. Regression equations and standard error are as follows.

2.2. Data Collection

A medical health check-up was performed, and collected data included age, gender, height, body weight, body mass index (BMI), and laboratory test results. Histories of hypertension, diabetes, and viral hepatitis were collected from the medical record and individual questionnaires.

2.3. Fibrosis-4 Index Calculation

Recent studies have shown that fibrotic burden in the liver is independently associated with sarcopenia. Therefore, the fibrosis-4 index (FIB-4) was calculated using the following formula: Age (years) × aspartate aminotransferase (AST) (U/L)/(platelets (10^9/L) × alanine aminotransferase (ALT) (U/L))$^{1/2}$ [26].

2.4. Measurements of Skeletal Muscle Area

Skeletal muscle area was measured at the mid-body level of the L3 vertebra in a supine position by a dual-source 128-slice CT scanner (Somatom Definition Flash, Siemens Healthcare, Forchheim, Germany), a 64-slice CT scanner (Somatom Sensation 64, Siemens Healthcare), a Discovery 710 PET-CT 128-slice scanner (General Electric Medical Systems, Milwaukee, WI, USA), a Biograph

TruePoint 40 PET-CT 40-slice scanner (Siemens Medical Solutions, Hoffman Estates, IL, USA), or a Discovery 600 PET-CT 16-slice scanner (General Electric Medical Systems, Milwaukee, WI, USA). The muscle area was identified using attenuation values between -29 to -150 Hounsfield units. Total lumbar skeletal muscle area (psoas, erector spinae, quadratus lumborum, transversus abdominus, external and internal obliques, and rectus abdominus) (cm^2) was defined as a region with density ranging from -29 to -150 Hounsfield units using Aquarius Intuition Viewer software, version 4.4.12 (Terarecon, San Mateo, CA, USA). Boundaries were corrected manually, as necessary. To minimize measurement error, the CT instruments are periodically tested and calibrated for spatial resolution, length measurement, alignment, and linearity of attenuation (CT number) using a standard phantom (AAPM CT Performance Phantom, 76-410). All tests are performed in compliance with the regulations of the Korean Institute for Accreditation of Medical Imaging. The lumbar skeletal muscle index (LSMI) was defined as $10,000 \times$ lumbar skeletal muscle area (LSMA, cm^2)/height^2 (m^2). Based on previous studies [2,10], we assumed that measurement of SMM by CT is more accurate.

The InBody 770 (Biospace Co., Seoul, Korea) measured body composition. Participants fasted for 12 h prior to testing. Participants wore a t-shirt and short pants on the day of testing, and provided their age, gender, and height at the time of measurement. Testing was conducted according to the manufacturer's instructions. Data were uploaded to the electronic medical record. The measurement was comprised of two combinations: z-axis at frequencies of 1, 5, 50, 250, and 500 kHz for impedance, and x-axis at frequencies of 5, 50, and 250 kHz for reactance. Impedance was measured for five body segments: Trunk, right and left arms, and right and left legs. We reviewed the medical records and measured appendicular skeletal muscle (ASM) (kg) through direct segmental multi-frequency BIA [27].

Muscle mass was determined by measuring electrical resistance [28] using four surface tactile electrodes placed on the dorsal surface of the hand and foot. Whole-body resistance (R_{sumx}) was calculated by summing the segmental resistances at frequency x, according to the following equation:

$$R_{sumx} = R_{RA} + R_{LA} + R_T + R_{RL} + R_{LL} \tag{1}$$

The index of R_{sumx} (RI_{sumx}) is calculated by using the following equation:

$$RI_{sumx} \text{ Height (cm)}^2 / R_{sumx} (\Omega) \tag{2}$$

$$\text{Appendicular muscle mass} = 0.236 \times \text{Height}^2/R_{RA} + 0.0109 \times \text{Hright}^{2/}R_T + 0.121 \times \text{Hright}^2/R_{RL} + 1.554 \tag{3}$$

Using the formula above, the muscle mass is automatically calculated in InBody.

2.5. Definition of Low SMM

The CT diagnostic criterion for low SMM was a lumbar skeletal mass index (LSMI) <1 standard deviation (SD) below the sex-specific mean of the study group. The BIA diagnostic criterion for low SMM was adopted from the Asian Working Group of Sarcopenia [6]: ASM/height^2 <7.0 kg/m^2 for men and <5.7 kg/m^2 for women [29].

We also used additional CT and BIA diagnostic criteria for low SMM. The additional criterion for CT was an LSMI ≤ 52.4 cm^2/m^2 for men and ≤ 38.5 cm^2/m^2 for women [30]. The additional criterion for BIA was adopted from The Foundation for the National Institutes of Health: ASM/BMI <0.79 for men and <0.51 for women [7]. We attached the relevant analysis using Supplementary Data.

2.6. Statistical Analysis

Statistical analyses were performed using Statistical Package for the Social Science (SPSS) version 23.0 for Windows (IBM Corp., Armonk, NY, USA). Continuous and categorical variables were expressed as mean $\pm$ standard deviation and n (%), respectively. p-Value < 0.05 was considered statistically significant. Simple and partial correlation analyses were used to analyze the relationship between CT and BIA muscle mass. The distribution between muscle mass by BIA and quartile stratification of muscle mass by CT was evaluated using the Mann-Whitney U test. The comparison between subjects with and without low SMM was performed using the chi-square test for categorical variables and Student's t-test for continuous variables. Multivariate analysis using binary logistic regression analysis was performed on variables that showed a p-value <0.05 and was used to determine the predictors of discordance in defining low SMM between CT and BIA.

3. Results

3.1. Patients

A total of 1191 subjects who underwent a comprehensive medical health check-up were considered eligible. However, 19 subjects were excluded due to a lack of BIA data, and an additional nine subjects were excluded due to poor-quality CT scans and a history of a major operations around the lumbar or appendicular skeletal muscle area. As a result, 1163 subjects were included in the statistical analysis, see Supplementary Figure S1.

Baseline characteristics of the study population (641 men and 521 women) are summarized in Table 1. The mean age of the patients was 57 years; 41.0% were over 60 years of age. The mean BMI of the patients was 24.0 kg/m^2. Of the study population, 41.0% of subjects ($n = 488$) had hypertension, 29.4% ($n = 314$) had diabetes, and 4.9% ($n = 57$) had viral hepatitis. Using CT scans, the mean whole-body fat-free mass and LSMI were 45.3 kg and 46.9 cm^2/m^2, respectively. Using BIA, the mean ASM, ASM index, and ASM/BMI ratio were 20.1 kg, 7.1 kg/m^2, and 0.82, respectively. The mean FIB-4 was 1.17.

Table 1. Baseline characteristics ($n = 1163$).

Variables	All
Demographic parameters	
Age, years	57 (18–92)
<40	59 (5.0)
40–49	182 (15.6)
50–59	445 (38.2)
60–69	296 (25.4)
>70	181 (15.5)
Female gender	521 (43.7)
Body mass index, kg/m^2	24.0 (15.4–43.9)
Hypertension	488 (41.0)
Diabetes mellitus	314 (26.4)
Viral hepatitis	57 (4.9)
Laboratory parameters	
Fasting glucose, mg/dL	96 (58–340)
Aspartate aminotransferase, IU/L	21 (8–140)
Alanine aminotransferase, IU/L	19 (3–196)
Serum albumin, mg/dL	4.3 (3.4–5.3)
Total bilirubin, mg/dL	0.7 (0.2–4.0)
Gamma glutamyl-transpeptidase, IU/L	23 (6–539)
Serum creatinine, mg/dL	0.8 (0.4–7.3)
Platelet count, 10^9/L	231 (89–846)
Prothrombin time, INR	0.9 (0.7–2.3)
Total cholesterol, mg/dL	187 (83–392)
Triglycerides, mg/dL	103 (31–815)
High-density lipoprotein cholesterol, mg/dL	48 (23–115)
Low-density lipoprotein cholesterol, mg/dL	109 (27–299)
HbA1c, %	5.8 (4.4–13.4)
Fibrosis-4 index	1.17 (0.20–5.47)
Muscle mass parameters	
By computed tomography	
Whole body fat-free mass, kg	45.3 (21.2–84.7)
Lumbar skeletal muscle index, cm^2/m^2	46.9 (20.0–85.6)
By bioimpedance analysis	
ASM, kg	20.1 (8.3–34.7)
ASM index, kg/m^2	7.1 (3.2–28.9)
ASM/body mass index	0.82 (0.43–1.23)

Variables are expressed as median (interquartile range) or n (%). INR, international normalized ratio; ASM, appendicular skeletal muscle mass; ASMI, appendicular skeletal mass index.

3.2. Association between SMM Assessed Using CT and BIA

The crude and BMI-adjusted SMM assessed by CT were significantly associated with those assessed by BIA ($p < 0.001$, correlation coefficient = 0.898 for crude SMM; $p < 0.001$, correlation coefficient = 0.858 for BMI-adjusted SMM), see Figure 1A. The association between crude SMM assessed by CT and BIA was statistically significant, regardless of gender ($p < 0.001$, correlation coefficient = 0.724 in men; $p < 0.001$, correlation coefficient = 0.645 in women), as shown in Figure 1. Linear regression results comparing CT and BIA assessed SMM were added to the Supplementary Table S6.

We divided the patients into four groups according to quartiles of SMM assessed by CT and BIA. SMM as assessed by BIA significantly increased according to the CT-assessed SMM quartile ($p < 0.001$), see Supplementary Figure S2.

3.3. Comparison between Subjects with and without Low SMM Assessed by CT

The baseline characteristics of subjects with and without CT-defined low SMM in Table 2. The cutoff value of low SMM was defined as less than one standard deviations sex-specific mean value of the participants. The sex-specific cut-off values of LSMI were 46.12 cm^2/m^2 in men and 34.18 c^2/m^2 in women.

Table 2. Comparison between subjects with and without low SMM assessed by CT.

Variables	without Low SMM	with Low SMM	p-Value
	(n = 988, 84.9%)	(n = 176, 15.1%)	
Demographic parameters			
Age, years	57 (19–92)	63 (18–92)	0.001
Female gender	435 (44.1)	86 (48.8)	0.017
Body mass index, kg/m^2	24.2 (16.5–43.8)	22.4 (15.4–28.9)	0.584
Hypertension	411 (41.5)	77 (43.7)	0.436
Diabetes mellitus	268 (27.1)	46 (26.1)	0.780
Viral hepatitis	45(4.5)	12 (6.8)	0.152
Laboratory parameters			
Fasting glucose, mg/dL	96 (58–340)	96 (65–325)	0.820
Aspartate aminotransferase, IU/L	21 (8–140)	20 (11–69)	0.964
Alanine aminotransferase, IU/L	19 (3–196)	18 (4–58)	0.756
Serum albumin, mg/dL	4.3 (3.4–5.3)	4.2 (3.5–4.8)	0.025
Total bilirubin, mg/dL	0.7 (0.2–4.0)	0.7 (0.2–2.8)	0.441
Gamma glutamyl-transpeptidase, IU/L	23 (7–398)	22 (6–539)	0.407
Serum creatinine, mg/dL	0.81 (0.38–7.3)	0.74 (0.41–2.74)	0.828
Platelet count, 10^9/L	232 (89–846)	229 (122–438)	0.654
Prothrombin time, INR	0.93 (0.78–2.28)	0.94 (0.73–2.15)	0.574
Total cholesterol, mg/dL	188 (83–392)	177 (98–302)	0.007
Triglycerides, mg/dL	105 (31–684)	84.5 (43–815)	0.825
High-density lipoprotein cholesterol, mg/dL	48 (24–100)	50 (23–115)	0.027
Low-density lipoprotein cholesterol, mg/dL	111 (27–299)	100 (43–213)	0.038
HbA1c, %	5.8 (4.4–13.4)	5.8 (4.7–12.4)	0.436
Fibrosis-4 index	1.15 (0.20–5.47)	1.31 (0.37–3.39)	0.825
Muscle mass parameters			
By computed tomography			
Whole body fat-free mass, kg	46.4 (23.9–84.7)	40.8 (21.2–79.3)	0.530
Lumbar skeletal muscle index, cm^2/m^2	48.7 (34.2–85.6)	39.9 (20.0–46.0)	<0.001
By bioimpedance analysis			
ASM, kg	20.3 (10.3–34.7)	18.1 (8.3–27.6)	0.973
ASM index, kg/m^2	7.30 (4.62–10.58)	6.39 (3.24–8.64)	<0.001
ASM/body mass index	0.81 (0.45–1.23)	0.82 (0.43–1.17)	0.044

Variables are expressed as median (interquartile range) or n (%). SMM, skeletal muscle mass; CT, computed tomography; INR, international normalized ratio; ASM, appendicular skeletal muscle mass; ASMI, appendicular skeletal mass index. * CT cutoff indicates <1 standard deviation (SD), sex–specific mean value of the participants.

When CT-defined cutoff values were used, subjects with low SMM were significantly older (median 63 vs. 57 years) and female gender (48.8% vs. 44.1%). Subjects with low SMM had significantly lower serum albumin levels (median 4.2 vs. 4.3 mg/dL), lower total cholesterol (median 177 vs.

188 mg/dL), higher high-density lipoprotein (HDL) cholesterol (median 50 vs. 48 mg/dL) and lower low-density lipoprotein (LDL) cholesterol (median 100 vs. 111 mg/dL) than those of subjects without low SMM (all $p < 0.05$). In addition, various muscle indexes were unfavorable in subjects with CT-defined low SMM.

We also analyzed additional diagnostic criteria for low SMM defined by CT (≤ 52.4 cm^2/m^2 for men and ≤ 38.5 cm^2/m^2 for women), see Supplementary Table S1.

3.4. Comparison between Subjects with and without Low SMM Assessed by BIA

The baseline characteristics of subjects with and without BIA-defined low SMM are shown in Table 3. The cutoff value of low SMM was defined previous study [6]. The Asian Working Group of Sarcopenia defined cutoff values appendicular lean mass (ALM)/height^2 of <7.0 kg/m^2 in men and <5.7 kg/m^2 in women.

Table 3. Comparison between subjects with and without low SMM assessed by BIA.

Variables	without Low SMM (n = 972, 83.6%)	with Low SMM (n = 191, 16.4%)	p-Value
Demographic parameters			
Age, years	57 (19–92)	60 (18–92)	<0.001
Female gender	392 (40.0)	129 (67.5)	<0.001
Body mass index, kg/m^2	24.2 (17.1–43.8)	21.8 (15.4–27.8)	0.005
Hypertension	411 (42.2)	77 (40.3)	0.474
Diabetes mellitus	273 (28.0)	41 (21.4)	0.339
Viral hepatitis	48 (4.9)	9 (4.7)	0.757
Laboratory parameters			
Fasting glucose, mg/dL	97 (58–340)	94 (65–265)	0.701
Aspartate aminotransferase, IU/L	21 (8–140)	20 (11–69)	0.604
Alanine aminotransferase, IU/L	20 (3–196)	17 (5–66)	0.683
Serum albumin, mg/dL	4.3 (3.4–5.2)	4.2 (3.5–5.3)	0.135
Total bilirubin, mg/dL	0.7 (0.2–4.0)	0.7 (0.3–2.5)	0.740
Gamma glutamyl-transpeptidase, IU/L	23 (6–398)	19 (7–539)	<0.001
Serum creatinine, mg/dL	0.82 (0.38–7.01)	0.69 (0.39–7.3)	0.016
Platelet count, 10^9/L	230 (89–846)	241 (122–458)	0.256
Prothrombin time, INR	0.93 (0.73–2.28)	0.94 (0.78–2.15)	0.027
Total cholesterol, mg/dL	185 (83–392)	194 (98–300)	0.918
Triglycerides, mg/dL	106 (31–815)	88 (36–435)	0.915
High-density lipoprotein cholesterol, mg/dL	47 (23–98)	53 (29–115)	0.082
Low-density lipoprotein cholesterol, mg/dL	108 (27–299)	112 (43–213)	0.968
HbA1c, %	5.8 (4.7–13.4)	5.8 (4.4–10.5)	0.386
Fibrosis-4 index	1.16 (0.32–5.47)	1.29 (0.20–4.82)	<0.001
Muscle mass parameters			
By computed tomography			
Whole body fat-free mass, kg	47.7 (21.2~84.7)	34.4 (23.5~54.2)	0.131
Lumbar skeletal muscle index, cm^2/m^2	48.5 (20.0–85.6)	38.0 (27.0–58.1)	<0.001
By bioimpedance analysis			
ASM, kg	21.3 (12.8–34.7)	14.0 (8.3–21.6)	<0.001
ASM index, kg/m^2	7.45 (5.70–10.58)	5.56 (3.24–6.99)	<0.001
ASMI/body mass index	0.83 (0.45–1.23)	0.76 (0.43–1.08)	0.568

Variables are expressed as median (interquartile range) or n (%). BIA Cutoff indicates AWGS index. SMM, skeletal muscle mass; BIA, bioimpedance analysis; INR, international normalized ratio; FNIH, The Foundation for the National Institutes of Health; ALM, appendicular lean mass; ASMI, appendicular skeletal mass index; BMI, body mass index; AWGS, Asian Working Group of Sarcopenia.

When BIA-defined cutoff values were used, subjects with low SMM were significantly older (median 60 vs. 57 years) and had a higher proportion of female subjects (67.5% vs. 40.0%), lower BMI (median 21.8 vs. 24.2 kg/m^2) (all $p < 0.05$). In addition, various muscle indices were unfavorable in subjects with BIA-defined low SMM.

We also analyzed additional diagnostic criteria for low SMM defined by BIA (ALM/BMI <0.79 for men and <0.51 for women), see Supplementary Table S2.

3.5. Prevalence and Predictors of Discordance in Defining Low SMM Assessed by CT and BIA

The proportion of non-discordant and discordant subjects, when different measuring methods were applied (CT vs. BIA), is described in Table 4. The proportion of subjects without low SMM by both CT and BIA was 72.3%, and that of subjects with low SMM ranged was 3.9%. The overall proportion of non-discordant subjects was 76.2%. The results of analysis using additional diagnostic criteria for low SMM are given in Supplementary Table S3.

Table 4. Distribution of subjects with and without low SMM assessed by CT and BIA.

Muscle Mass Assessed by CT	Muscle Mass Assessed by BIA	
	* BIA Cutoff	
	without Low SMM	with Low SMM
	(n = 972, 83.6%)	(n = 191, 16.4%)
** CT cutoff		
Without low SMM (n = 987, 84.9%)	841 (72.3)	146 (12.6)
With low SMM (n = 176, 15.1%)	131 (11.3)	45 (3.9)

Variables are expressed as n (%). * BIA cutoff indicates AWGS index (ASMI, ALM/height^2) of <7.0 kg/m^2 in men and <5.7 kg/m^2. ** CT cutoff indicates <1 SD, sex-specific mean value of the participants. SMM, skeletal muscle mass; CT, computed tomography; BIA, bioimpedance analysis; FNIH, The Foundation for the National Institutes of Health; ALM, appendicular lean mass; ASMI, appendicular skeletal mass index; BMI, body mass index; AWGS, Asian Working Group of Sarcopenia.

To identify the predictors of discordant results by CT and BIA, univariate analysis was performed, see Table 5. Older age (HR = 1.05), female sex (HR = 1.48), lower BMI (HR = 0.73), lower serum albumin level (HR = 0.58), and higher GGT (HR = 1.01) were significantly predictive of discordance between CT- and BIA-defined low SMM (p < 0.05). The results of analyses using the additional diagnostic criteria for low SMM are listed in Supplementary Table S4. The results of basic demographic characteristics, specificity and sensitivity of the low SMM defined by the BIA compared to the low SMM defined by the CT as diagnostic standard criteria, added to Supplementary Table S5.

Among selected independent predictors of the presence of discordance, age, female gender, and BMI were selected for multivariate analysis. Thus, we stratified our study population into two groups according to these three independent variables to check the prevalence of discordance, see Figure 2. Older age (>65 years) (22.3% vs. 12.2%), female gender (20.9% vs. 9.8%), and lower BMI (<25 kg/m^2) (20.1%% vs. 3.5%) had a significantly higher risk of discordance than the counterparts (all p < 0.001). The results of analysis using additional diagnostic criteria for low SMM are given in Supplementary Figure S3.

Table 5. Predictors of discordance between CT and BIA-based low SMM.

Variables	Discordance between CT and BIA-Based Low SMM		
	Univariate	Multivariate	
	p-Value	*p*-Value	OR (95% CI)
Demographic parameters			
Age, years	<0.001	<0.001	1.050 (1.035–1.069)
Female gender	<0.001	0.044	1.480 (1.012–2.303)
Body mass index, kg/m^2	<0.001	<0.001	0.725 (0.668–0.790)
Hypertension	0.420	-	-
Diabetes mellitus	0.219	-	-
Viral hepatitis	0.875	-	-
Laboratory parameters			
Fasting glucose, mg/dL	0.728	-	-
Aspartate aminotransferase, IU/L	0.734	-	-
Alanine aminotransferase, IU/L	0.092	0.021	0.977 (0.955–0.996)
Serum albumin, mg/dL	0.020	0.097	0.581 (0.264–1.117)
Total bilirubin, mg/dL	0.691	-	-
Gamma glutamyl-transpeptidase, IU/L	0.002	<0.001	1.009 (1.004–1.014)
Serum creatinine, mg/dL	0.803	-	-
Platelet count, 10^9/L	0.759	-	-
Prothrombin time, INR	0.084	0.153	3.580 (0.629–19.312)
Total cholesterol, mg/dL	0.277	-	-
Triglycerides, mg/dL	0.096	0.128	1.003 (0.999–1.005)
High-density lipoprotein cholesterol, mg/dL	0.096	0.280	1.011 (0.993–1.023)
Low-density lipoprotein cholesterol, mg/dL	0.172	-	-
HbA1c, %	0.696	-	-
Fibrosis-4 index	0.615	-	-

CT cutoff indicates <1 SD, sex-specific mean value of the participants. BIA cutoff indicates AWGS index (ASMI, ALM/height^2) of <7.0 kg/m^2 in men and <5.7 kg/m^2. SMM, skeletal muscle mass; CT, computed tomography; BIA, bioimpedance analysis; OR, odds ratio; CI, confidence interval; INR, international normalized ratio; FNIH, The Foundation for the National Institutes of Health; ALM, appendicular lean mass; ASMI, appendicular skeletal mass index; BMI, body mass index; AWGS, Asian Working Group of Sarcopenia.

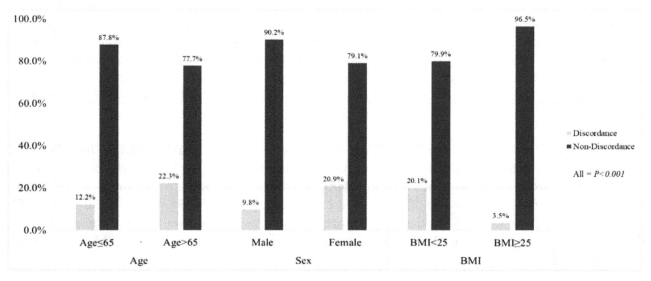

Figure 2. Percentage of subjects with non-discordance and those with discordance in diagnosing low SMM using CT and BIA according to identified independent predictors. Participants with age > 65 years, female gender and BMI < 25 kg/m^2 had a significantly higher proportion of discordance than the counterparts (all *p* < 0.001). CT cutoff indicates < 1 SD. BIA cutoff indicates AWGS index (ASMI, ALM/height^2) of <7.0 kg/m^2 in men and <5.7 kg/m^2. BMI, body mass index; ALM, appendicular lean mass; ASMI, appendicular skeletal mass index; AWGS, Asian Working Group of Sarcopenia.

4. Discussion

The diagnostic criteria for sarcopenia have not yet been definitively established, even though it is one of the most important public health concerns [31]. Varying diagnostic criteria for sarcopenia based on several assessment modalities, which include CT and BIA, are available [2,3,10], and the criteria are different between Asian and Western countries [6,7,32]. Ethnicity is an important factor for the diagnosis of sarcopenia [33]. Several recent research groups have published diagnostic guidelines for sarcopenia, which have emphasized the importance of ethnicity [34,35]. The BIA and CT diagnostic criteria differ according to ethnicity [3,6,7,35]. According to our knowledge, no comparison of BIA and SMM measured by CT at the L3 level has been performed. Therefore, our findings will facilitate the establishment of diagnostic cutoff values for Asian patients.

Our data show a significant association in crude and BMI-adjusted SMM assessed by CT and BIA, although the area assessed was different for each method. Similar to previous studies [3,11,32,36–39], the proportion of subjects with low SMM in our study varied from 15.1% to 16.4% when CT or BIA was used to assess SMM, and the risk factors for discordant results between the methodologies were advanced age, female gender, and lower BMI.

We believe the identified risk factors for discordant results can be explained in several ways: Total fat mass tends to be higher in older adults [40], and BIA can overestimate SMM when the subject has a high fat mass [41]; assessment of SMM using BIA can be overestimated in female subjects who have a higher probability of increased body fat [41]; and there is a weaker correlation between SMM in the limb and L3 area among subjects with a lower BMI [42,43]. All of these factors suggest that CT may be required for a more accurate assessment of SMM in subjects with advanced age, female gender, and low BMI.

Our study has several strengths. First, the overall sample size was over 1100, which ensures the statistical power and precision of our results. We adopted several cutoff values for CT and BIA when defining low SMM, and we found the three factors of age, gender, and BMI to be associated with discordance between CT- and BIA-based SMM assessments. Second, we focused on the general population instead of medically vulnerable subjects, such as only older adults, or those with liver cirrhosis or cancers for whom sarcopenia already showed clinical implications. Similar to our study, several recent studies proved the clinical significance of assessing sarcopenia in the general population and non-alcoholic fatty liver disease (NAFLD) subjects [44,45]. Thus, our study provides information that helps to identify optimal subjects for CT-based assessment of sarcopenia. Third, in contrast to most previous studies [7,11,27,46], we adopted several cutoff values for SMM assessed by CT and BIA. Although the predictors of discordance were not exactly the same, we obtained relatively consistent results regardless of the cutoff value used. Fourth, several studies have compared DXA and BIA, but few have directly compared CT and BIA to assess SMM [46,47]. In our study, SMM using CT and BIA was measured on the same day, in contrast to most previous studies [9,25,46]. As a result, any bias caused by different time points of SMM assessments may have been prevented. Lastly, because there are significant differences in SMM between Western and Asian populations, focusing on a single ethnicity may be important. Thus, the results of our study could be optimized for an Asian population.

Several issues remain unresolved in our study. First, although we adopted several known cutoff values for CT and BIA, the results of our study should be further validated based on existing diagnostic criteria for sarcopenia. Second, recent studies have insisted that other factors, such as muscle strength and walking speed, should be considered when diagnosing sarcopenia. However, our study was retrospectively performed based on the clinical information of the subjects who underwent a comprehensive medical health check-up, and we only used SMM to define sarcopenia. Further studies with additional markers of sarcopenia should validate our results. Third, our study only included subjects who were willing to receive and could afford a medical health check-up. The prevalence of hypertension (29.1%) and diabetes (11.3%) in the general Korean population in 2016 (Korean Center for Disease Control and Prevention; Ministry of Health and Welfare) [48], were lower than those in this study (41.0% and 26.4%, respectively). In Korea, individuals >40 years of age are eligible for basic health check-ups; those with chronic diseases such as hypertension and diabetes receive health checkups more frequently. The mean age of our patients was 57 years, and 40.9% were >60 years of age. Because of this potential selection bias, our results may not be fully applicable to the general population, but this can be resolved in future studies. Fourth, SMM measured by BIA is affected by the hydration status [12]. The patients were admitted to the health check-up unit and fasted overnight. Thus, the hydration status of all of the patients should have been similar. Lastly, when discordant results between CT- and BIA-based SMM assessments were obtained, we did not know which diagnostic modality to accept. For patients with discordant CT and BIA results, it is important to decide which results should be used. However, a definitive diagnostic method for sarcopenia has not been established. This issue should be explored in future longitudinal follow-up studies that use solid end-points, such as mortality. This issue should be explored in future longitudinal follow-up studies that use solid end-points such as mortality, which might propose the right direction toward CT or BIA.

In conclusion, the significant association between CT and BIA for SMM assessment suggests that BIA could be used to assess sarcopenia in clinical practice. However, because advanced age, female gender, and low BMI were risk factors for discordant results between CT and BIA, BIA assessment should be interpreted cautiously in subjects with these risk factors and, if possible, CT or other modalities should be considered as an alternative diagnostic tool to assess SMM to define sarcopenia.

Supplementary Materials:
Supplementary Figure S1: Flow chart depicting selection of the study population. Supplementary Figure S2: Distribution of skeletal muscle mass assessed by BIA according to quartile stratification of skeletal muscle mass assessed by CT. Supplementary Figure S3. Percentage of subjects with non-discordance and those with discordance in diagnosing low skeletal muscle mass assessed using CT and BIA according to identified independent predictors. Participants with Age>65 years (A), female gender (B) and BMI<25 kg/m^2 (C). Supplementary Table S1: Comparison between subjects with and without low skeletal muscle mass assessed by CT. Supplementary Table S2: Comparison between subjects with and without low skeletal muscle mass assessed by BIA. Supplementary Table S3: Distribution of subjects with and without low skeletal muscle mass according to CT and BIA. Supplementary Table S4: Predictors of discordance in defining low skeletal muscle mass assessed by CT and BIA Supplementary Table S5: Basic demographic characteristics, specificity and sensitivity of the low SMM defined by the BIA compared to the low SMM defined by the CT as diagnostic standard criteria. Supplementary Table S1: Linear regression results of comparing SMM evaluated by CT and BIA.

Author Contributions: Conceptualization, M.H.J. and S.U.K.; methodology, M.H.J., T.S.L., M.Y.J. and S.U.K.; participation in patient management and data collection; H.W.L., B.K.K., J.Y.P., D.Y.K., S.H.A., K.-H.H. and S.U.K.; contribution to the data acquisition, responsibility for writing the paper, and statistical analysis: M.H.J. and S.U.K.; All authors reviewed the paper and approved the final version.

Acknowledgments: This study was supported by the Liver Cirrhosis Clinical Research Center, in part by a grant from the Korea Healthcare technology R & D project, Ministry of Health and Welfare, Republic of Korea (no. HI10C2020). The funders had no role in study design, data collection and analysis, decision to publish, or preparation of the manuscript.

References

1.   Roubenoff, R. Origins and clinical relevance of sarcopenia. *Can. J. Appl. Physiol.* **2001**, *26*, 78–89. [CrossRef] [PubMed]

2.   Cruz-Jentoft, A.J.; Baeyens, J.P.; Bauer, J.M.; Boirie, Y.; Cederholm, T.; Landi, F.; Martin, F.C.; Michel, J.P.; Rolland, Y.; Schneider, S.M.; et al. Sarcopenia: European consensus on definition and diagnosis: Report of the european working group on sarcopenia in older people. *Age Ageing* **2010**, *39*, 412–423. [CrossRef] [PubMed]

3.   Janssen, I. The epidemiology of sarcopenia. *Clin. Geriatr. Med.* **2011**, *27*, 355–363. [CrossRef] [PubMed]

4.   Cesari, M.; Pahor, M.; Lauretani, F.; Zamboni, V.; Bandinelli, S.; Bernabei, R.; Guralnik, J.M.; Ferrucci, L. Skeletal muscle and mortality results from the inchianti study. *J. Gerontol. A. Biol. Sci. Med. Sci.* **2009**, *64*, 377–384. [CrossRef] [PubMed]

5.	Newman, A.B.; Kupelian, V.; Visser, M.; Simonsick, E.M.; Goodpaster, B.H.; Kritchevsky, S.B.; Tylavsky, F.A.; Rubin, S.M.; Harris, T.B. Strength, but not muscle mass, is associated with mortality in the health, aging and body composition study cohort. *J. Gerontol. A. Biol. Sci. Med. Sci.* **2006**, *61*, 72–77. [CrossRef] [PubMed]

6.	Chen, L.K.; Liu, L.K.; Woo, J.; Assantachai, P.; Auyeung, T.W.; Bahyah, K.S.; Chou, M.Y.; Chen, L.Y.; Hsu, P.S.; Krairit, O.; et al. Sarcopenia in Asia: Consensus report of the asian working group for sarcopenia. *J. Am. Med. Dir. Assoc.* **2014**, *15*, 95–101. [CrossRef] [PubMed]

7.	Studenski, S.A.; Peters, K.W.; Alley, D.E.; Cawthon, P.M.; McLean, R.R.; Harris, T.B.; Ferrucci, L.; Guralnik, J.M.; Fragala, M.S.; Kenny, A.M.; et al. The fnih sarcopenia project: Rationale, study description, conference recommendations, and final estimates. *J. Gerontol. A. Biol. Sci. Med. Sci.* **2014**, *69*, 547–558. [CrossRef] [PubMed]

8.	Vellas, B.; Fielding, R.A.; Bens, C.; Bernabei, R.; Cawthon, P.M.; Cederholm, T.; Cruz-Jentoft, A.J.; Del Signore, S.; Donahue, S.; Morley, J.; et al. Implications of ICD-10 for sarcopenia clinical practice and clinical trials: Report by the international conference on frailty and sarcopenia research task force. *J. Frailty Aging* **2018**, *7*, 2–9. [PubMed]

9.	Proctor, D.N.; O'Brien, P.C.; Atkinson, E.J.; Nair, K.S. Comparison of techniques to estimate total body skeletal muscle mass in people of different age groups. *Am. J. Physiol.* **1999**, *277*, 489–495. [CrossRef] [PubMed]

10.	Lee, R.C.; Wang, Z.M.; Heymsfield, S.B. Skeletal muscle mass and aging: Regional and whole-body measurement methods. *Can. J. Appl. Physiol.* **2001**, *26*, 102–122. [CrossRef] [PubMed]

11.	Chien, M.Y.; Huang, T.Y.; Wu, Y.T. Prevalence of sarcopenia estimated using a bioelectrical impedance analysis prediction equation in community-dwelling elderly people in taiwan. *J. Am. Geriatr. Soc.* **2008**, *56*, 1710–1715. [CrossRef] [PubMed]

12.	Chumlea, W.C.; Guo, S.S. Bioelectrical impedance and body composition: Present status and future directions. *Nutr. Rev.* **1994**, *52*, 123–131. [CrossRef] [PubMed]

13.	Batsis, J.A.; Mackenzie, T.A.; Barre, L.K.; Lopez-Jimenez, F.; Bartels, S.J. Sarcopenia, sarcopenic obesity and mortality in older adults: Results from the national health and nutrition examination survey III. *Eur. J. Clin. Nutr.* **2014**, *68*, 1001–1007. [CrossRef] [PubMed]

14.	Janssen, I.; Heymsfield, S.B.; Baumgartner, R.N.; Ross, R. Estimation of skeletal muscle mass by bioelectrical impedance analysis. *J. Appl. Physiol.* **2000**, *89*, 465–471. [CrossRef] [PubMed]

15.	Kyle, U.G.; Genton, L.; Hans, D.; Pichard, C. Validation of a bioelectrical impedance analysis equation to predict appendicular skeletal muscle mass (ASMM). *Clin. Nutr.* **2003**, *22*, 537–543. [CrossRef]

16.	Sergi, G.; De Rui, M.; Veronese, N.; Bolzetta, F.; Berton, L.; Carraro, S.; Bano, G.; Coin, A.; Manzato, E.; Perissinotto, E. Assessing appendicular skeletal muscle mass with bioelectrical impedance analysis in free-living caucasian older adults. *Clin. Nutr.* **2015**, *34*, 667–673. [CrossRef] [PubMed]

17.	Scafoglieri, A.; Clarys, J.P.; Bauer, J.M.; Verlaan, S.; Van Malderen, L.; Vantieghem, S.; Cederholm, T.; Sieber, C.C.; Mets, T.; Bautmans, I.; et al. Predicting appendicular lean and fat mass with bioelectrical impedance analysis in older adults with physical function decline - the provide study. *Clin. Nutr.* **2017**, *36*, 869–875. [CrossRef] [PubMed]

18.	Karelis, A.D.; Chamberland, G.; Aubertin-Leheudre, M.; Duval, C.; Ecological mobility in Aging and Parkinson (EMAP) Group. Validation of a portable bioelectrical impedance analyzer for the assessment of body composition. *Appl. Physiol. Nutr. Metab.* **2013**, *38*, 27–32. [CrossRef] [PubMed]

19.	Ling, C.H.; de Craen, A.J.; Slagboom, P.E.; Gunn, D.A.; Stokkel, M.P.; Westendorp, R.G.; Maier, A.B. Accuracy of direct segmental multi-frequency bioimpedance analysis in the assessment of total body and segmental body composition in middle-aged adult population. *Clin. Nutr.* **2011**, *30*, 610–615. [CrossRef] [PubMed]

20.	Kim, H.; Kim, C.H.; Kim, D.W.; Park, M.; Park, H.S.; Min, S.S.; Han, S.H.; Yee, J.Y.; Chung, S.; Kim, C. External cross-validation of bioelectrical impedance analysis for the assessment of body composition in korean adults. *Nutr. Res. Pract.* **2011**, *5*, 246–252. [CrossRef] [PubMed]

21.	Gibson, A.L.; Holmes, J.C.; Desautels, R.L.; Edmonds, L.B.; Nuudi, L. Ability of new octapolar bioimpedance spectroscopy analyzers to predict 4-component-model percentage body fat in hispanic, black, and white adults. *Am. J. Clin. Nutr.* **2008**, *87*, 332–338. [CrossRef] [PubMed]

22.	Malavolti, M.; Mussi, C.; Poli, M.; Fantuzzi, A.L.; Salvioli, G.; Battistini, N.; Bedogni, G. Cross-calibration of eight-polar bioelectrical impedance analysis versus dual-energy x-ray absorptiometry for the assessment of total and appendicular body composition in healthy subjects aged 21–82 years. *Ann. Hum. Biol.* **2003**, *30*, 380–391. [CrossRef] [PubMed]

23. Ward, L.C. Segmental bioelectrical impedance analysis: An update. *Curr. Opin. Clin. Nutr. Metab. Care* **2012**, *15*, 424–429. [CrossRef] [PubMed]

24. Hanaoka, M.; Yasuno, M.; Ishiguro, M.; Yamauchi, S.; Kikuchi, A.; Tokura, M.; Ishikawa, T.; Nakatani, E.; Uetake, H. Morphologic change of the psoas muscle as a surrogate marker of sarcopenia and predictor of complications after colorectal cancer surgery. *Int. J. Colorectal Dis.* **2017**, *32*, 847–856. [CrossRef] [PubMed]

25. Mourtzakis, M.; Prado, C.M.; Lieffers, J.R.; Reiman, T.; McCargar, L.J.; Baracos, V.E. A practical and precise approach to quantification of body composition in cancer patients using computed tomography images acquired during routine care. *Appl. Physiol. Nutr. Metab.* **2008**, *33*, 997–1006. [CrossRef] [PubMed]

26. Vallet-Pichard, A.; Mallet, V.; Nalpas, B.; Verkarre, V.; Nalpas, A.; Dhalluin-Venier, V.; Fontaine, H.; Pol, S. Fib-4: An inexpensive and accurate marker of fibrosis in hcv infection. Comparison with liver biopsy and fibrotest. *Hepatology* **2007**, *46*, 32–36. [CrossRef] [PubMed]

27. Buckinx, F.; Reginster, J.Y.; Dardenne, N.; Croisiser, J.L.; Kaux, J.F.; Beaudart, C.; Slomian, J.; Bruyere, O. Concordance between muscle mass assessed by bioelectrical impedance analysis and by dual energy x-ray absorptiometry: A cross-sectional study. *BMC Musculoskelet Disord.* **2015**, *16*, 60. [CrossRef] [PubMed]

28. Forslund, A.H.; Johansson, A.G.; Sjodin, A.; Bryding, G.; Ljunghall, S.; Hambraeus, L. Evaluation of modified multicompartment models to calculate body composition in healthy males. *Am. J. Clin. Nutr.* **1996**, *63*, 856–862. [CrossRef] [PubMed]

29. Han, D.S.; Chang, K.V.; Li, C.M.; Lin, Y.H.; Kao, T.W.; Tsai, K.S.; Wang, T.G.; Yang, W.S. Skeletal muscle mass adjusted by height correlated better with muscular functions than that adjusted by body weight in defining sarcopenia. *Sci. Rep.* **2016**, *6*, 19457. [CrossRef] [PubMed]

30. Montano-Loza, A.J.; Meza-Junco, J.; Prado, C.M.; Lieffers, J.R.; Baracos, V.E.; Bain, V.G.; Sawyer, M.B. Muscle wasting is associated with mortality in patients with cirrhosis. *Clin. Gastroenterol. Hepatol.* **2012**, *10*, 166–173. [CrossRef] [PubMed]

31. Dasarathy, S.; Merli, M. Sarcopenia from mechanism to diagnosis and treatment in liver disease. *J. Hepatol.* **2016**, *65*, 1232–1244. [CrossRef] [PubMed]

32. Baumgartner, R.N.; Koehler, K.M.; Gallagher, D.; Romero, L.; Heymsfield, S.B.; Ross, R.R.; Garry, P.J.; Lindeman, R.D. Epidemiology of sarcopenia among the elderly in new mexico. *Am. J. Epidemiol.* **1998**, *147*, 755–763. [CrossRef] [PubMed]

33. Shafiee, G.; Keshtkar, A.; Soltani, A.; Ahadi, Z.; Larijani, B.; Heshmat, R. Prevalence of sarcopenia in the world: A systematic review and meta- analysis of general population studies. *J. Diabetes Metab. Disord* **2017**, *16*, 21. [CrossRef] [PubMed]

34. Dent, E.; Morley, J.E.; Cruz-Jentoft, A.J.; Arai, H.; Kritchevsky, S.B.; Guralnik, J.; Bauer, J.M.; Pahor, M.; Clark, B.C.; Cesari, M.; et al. International clinical practice guidelines for Sarcopenia (ICFSR): Screening, Diagnosis and Management. *J. Nutr. Health. Aging* **2018**, *22*, 1148–1161. [CrossRef] [PubMed]

35. Cruz-Jentoft, A.J.; Bahat, G.; Bauer, J.; Boirie, Y.; Bruyere, O.; Cederholm, T.; Cooper, C.; Landi, F.; Rolland, Y.; Sayer, A.A.; et al. Sarcopenia: Revised European consensus on definition and diagnosis. *Age Ageing* **2019**, *48*, 16–31. [CrossRef] [PubMed]

36. Kim, T.N.; Park, M.S.; Yang, S.J.; Yoo, H.J.; Kang, H.J.; Song, W.; Seo, J.A.; Kim, S.G.; Kim, N.H.; Baik, S.H.; et al. Prevalence and determinant factors of sarcopenia in patients with type 2 diabetes: The Korean Sarcopenic Obesity Study (KSOS). *Diabetes Care* **2010**, *33*, 1497–1499. [CrossRef] [PubMed]

37. Kim, T.N.; Yang, S.J.; Yoo, H.J.; Lim, K.I.; Kang, H.J.; Song, W.; Seo, J.A.; Kim, S.G.; Kim, N.H.; Baik, S.H.; et al. Prevalence of sarcopenia and sarcopenic obesity in Korean adults: The Korean sarcopenic obesity study. *Int. J. Obes.* **2009**, *33*, 885–892. [CrossRef] [PubMed]

38. Lau, E.M.; Lynn, H.S.; Woo, J.W.; Kwok, T.C.; Melton, L.J., 3rd. Prevalence of and risk factors for sarcopenia in elderly Chinese men and women. *J. Gerontol. A Biol. Sci. Med. Sci.* **2005**, *60*, 213–216. [CrossRef] [PubMed]

39. Lim, S.; Kim, J.H.; Yoon, J.W.; Kang, S.M.; Choi, S.H.; Park, Y.J.; Kim, K.W.; Lim, J.Y.; Park, K.S.; Jang, H.C. Sarcopenic obesity: Prevalence and association with metabolic syndrome in the Korean Longitudinal Study on Health and Aging (KLoSHA). *Diabetes Care* **2010**, *33*, 1652–1654. [CrossRef] [PubMed]

40. Baumgartner, R.N.; Stauber, P.M.; McHugh, D.; Koehler, K.M.; Garry, P.J. Cross-sectional age differences in body composition in persons 60+ years of age. *J. Gerontol. A Biol. Sci. Med. Sci.* **1995**, *50*, M307–M316. [CrossRef] [PubMed]

41. Lloret Linares, C.; Ciangura, C.; Bouillot, J.L.; Coupaye, M.; Decleves, X.; Poitou, C.; Basdevant, A.; Oppert, J.M. Validity of leg-to-leg bioelectrical impedance analysis to estimate body fat in obesity. *Obes. Surg.* **2011**, *21*, 917–923. [CrossRef] [PubMed]

42. Pomeroy, E.; Macintosh, A.; Wells, J.C.K.; Cole, T.J.; Stock, J.T. Relationship between body mass, lean mass, fat mass, and limb bone cross-sectional geometry: Implications for estimating body mass and physique from the skeleton. *Am. J. Phys. Anthropol.* **2018**, *166*, 56–69. [CrossRef] [PubMed]

43. Bosy-Westphal, A.; Muller, M.J. Identification of skeletal muscle mass depletion across age and BMI groups in health and disease—There is need for a unified definition. *Int. J. Obes.* **2015**, *39*, 379–386. [CrossRef] [PubMed]

44. Lee, Y.H.; Jung, K.S.; Kim, S.U.; Yoon, H.J.; Yun, Y.J.; Lee, B.W.; Kang, E.S.; Han, K.H.; Lee, H.C.; Cha, B.S. Sarcopaenia is associated with NAFLD independently of obesity and insulin resistance: Nationwide surveys (KNHANES 2008-2011). *J. Hepatol.* **2015**, *63*, 486–493. [CrossRef] [PubMed]

45. Lee, Y.H.; Kim, S.U.; Song, K.; Park, J.Y.; Kim, D.Y.; Ahn, S.H.; Lee, B.W.; Kang, E.S.; Cha, B.S.; Han, K.H. Sarcopenia is associated with significant liver fibrosis independently of obesity and insulin resistance in nonalcoholic fatty liver disease: Nationwide surveys (KNHANES 2008–2011). *Hepatology* **2016**, *63*, 776–786. [CrossRef] [PubMed]

46. Lee, S.Y.; Ahn, S.; Kim, Y.J.; Ji, M.J.; Kim, K.M.; Choi, S.H.; Jang, H.C.; Lim, S. Comparison between dual-energy X-ray absorptiometry and bioelectrical impedance analyses for accuracy in measuring whole body muscle mass and appendicular skeletal muscle mass. *Nutrients* **2018**, *10*. [CrossRef] [PubMed]

47. Vermeiren, S.; Beckwee, D.; Vella-Azzopardi, R.; Beyer, I.; Knoop, V.; Jansen, B.; Delaere, A.; Antoine, A.; Bautmans, I.; Scafoglieri, A.; et al. Evaluation of appendicular lean mass using bio impedance in persons aged 80+: A new equation based on the BUTTERFLY-study. *Clin. Nutr.* **2018**. [CrossRef] [PubMed]

48. National Health Statistics. Available online: http://www.index.go.kr/potal/main/EachDtlPageDetail.do?idx_cd=1438 (accessed on 10 December 2018).

Evaluation of Transfer Learning with Deep Convolutional Neural Networks for Screening Osteoporosis in Dental Panoramic Radiographs

Ki-Sun Lee [1,2,3,*], **Seok-Ki Jung** [4], **Jae-Jun Ryu** [5], **Sang-Wan Shin** [6,7] **and Jinwook Choi** [1,8,*]

[1] Department of Biomedical Engineering, College of Medicine, Seoul National University, Seoul 03080, Korea
[2] Department of Clinical Dentistry, College of Medicine, Korea University, Seoul 02841, Korea
[3] Department of Prosthodontics, Korea University An-san Hospital, Gyung-gi do 15355, Korea
[4] Department of Orthodontics, Korea University Ansan Hospital, Gyung-gi do 15355, Korea; jgosggg@korea.ac.kr
[5] Department of Prosthodontics, Korea University Anam Hospital, Seoul 02841, Korea; koprosth@unitel.co.kr
[6] Department of Advanced Prosthodontics, Graduate School of Clinical Dentistry, Korea University, Seoul 02841, Korea; swshin@korea.ac.kr
[7] Institute of Clinical Dental Research, Korea University, Seoul 02841, Korea
[8] Institute of Medical & Biological Engineering, Medical Research Center, Seoul 03080, Korea
* Correspondence: kisuns@gmail.com (K.-S.L.); jinchoi@snu.ac.kr (J.C.)

Abstract: Dental panoramic radiographs (DPRs) provide information required to potentially evaluate bone density changes through a textural and morphological feature analysis on a mandible. This study aims to evaluate the discriminating performance of deep convolutional neural networks (CNNs), employed with various transfer learning strategies, on the classification of specific features of osteoporosis in DPRs. For objective labeling, we collected a dataset containing 680 images from different patients who underwent both skeletal bone mineral density and digital panoramic radiographic examinations at the Korea University Ansan Hospital between 2009 and 2018. Four study groups were used to evaluate the impact of various transfer learning strategies on deep CNN models as follows: a basic CNN model with three convolutional layers (CNN3), visual geometry group deep CNN model (VGG-16), transfer learning model from VGG-16 (VGG-16_TF), and fine-tuning with the transfer learning model (VGG-16_TF_FT). The best performing model achieved an overall area under the receiver operating characteristic of 0.858. In this study, transfer learning and fine-tuning improved the performance of a deep CNN for screening osteoporosis in DPR images. In addition, using the gradient-weighted class activation mapping technique, a visual interpretation of the best performing deep CNN model indicated that the model relied on image features in the lower left and right border of the mandibular. This result suggests that deep learning-based assessment of DPR images could be useful and reliable in the automated screening of osteoporosis patients.

Keywords: osteoporosis screening; artificial intelligence; convolutional neural networks; dental panoramic radiographs

1. Introduction

Osteoporosis is a systemic disease characterized by low bone mineral density (BMD) and micro-architectural deterioration of bone structure, thereby leading to compromised bone strength and, consequently, an increased risk of fracture [1]. Hip, spine, and wrist fractures caused by osteoporosis often lead to disorders that reduce the quality of life of the patient and, in severe cases, increase the risk of mortality [2,3]. With fast population aging and an increase in life expectancy, osteoporosis is increasingly becoming a global public health issue; it has been estimated that more than 200 million people are suffering from osteoporosis [4]. According to recent statistics from the International Osteoporosis Foundation, approximately one in three women over the age of 50 will experience osteoporotic fractures, as will one in five men over the age of 50 [4–7]. Moreover, it is expected that more people will be affected by osteoporosis in the future and, consequently, the rate of osteoporotic fractures will increase [8]. This is because the disease initially develops without any symptoms, remains undiagnosed due to scarce symptomatology, and its first manifestation is often a low-energy fracture of long bones or vertebrae [9].

Generally, osteoporosis is diagnosed by evaluating bone mineral density (BMD) measurements (expressed as a T-score) using dual-energy X-ray absorptiometry (DXA), which is considered as the reference-standard examination for BMD assessment [10,11]. However, this technique is complex, expensive, and the availability is limited for overall population diagnosis [12]. Recently, digital images of dental panoramic radiographs (DPRs) have been evaluated as cost-effective and important image data for osteoporosis screening. This is because the widespread use of panoramic radiation in dental care for elderly patients with increased life expectancy and a number of studies have demonstrated the feasibility of BMD estimation and osteoporosis screening using panoramic radiography [13–23].

However, previous approaches primarily relied on manually categorized feature indexes [13–23], such as the Gonion index, mandibular cortical index, mental index, and panoramic mandibular index, and traditional classifier called machine learning (ML) algorithms, such as support vector machine (SVM) [22] and fuzzy classifiers [23], for screening osteoporosis. Although the previously handcrafted feature indexes provided sufficient evidence for assisting osteoporosis screening using panoramic radiographs, these methods for discriminating features are of a low order and do not fully characterize the heterogeneous pattern in radiographic images. In addition, most previous studies require tedious and manual operations, such as extensive preprocessing, image normalization, and region of interest (ROI) segmentation, which can significantly affect the repeatability of the classification method.

In the last few years, deep learning algorithms, particularly deep convolutional neural networks (CNNs) architecture, have been widely recognized as a reliable approach to learn the classification of the characteristics of features directly from original medical images [24,25]. As opposed to ML approaches that rely on explicitly classified features, deep CNNs are a class of deep neural networks that can learn high dimensional features to maximize the networks ability to discriminate abnormalities among images [26]. There are many different CNN architectures that have been designed to perform image classifications and recognitions. Each of these architectures differ in specific aspects, including the number and size of layers, the connections between these layers, and the overall network depth. Because different network architectures are best suited for different problems, and it is difficult to know in advance which architecture is the right choice for a given task, empirical examination is often recognized as the best way to make these decisions [27].

Although deep CNNs have been recognized as efficient tools for image classification, they require a large amount of training data, which can be difficult to apply to medical radiographic image data. When the target dataset is significantly smaller than the base dataset, transfer learning is considered a powerful technique for training deep CNNs without overfitting [28,29]. The general process of transfer learning is performed through the use of pretrained models in a two-step method as follows: First, copying the first n layers of pretrained base network on a general large dataset to the first n layers of a target network and secondly, the remaining layers of the target network are then randomly initialized and trained on a small local dataset toward the target task [28]. On the basis of the transfer learning techniques, several state-of-the-art results showed outperformance in both general image classification [30–32] and medical image classification [33–36]. However, a few studies have been done to develop and evaluate transfer learning-based deep CNN models for predicting osteoporosis in DPRs.

The aim of this study is to develop and evaluate the deep learning approaches for screening osteoporosis with DPR images. Using the classified panoramic radiograph images based on the BMD value (T-score), this study evaluated several different CNN models based on osteoporosis discriminating accuracy. In addition, we quantitatively evaluated the effect of transfer learning and fine-tuning of a deep CNN model on classifying performance.

2. Patients and Methods

2.1. Patients

The study was done on a total of 680 panoramic radiograph images from 680 different patients who visited the Korea University Ansan Hospital. The patients simultaneously underwent skeletal BMD examinations and digital panoramic radiography evaluations within four months, between 2009 and 2018. The subjects were classified into a non-osteoporosis group (T-score ≥ -2.5) or osteoporosis group (T-score < -2.5), according to the World Health Organization criteria [37], into which 380 and 300 subjects were assigned, respectively. The dataset was divided into training and test sets as follows: The radiographs were selected randomly, and 136 radiographs (20% of the total), 68 each from the osteoporosis and non-osteoporosis groups, were set aside as a test set. This ensured that the testing data set only contained images of novel radiographs that had not been encountered by the model during training. The remaining 544 radiographs were used for the training and validation set. This study protocol was approved by the institutional review board of the Korea University Ansan Hospital (no. 2019AS0126).

2.2. Data Preprocessing

The dimensions of the collected dental X-ray images varied from 1348 to 2820 pixels in width and 685 to 1348 pixels in height. For consistency of image preprocessing, the images were downsampled to a uniform size of 1200×630 pixels, using bilinear interpolation. The final ROI was restricted to the lower part of the mandible, below the teeth-containing alveolar bone, for an image size of 700×140 pixels (Figure 1). This included the most ROI areas of previous studies [13–23] that applied various classification techniques by detailed and specifically indexing the image feature characteristics of the limited small region of mandible. By setting the ROI to include most of the mandible instead of the specific area of it, this study evaluated the area that plays the most distinctive role in osteoporosis classification through explainable deep learning techniques.

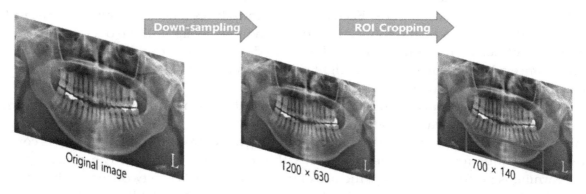

Figure 1. Image preprocessing for this study. The original DPRs were downsampled, and the ROI is restricted to the mandibular region below the teeth (region inside the bounding box). DPR, dental panoramic radiograph; ROI, region of interest.

2.3. Convolutional Neural Networks

This study employed four study groups of CNN as follows: a basic CNN model with three convolutional layers (CNN3), a visual geometry group deep CNN model with no pre-trained weights (VGG16), a transfer learning model from VGG16 with pre-trained weights (VGG16-TF), and a transfer learning and fine-tuning model from VGG16 with pre-trained weights (VGG16-TF-FT). The preceding architectures, along with the four variant CNN models (CNN3, VGG16, VGG16-TR, and VGG16-TR-FT) used in this study, are depicted in the block diagram in Figure 2.

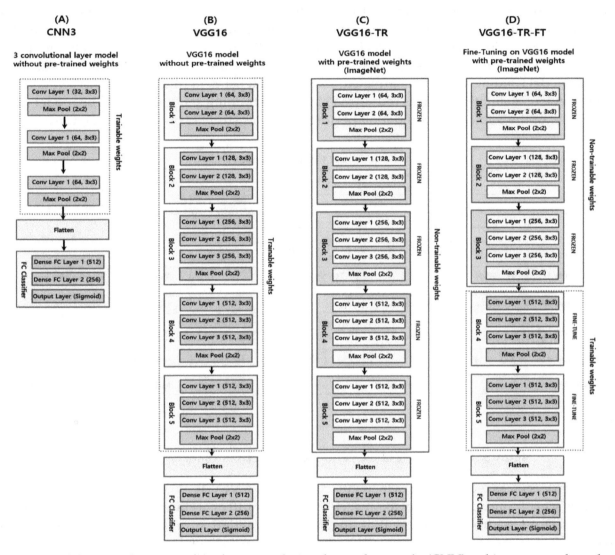

Figure 2. Schematic diagrams of the four convolutional neural networks (CNN) architectures evaluated in this study.

The reason for choosing VGG16 [31] architecture was that it had been widely adopted and recognized as state-of-the-art in both general and medical image classification tasks [24]. Additionally, it has been trained on large-scale datasets, so that a transfer learning approach could be adopted for large-scale image recognition [38]. For the VGG16 architecture under consideration, the following three different experimental groups were evaluated: the native group (VGG16), transfer learning group (VGG16-TR), and transfer learning with fine-tuning group (VGG16-TR-TF). In the native version, model weights were randomly initialized, and training was conducted using only the DPR data described in this study. In the transfer learning version, model weights were fixed, based on pre-training with a general image dataset, except for the final, fully connected layers, which were randomly initialized. In the transfer learning with fine-tuning version, model weights were initialized based on pre-training on a general image dataset, the same as previous versions, except that some of the last blocks were unfrozen so that their weights were updated in each training step. In this study, the last two transfer learning version models (VGG16-TR and VGG16-TR-FT) employed pre-trained weights using the ImageNet database [38]. ImageNet is an image dataset containing thousands of different objects used to train and evaluate image classification models.

2.4. Model Training

The 544 images selected as the training dataset were randomly divided into five folds. This was done to perform 5-fold cross validation to evaluate the model training, while avoiding overfitting or bias [39]. Within each fold, the dataset was partitioned into independent training and validation sets, using an 80 to 20 percentage split. The selected validation set was a completely independent fold from the other training folds and it was used to evaluate the training status during the training. After one model training step was completed, the other independent fold was used as a validation set and the previous validation set was reused, as part of the training set, to evaluate the model training. An overview of the 5-fold cross validation performed in this study is presented in Figure 3.

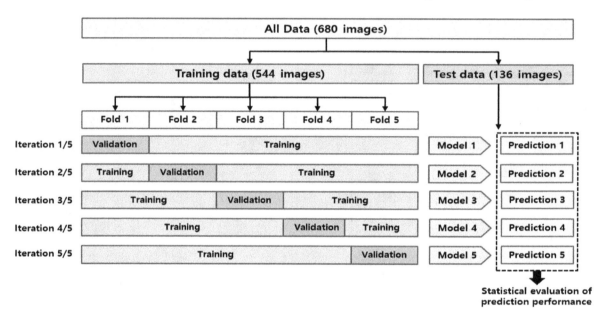

Figure 3. The overview of the performed 5-fold cross validation in this study.

This process was repeated for each architecture (CNN3, VGG16, VGG16-TR, and VGG16-TR-FT). All models were trained and evaluated on a 64-bit Windows 10 operating system, with 64 GB memory and an NVIDIA Quadro P4000 GPU. Building, training, validation, and prediction of deep learning models were performed using the Keras [40] library and TensorFlow [41] backend engine.

2.5. Performance Evaluation

The evaluation of the screening performance of the CNN models was performed with the independent test dataset in each cross-validation fold. To comprehensively evaluate the screening performance on the test dataset, the accuracy, sensitivity, specificity, receiver operating characteristic (ROC) curve, and precision recall (PR) curve were calculated. The accuracy, sensitivity, and specificity score can be calculated as follows:

$$accuracy = \frac{TP + TN}{TP + TN + FN + FP}$$

$$sensitivity = \frac{TP}{TP + FN}$$

$$specificity = \frac{TN}{TN + FP}$$

TP and FP are the number of correctly and incorrectly predicted images, respectively. Similarly, TN and FN represent the number of correctly and incorrectly predicted images, respectively. The area under the ROC curve (AUC) was also calculated.

2.6. Visualizing Model Decisions

Deep learning models have often been referred to as non-interpretable black boxes because it is difficult to know the process by which they make predictions. To know the decision-making process of the model, and which features are most important for the model to screen osteoporosis in DPR images, this study employed the gradient-weighted class activation mapping technique (Grad-CAM) [42] and the most significant regions for screening osteoporosis in DPR images were highlighted.

3. Results

3.1. Baseline Clinical and Demographic Characteristics of the Subjects

The patients were 565 female and 115 male, with an age range from 27 to 90 years (mean age of 63.0 years). There were 380 patients (mean age 58.5) without osteoporosis (T-score ≥ -2.5) and 300 patients (mean age 68.6) with osteoporosis (T-score < -2.5). The clinical characteristics of the DPR dataset used in this study are summarized in Table 1.

Table 1. Clinical and demographic characteristics of the dental panorama radiographs (DPRs) dataset in this study.

Parameter	Without Osteoporosis (T-Score ≥ -2.5)	With Osteoporosis (T-Score < -2.5)	Total
Number of patients	380	300	680
Number of female/male	332/48	233/67	565/115
Mean age (±SD)	58.5 (±11.8)	68.4 (±8.4)	63.0 (±11.6)

3.2. Prediction Performance

The CNN models of this study were trained using a cross-entropy loss function on the selected training image dataset. The screening performances of the four CNN models tested in this study are displayed in Table 2. It was observed that the transfer learning and fine tuning VGG16 model with pre-trained weights (VGG16-TR-FT) achieved the top performance, with the highest AUC of 0.858 (95% CI 0.865 to 0.850), sensitivity of 0.900 (95% CI 0.919 to 0.881), specificity of 0.815 (95% CI 0.847 to 0.783), and accuracy of 0.840 (95% CI 0.857 to 0.822). The screening performances of the other models that applied transfer learning techniques, but did not apply fine tuning, one with pre-trained weights (VGG-TR) and the other without pre-trained weights (VGG16), were slightly degraded. The arbitrarily established model with three convolutional layers (CNN3) achieved the lowest performance, with an AUC of 0.667 (95% CI 0.708 to 0.626), sensitivity of 0.684 (95% CI 0.889 to 0.480), specificity of 0.649 (95% CI 0.813 to 0.486), and accuracy of 0.660 (95% CI 0.725 to 0.594).

Table 2. Osteoporosis screening accuracy of convolutional neural network models in this research.

Model	AUC (95% CI)	Sensitivity (95% CI)	Specificity (95% CI)	Accuracy (95% CI)
CNN3	0.667 (±0.041)	0.684 (±0.204)	0.649 (±0.164)	0.660 (±0.066)
VGG16	0.742 (±0.018)	0.674 (±0.048)	0.811 (±0.034)	0.771 (±0.018)
VGG16-TR	0.782 (±0.006)	0.737 (±0.046)	0.828 (±0.052)	0.802 (±0.024)
VGG16-TR-TF	0.858 (±0.008)	0.900 (±0.019)	0.815 (±0.032)	0.840 (±0.018)

Figure 4 shows the ROC curves of all tested models. The VGG16-TR-FT models achieved the highest AUC of 0.86, while the CNN3 model achieved the lowest AUC of 0.61. Figure 5 shows the PR curves of the tested CNN models. It was also observed that the VGG16-TR-FT models achieved the highest PR of 0.86, while the CNN3 model achieved the lowest PR of 0.61.

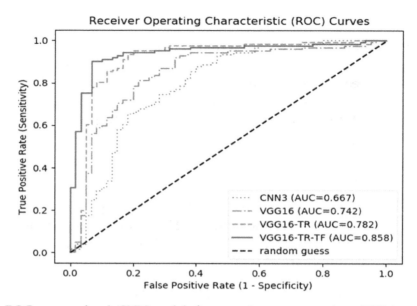

Figure 4. Mean ROC curves of each CNN models for screening osteoporosis on DPR images in this study.

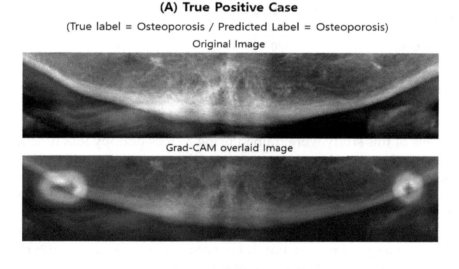

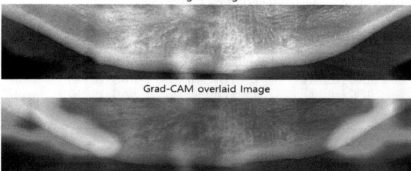

Figure 5. Original and Grad-CAM sample images of correctly predicted by the best-performing deep CNN model (VGG16-TR-TF) for DPR image-based osteoporosis screening are illustrated. Below each original sample images, a Grad-CAM image is superimposed over the original image. The bright red in each Grad-CAM image indicate the region that has the greatest impact on screening osteoporosis patients.

3.3. Visualizing Model Decisions

Figures 5 and 6 illustrate the case examples of predictions using the best predictive VGG16-TR-FT model as compared with ground truth. Each case example employed a Grad-CAM technique to perform a visual interpretation to determine which areas affected the deep CNN's class classification. In the case of screening correctly for osteoporosis (Figure 5A), the region showing the weak lower border of the mandibular cortical bone and the less dense, spongy bone texture at its periphery was extracted as the main image feature of the classification. In correctly screened cases of no osteoporosis (Figure 5B), the region showing the strong lower boundary of the mandible cortical bone and the dense texture around its periphery was extracted as the main image feature of the classification. However, in the case of incorrectly screened cases, i.e., the non-osteoporosis case predicted as osteoporosis (Figure 6A) or the osteoporosis case predicted as non-osteoporosis (Figure 6B), the central region of the mandible or the ghost images of the hyoid bone was extracted as the main image feature.

(A) False Positive Case

(True label = Non-osteoporosis / Predicted Label = Osteoporosis)
Original Image

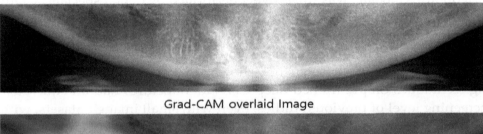

Grad-CAM overlaid Image

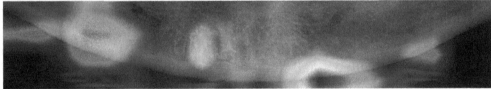

(B) False Negative Case

(True label = Osteoporosis / Predicted Label = Non-osteoporosis)
Original Image

Grad-CAM overlaid Image

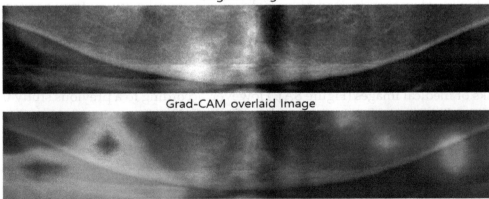

Figure 6. Original and Grad-CAM sample images of incorrectly predicted by the best-performing deep CNN model (VGG16-TR-TF) for DPR image-based osteoporosis screening are illustrated. Below each original sample images, a Grad-CAM image is superimposed over the original image. The bright red in each Grad-CAM image indicate the region that has the greatest impact on screening osteoporosis patients.

4. Discussion

Although DPRs are commonly performed for the evaluation of dentition and adjacent structures of the jaw, some clinical assistant diagnosis (CAD) systems based on DPRs have been suggested for screening systemic diseases, such as osteoporosis and carotid artery calcification [13–23,43]. However, the approaches of most previous studies are only valid when image features are accurately extracted, using sophisticated and manual image preprocessing algorithms or techniques. If a DPR image is imported from an unfamiliar environment or unexpected noise is added to the image, the prediction can easily be distorted. The neural network algorithm can resolve this problem. All the knowledge necessary for diagnosis is established only with the given training image data, without complicated or sophisticated image preprocessing. In recent years, a cutting-edge neural network technology, called deep learning, has been applied to medical imaging analysis and has shown a level of performance that is equal to or better than a clinician. As mentioned above, most previous CAD system studies, which used manual or sophisticated image preprocessing and machine learning algorithms for the screening of osteoporosis based on DPRs, presented variable diagnostic performances, in terms of sensitivity and specificity [13–23]. Recently, a deep learning-based osteoporosis prescreening study, which resulted in a very high AUC score (0.9763 to 0.9991) and accuracy (92.5% to 98.5%), was published [44]. However, in that study, osteoporosis labeling was subjectively performed by dental specialists, rather than BMD score (T-score) which is the gold standard for diagnosing osteoporosis. In addition, the study did not visually interpret the decision of the trained CNN model, and using five arbitrarily established convolutional layers, there is a limitation to the reproducibility of the deep CNN model.

The first major findings of the present study showed that applying appropriate transfer learning and fine-tuning techniques on pre-trained deep CNN architectures had an equivalent DPR-based osteoporosis screening level of previous studies, even with small image datasets, without complex image preprocessing and image ROI settings. According to Table 2 and Figure 4, the CNN3 group, having only arbitrary established three convolutional layers, showed the lowest true-positive screening performance and accuracy among the experimental groups. On the basis of these results, it can be estimated that a CNN model with a small number of convolutional layers can have limitation in learning the true data distribution from a small number of datasets.

Comparing models that used pre-trained weights (VGG16-TR and VGG16-TR-FT) to those that did not (VGG16), also revealed that deep CNNs initialized with large-scale pre-trained weights outperformed those directly learnt from small-scale data, with AUC improvements between 7% to 11%. Thus, in the case of having a small-scale image dataset, this study also suggests that the use of transfer learning on deep CNN models with pre-trained weights can be an efficient solution for the classification of medical images, instead of learning a deep neural network from scratch.

Moreover, as shown in Table 2 and Figure 7, the results of this study also indicated an improvement in screening performance when using fine-tuning on some convolutional blocks in deep CNN layers. In general, the deep CNN model learned from pre-trained deep neural networks on a large natural image dataset could be used to classify common images but cannot be well utilized for specific classifying tasks of medical images (Figure 8A). However, according to a previous study that described the effects and mechanisms of fine tuning on deep CNNs [45], when certain convolutional blocks of a deep CNN model were fine-tuned, the deep CNN model could be further specialized for specific classifying tasks (Figure 8B). More specifically, earlier layers of a deep CNN contain generic features that should be useful to many classification tasks, but later layers progressively contain more specialized features to the details of the classes contained in the original dataset (i.e., the large natural image dataset on which the deep CNN was originally trained). Using this property, when the parameters of the early layers are preserved and the parameters in later layers are updated during training new datasets, the deep CNN model can be effectively used in new classification tasks. In conclusion, fine-tuning uses the parameters learned from a previous training of the network on a large dataset and, then, adjusts the parameters in later layers from the new dataset, improving the performance and accuracy in the new classification task. As with the previous study, the fine-tuning technique, which freezes the weight parameters of some initial convolutional blocks in the deep CNN model called VGG16, and, then, updates the weight parameters of the later convolutional blocks (Figure 8B), show higher performance than other experimental groups. The conceptual diagram of the fine-tuning technique mentioned above can be seen in Figure 8.

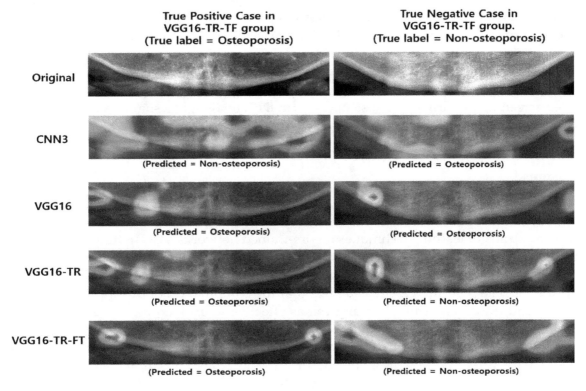

Figure 7. Comparison of grad-CAM images from other groups against some original images showing true positive and true negative in the best performing VGG16-TR-TF group.

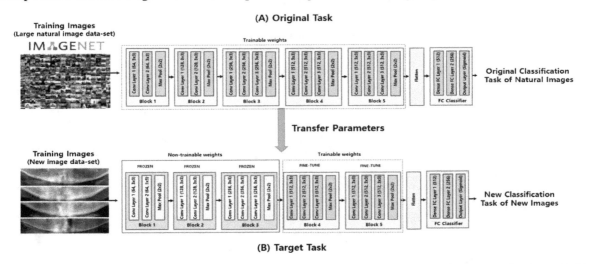

Figure 8. The conceptual diagram of the fine-tuning technique in the transfer learning of a deep CNN.

The second major result of this study was to identify areas where image feature differences occurred when screening osteoporosis in DPR images using the Grad-CAM technique. To understand and visualize the decision of deep CNN models, some samples of the correctly and incorrectly screened examples were reviewed (Figures 5 and 6). For additional insight to model decisions, a Grad-CAM technique was performed in this study. This technique identified the areas of input images that had the greatest impact on model classification. According to this additional review, the model does seem to identify the feature characteristics of osteoporosis in DPR images (e.g., cortical bone thinning). According to the Grad-CAM evaluation of this study, DPR-based screening performances of osteoporosis were high when the image features were specified in the middle region of the left and right side of the mandibular lower border. This region is also consistent with the regions used to discriminate osteoporosis using DPR images, in most previous studies [13–23], although the measurement algorithm was different. This indicates that most osteoporosis patients have image feature characteristics, on DPR images, at the lower border of the cortical bone in the mandible. However, image quality issues, such as blurring, low contrast, and ghost images of adjacent objects can cause incorrect predictions. When the image features were specified in the center region of the mandible, or when the ghost images of the hyoid bone were in the ROI region, the accuracy was reduced. Therefore, to improve the deep CNN-based screening performance of osteoporosis in DPR images, it is suggested that the ROI setting be limited to the area around the middle of the left and right side of the lower border of the mandible.

5. Conclusions

This study presents the usefulness of transfer learning and fine tuning with a deep CNN for the screening of osteoporosis in DPR images, in cases with a limited training dataset. We have applied various transfer learning techniques on pre-trained networks VGG16 for the discrimination of osteoporosis using a DPR image dataset, labeled based on T-score. The experimental results showed that transfer learning with pre-trained weights and fine-tuning techniques achieved the highest overall accuracy of 84%. The presented results suggest that the combination of the appropriate deep CNN architectures and transfer learning techniques has effectively resolved the issue of a small training set of images and that DPR images have the potential for osteoporosis prescreening. In addition, using the Grad-CAM technique, this study performed a deep learning-based visual explanation for the area where the image feature difference occurred. Therefore, this study confirmed the previous osteoporosis screening studies using DPR images that set the ROI at the middle of the left and right side of the lower border of the mandible. Given the increasing burden of osteoporosis on the global healthcare system, as our population ages, and the proliferation of dental panoramic image devices, the results presented in this study suggest that deep learning-based image analysis of DPRs could serve an important role in cost-effective prescreening for patients unaware of osteoporosis. To further improve screening performance, future research is needed, using different deep CNN architectures and deep learning techniques, more validated and qualified labeled image dataset, the appropriate number of datasets, and automated configuration techniques for more limited range of ROI.

Author Contributions: Conceptualization, K.-S.L., J.-J.R. and S.-W.S.; Data curation, K.-S.L. and S.-K.J.; Formal analysis, K.-S.L.; Funding acquisition, K.-S.L.; Investigation, K.-S.L.; Methodology, K.-S.L.; Project administration, K.-S.L. and J.C.; Software, K.-S.L.; Supervision, J.C.; Validation, S.-K.J. and J.C.; Visualization, K.-S.L.; Writing—original draft, K.-S.L.; Writing—review & editing, K.-S.L. and J.C. All authors have read and agreed to the published version of the manuscript.

References

1.   NIH Consensus Development Panel on Osteoporosis Prevention, Diagnosis, and Therapy, March 7–29, 2000: Highlights of the conference. *South. Med. J.* **2001**, *94*, 569–573.

2.   Cauley, J.A. Public health impact of osteoporosis. *J. Gerontol. A Biol. Sci. Med. Sci.* **2013**, *68*, 1243–1251. [CrossRef]

3.   Bliuc, D.; Nguyen, N.D.; Nguyen, T.V.; Eisman, J.A.; Center, J.R. Compound risk of high mortality following osteoporotic fracture and refracture in elderly women and men. *J. Bone Miner. Res.* **2013**, *28*, 2317–2324. [CrossRef] [PubMed]

4.   Sozen, T.; Ozisik, L.; Basaran, N.C. An overview and management of osteoporosis. *Eur. J. Rheumatol.* **2017**, *4*, 46–56. [CrossRef] [PubMed]

5.   Melton, L.J., 3rd; Chrischilles, E.A.; Cooper, C.; Lane, A.W.; Riggs, B.L. Perspective. How many women have osteoporosis? *J. Bone Miner. Res.* **1992**, *7*, 1005–1010. [CrossRef]

6.   Melton, L.J., 3rd; Atkinson, E.J.; O'Connor, M.K.; O'Fallon, W.M.; Riggs, B.L. Bone density and fracture risk in men. *J. Bone Miner. Res.* **1998**, *13*, 1915–1923. [CrossRef]

7.   Kanis, J.A.; Johnell, O.; Oden, A.; Sembo, I.; Redlund-Johnell, I.; Dawson, A.; De Laet, C.; Jonsson, B. Long-term risk of osteoporotic fracture in Malmo. *Osteoporos. Int.* **2000**, *11*, 669–674. [CrossRef]

8.   Kalinowski, P.; Rozylo-Kalinowska, I.; Piskorz, M.; Bojakowska-Komsta, U. Correlations between periodontal disease, mandibular inferior cortex index and the osteoporotic fracture probability assessed by means of the fracture risk assessment body mass index tool. *BMC Med. Imaging* **2019**, *19*, 41. [CrossRef]

9.   Marcucci, G.; Brandi, M.L. Rare causes of osteoporosis. *Clin. Cases Miner. Bone Metab.* **2015**, *12*, 151–156. [CrossRef]

10. Kanis, J.A.; Johnell, O. Requirements for DXA for the management of osteoporosis in Europe. *Osteoporos. Int.* **2005**, *16*, 229–238. [CrossRef]

11. Kanis, J.A. Diagnosis of osteoporosis and assessment of fracture risk. *Lancet* **2002**, *359*, 1929–1936. [CrossRef]

12. Mithal, A.; Bansal, B.; Kyer, C.S.; Ebeling, P. The Asia-Pacific Regional Audit-Epidemiology, Costs, and Burden of Osteoporosis in India 2013: A report of International Osteoporosis Foundation. *Indian J. Endocrinol. Metab.* **2014**, *18*, 449–454. [CrossRef] [PubMed]

13. Taguchi, A.; Suei, Y.; Ohtsuka, M.; Otani, K.; Tanimoto, K.; Ohtaki, M. Usefulness of panoramic radiography in the diagnosis of postmenopausal osteoporosis in women. Width and morphology of inferior cortex of the mandible. *Dentomaxillofac. Radiol.* **1996**, *25*, 263–267. [CrossRef] [PubMed]

14. Ledgerton, D.; Horner, K.; Devlin, H.; Worthington, H. Radiomorphometric indices of the mandible in a British female population. *Dentomaxillofac. Radiol.* **1999**, *28*, 173–181. [CrossRef]

15. White, S.C.; Taguchi, A.; Kao, D.; Wu, S.; Service, S.K.; Yoon, D.; Suei, Y.; Nakamoto, T.; Tanimoto, K. Clinical and panoramic predictors of femur bone mineral density. *Osteoporos. Int.* **2005**, *16*, 339–346. [CrossRef]

16. Yasar, F.; Akgunlu, F. The differences in panoramic mandibular indices and fractal dimension between patients with and without spinal osteoporosis. *Dentomaxillofac. Radiol.* **2006**, *35*, 1–9. [CrossRef]

17. Taguchi, A.; Ohtsuka, M.; Tsuda, M.; Nakamoto, T.; Kodama, I.; Inagaki, K.; Noguchi, T.; Kudo, Y.; Suei, Y.; Tanimoto, K. Risk of vertebral osteoporosis in post-menopausal women with alterations of the mandible. *Dentomaxillofac. Radiol.* **2007**, *36*, 143–148. [CrossRef]

18. Devlin, H.; Karayianni, K.; Mitsea, A.; Jacobs, R.; Lindh, C.; van der Stelt, P.; Marjanovic, E.; Adams, J.; Pavitt, S.; Horner, K. Diagnosing osteoporosis by using dental panoramic radiographs: The OSTEODENT project. *Oral Surg. Oral Med. Oral Pathol. Oral Radiol. Endod.* **2007**, *104*, 821–828. [CrossRef]

19. Okabe, S.; Morimoto, Y.; Ansai, T.; Yoshioka, I.; Tanaka, T.; Taguchi, A.; Kito, S.; Wakasugi-Sato, N.; Oda, M.; Kuroiwa, H.; et al. Assessment of the relationship between the mandibular cortex on panoramic radiographs and the risk of bone fracture and vascular disease in 80-year-olds. *Oral Surg. Oral Med. Oral Pathol. Oral Radiol. Endod.* **2008**, *106*, 433–442. [CrossRef]

20. Taguchi, A. Triage screening for osteoporosis in dental clinics using panoramic radiographs. *Oral Dis.* **2010**, *16*, 316–327. [CrossRef]

21. Al-Dam, A.; Blake, F.; Atac, A.; Amling, M.; Blessmann, M.; Assaf, A.; Hanken, H.; Smeets, R.; Heiland, M. Mandibular cortical shape index in non-standardised panoramic radiographs for identifying patients with osteoporosis as defined by the German Osteology Organization. *J. Craniomaxillofac. Surg.* **2013**, *41*, e165–e169. [CrossRef] [PubMed]

22. Kavitha, M.S.; Asano, A.; Taguchi, A.; Kurita, T.; Sanada, M. Diagnosis of osteoporosis from dental panoramic radiographs using the support vector machine method in a computer-aided system. *BMC Med. Imaging* **2012**, *12*, 1. [CrossRef] [PubMed]

23. Kavitha, M.S.; Ganesh Kumar, P.; Park, S.Y.; Huh, K.H.; Heo, M.S.; Kurita, T.; Asano, A.; An, S.Y.; Chien, S.I. Automatic detection of osteoporosis based on hybrid genetic swarm fuzzy classifier approaches. *Dentomaxillofac. Radiol.* **2016**, *45*, 20160076. [CrossRef]

24. Litjens, G.; Kooi, T.; Bejnordi, B.E.; Setio, A.A.A.; Ciompi, F.; Ghafoorian, M.; van der Laak, J.; van Ginneken, B.; Sanchez, C.I. A survey on deep learning in medical image analysis. *Med. Image Anal.* **2017**, *42*, 60–88. [CrossRef] [PubMed]

25. Park, C.; Took, C.C.; Seong, J.K. Machine learning in biomedical engineering. *Biomed. Eng. Lett.* **2018**, *8*, 1–3. [CrossRef] [PubMed]

26. LeCun, Y.; Bengio, Y.; Hinton, G. Deep learning. *Nature* **2015**, *521*, 436–444. [CrossRef]

27. Baker, B.; Gupta, O.; Naik, N.; Raskar, R. Designing neural network architectures using reinforcement learning. *arXiv* **2016**, arXiv:1611.02167.

28. Yosinski, J.; Clune, J.; Bengio, Y.; Lipson, H. How transferable are features in deep neural networks? *arXiv* **2014**, arXiv:1411.1792.

29. Pan, S.J.; Yang, Q. A survey on transfer learning. *IEEE Trans. Knowl. Data Eng.* **2009**, *22*, 1345–1359. [CrossRef]

30. He, K.; Zhang, X.; Ren, S.; Sun, J. Deep residual learning for image recognition. *arXiv* **2015**, arXiv:1512.03385.

31. Simonyan, K.; Zisserman, A. Very deep convolutional networks for large-scale image recognition. *arXiv* **2014**, arXiv:1409.1556.

32. Krizhevsky, A.; Sutskever, I.; Hinton, G.E. Imagenet classification with deep convolutional neural networks. In Proceedings of the 25th International Conference on Neural Information Processing Systems, Lake Tahoe, Nevada, 3–8 December 2012; Curran Associates Inc.: Red Hook, NY, USA, 2012; Volume 1, pp. 1097–1105.

33. Han, Z.; Wei, B.; Zheng, Y.; Yin, Y.; Li, K.; Li, S. Breast cancer multi-classification from histopathological images with structured deep learning model. *Sci. Rep.* **2017**, *7*, 4172. [CrossRef] [PubMed]

34. Christopher, M.; Belghith, A.; Bowd, C.; Proudfoot, J.A.; Goldbaum, M.H.; Weinreb, R.N.; Girkin, C.A.; Liebmann, J.M.; Zangwill, L.M. Performance of Deep Learning Architectures and Transfer Learning for Detecting Glaucomatous Optic Neuropathy in Fundus Photographs. *Sci. Rep.* **2018**, *8*, 16685. [CrossRef] [PubMed]

35. Shin, H.-C.; Roth, H.R.; Gao, M.; Lu, L.; Xu, Z.; Nogues, I.; Yao, J.; Mollura, D.; Summers, R.M. Deep convolutional neural networks for computer-aided detection: CNN architectures, dataset characteristics and transfer learning. *IEEE Trans. Med. Imaging* **2016**, *35*, 1285–1298. [CrossRef] [PubMed]

36. Ravishankar, H.; Sudhakar, P.; Venkataramani, R.; Thiruvenkadam, S.; Annangi, P.; Babu, N.; Vaidya, V. Understanding the mechanisms of deep transfer learning for medical images. *arXiv* **2017**, arXiv:1704.06040.

37. Kanis, J.A. Assessment of fracture risk and its application to screening for postmenopausal osteoporosis: Synopsis of a WHO report. WHO Study Group. *Osteoporos. Int.* **1994**, *4*, 368–381. [CrossRef]

38. Russakovsky, O.; Deng, J.; Su, H.; Krause, J.; Satheesh, S.; Ma, S.; Huang, Z.; Karpathy, A.; Khosla, A.; Bernstein, M. Imagenet large scale visual recognition challenge. *Int. J. Compute. Vis.* **2015**, *115*, 211–252. [CrossRef]

39. Stone, M. Cross-validatory choice and assessment of statistical predictions. *J. R. Stat. Soc. Ser. B Methodol.* **1974**, *36*, 111–133. [CrossRef]

40. Chollet, F. Keras: Deep Learning Library for Theano and Tensorflow. 2015, 7, p. T1. Available online: https://keras.io (accessed on 30 January 2020).

41. Abadi, M.; Agarwal, A.; Barham, P.; Brevdo, E.; Chen, Z.; Citro, C.; Corrado, G.S.; Davis, A.; Dean, J.; Devin, M. Tensorflow: Large-scale machine learning on heterogeneous distributed systems. *arXiv* **2016**, arXiv:1603.04467.

42. Selvaraju, R.R.; Cogswell, M.; Das, A.; Vedantam, R.; Parikh, D.; Batra, D. Grad-CAM: Visual explanations from deep networks via gradient-based localization. *arXiv* **2016**, arXiv:1610.02391.

43. Sawagashira, T.; Hayashi, T.; Hara, T.; Katsumata, A.; Muramatsu, C.; Zhou, X.; Iida, Y.; Katagi, K.; Fujita, H. An automatic detection method for carotid artery calcifications using top-hat filter on dental panoramic radiographs. *IEICE Trans. Inf. Syst.* **2013**, *96*, 1878–1881. [CrossRef]

44. Lee, J.-S.; Adhikari, S.; Liu, L.; Jeong, H.-G.; Kim, H.; Yoon, S.-J. Osteoporosis detection in panoramic radiographs using a deep convolutional neural network-based computer-assisted diagnosis system: A preliminary study. *Dentomaxillofac. Radiol.* **2019**, *48*, 20170344. [CrossRef] [PubMed]

45. Nogueira, K.; Penatti, O.A.; Dos Santos, J.A. Towards better exploiting convolutional neural networks for remote sensing scene classification. *Pattern Recognit.* **2017**, *61*, 539–556. [CrossRef]

A Scoping Review of the Efficacy of Virtual Reality and Exergaming on Patients of Musculoskeletal System Disorder

Hui-Ting Lin [1], Yen-I Li [1], Wen-Pin Hu [2], Chun-Cheng Huang [3] and Yi-Chun Du [4,*]

[1] Department of Physical Therapy, I-Shou University No. 8, Yida Road, Yan-chao District, Kaohsiung 82445, Taiwan; huitinglin@isu.edu.tw (H.-T.L.); ssttaarrtt7616274@gmail.com (Y.-I.L.)

[2] Department of Bioinformatics and Medical Engineering, Asia University. 500, Lioufeng Road, Wufeng, Taichung 41354, Taiwan; wenpinhu@asia.edu.tw

[3] Department of Rehabilitation, E-DA Hospital, No.1, Yida Road, Yan-chao District, Kaohsiung 82445, Taiwan; ed109049@edah.org.tw

[4] Department of Electrical Engineering, Southern Taiwan University of Science and Technology, No. 1, Nan-Tai Street, Yungkang District, Tainan 71005, Taiwan

* Correspondence: terrydu@stust.edu.tw

Abstract: To assess the effects of virtual reality on patients with musculoskeletal disorders by means of a scoping review of randomized controlled trials (RCTs). The databases included PubMed, IEEE, and the MEDLINE database. Articles involving RCTs with higher than five points on the Physiotherapy Evidence Database (PEDro) scale were reviewed for suitability and inclusion. The methodological quality of the included RCT was evaluated using the PEDro scale. The three reviewers extracted relevant information from the included studies. Fourteen RCT articles were included. When compared with simple usual care or other forms of treatment, there was significant pain relief, increased functional capacity, reduced symptoms of the disorder, and increased joint angles for the virtual reality treatment of chronic musculoskeletal disorders. Furthermore, burn patients with acute pain were able to experience a significant therapeutic effect on pain relief. However, virtual reality treatment of patients with non-chronic pain such as total knee replacement, ankle sprains, as well as those who went through very short virtual reality treatments, did not show a significant difference in parameters, as compared with simple usual care and other forms of treatment. Current evidence supports VR treatment as having a significant effect on pain relief, increased joint mobility, or motor function of patients with chronic musculoskeletal disorders. VR seems quite effective in relieving the pain of patients with acute burns as well.

Keywords: virtual reality; musculoskeletal disorders; randomized controlled tria

1. Introduction

Virtual reality (VR) of players using body movement to interact with a computer is a new form of treatment in rehabilitation settings. It generates a virtual world in three-dimensional space through a computer simulation that stimulates user senses, such as sight and hearing, making users feel as if they are immersed in it. VR has three elements: Interaction, Immersion, and Imagination [1]. It can be used in the teaching of human anatomy, online navigation of museums, 3D game teaching, flight training, and rehabilitation [2]. VR has become a therapeutic tool in many medical and rehabilitation fields. Due to the cost decline and ease of use of this technology, it has become an effective tool and trend in various fields.

However, its greatest obstacles lie in the lack of space, time, support staff, appropriate customer and customer incentives, therapist knowledge, and management support. The clinical use of VR often depends on the motivation and attitude of the therapist [3,4].

In the clinical investigations on the VR experience and perception of physical therapists (PTs) and occupational therapists (OTs) in Canada conducted by Levac et al., it was found that VR treatment is most commonly used for stroke (25.8%), brain injury (15.3%), musculoskeletal disorder (14.9%), cerebral palsy (10.5%), and neurodevelopmental disorders (6.3%) [3]. Most of the clinical applications of VR are for neurological problems. Moreover, numerous literature shows that VR is used to treat patients with stroke, cerebral palsy, Parkinson's disease, etc. [5–10]. Most researches in VR medical applications are used to the upper limb movement rehabilitation for stroke patients. The upper limb virtual reality rehabilitation systems were developed for the stroke group. The patient grasped and released the characteristic objects in the virtual environment, and finger movement control of the stroke patients after 4–6 weeks of VR intervention was improved [6,10]. Some scholars used Kinect and customized games to train the children with cerebral palsy (CP). The evidence appears to support the use of VR as a promising tool to be incorporated into the rehabilitation process of CP [7,11,12].

According to the World Heath Organization (WHO), musculoskeletal conditions affect muscles, bones, joints and associated tissues such as tendons and ligaments. To patients, musculoskeletal conditions are typically characterized by pain and limitations in mobility or functional ability.... Pain and restricted mobility are the consistent features of the range of musculoskeletal conditions. Musculoskeletal conditions are the second largest contributor to disability worldwide [13]. However, at present, there is less evidence on the therapeutic effect of VR on patients with musculoskeletal system disorder [14–18]. In addition, studies have shown that VR is beneficial in pain management, for example, in pain relief during dressing changes of burn patients [19]. VR can also reduce anxiety, distract from the fear of pain, and alleviate stress [20]. It can divert the attention of patients who are afraid of moving because of pain.

So far, there are no integrated and first-rate studies that explore which musculoskeletal disorders are suitable for VR treatment. The comparison of the effects of VR games and other treatments (e.g., traditional treatment, instrumental therapy, exercise) on patients with musculoskeletal disorder is inconclusive. Therefore, this article integrates the results of studies made in recent years into a scoping review to: (1) Compare the effectiveness of VR and other treatment interventions for patients with musculoskeletal disorder; (2) further explore whether there is any consistency in the VR treatment of patients with musculoskeletal system disorder, so as to give recommendations based on the highest level of evidence. This review only contains RCT articles with a PEDro Scale score ≥5 points.

2. Materials and Methods

2.1. Determination and Selection of Articles

The methodology of this scoping review was based on the Preferred Reporting Items for Systematic Reviews and Meta-Analyses (PRISMA) guidelines because the main aim of this work is mapping all the available literature in the musculoskeletal field [21]. The use of the checklists based on PRISMA statement improve the quality and transparency of the scoping reviews [17]. Search was made in the PubMed, IEEE, and the MEDLINE library for reference literature using keywords and synonyms of "virtual reality", "pain", and "musculoskeletal". After performing a journal search, RCT (randomized controlled trial) journals that were written in English within the last 10 years (January 2008 to August 2018) were selected, and non-musculoskeletal diseases such as "stroke", "neurological", and "cognitive" were excluded using the Physiotherapy Evidence Database (PEDro) scale (http://www.pedro.org.au/). When reference materials could not be found on the PEDro website, scores were independently made by two authors who have completed the PEDro Scale training tutorial on the Physiotherapy Evidence Database.

When the scores were different, the clinical physiotherapist with more than five years of experience, and who completed the PEDro assessment training, was asked to conduct another assessment. When issues such as disagreement or ambiguity arose, they were resolved through discussions. Finally, literature with very low PEDro scores (<5/10) was excluded. The search process is shown in Figure 1. Since there are few studies on VR for musculoskeletal disorders, we do not explore the virtual reality (VR) outcomes for any specific pathology in our study, but explore the VR treatment effects, such as pain relief, joint mobility, function, range of motion (ROM), muscle strength, angular velocity and self-satisfaction for all musculoskeletal disorders.

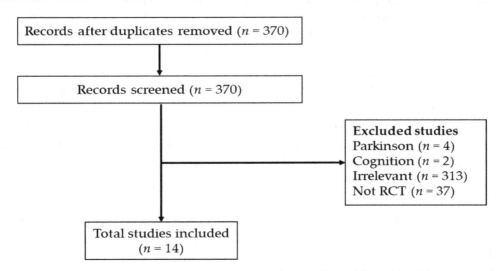

Figure 1. Flow chart displaying the screening process for studies included in this systematic review.

2.2. Data Extraction and Quality Assessment

Initially, the two authors completed the abstract review independently. When it was not possible to know whether an article could be included in the scoping review from its abstract, an assessment of the full article was made. All of the articles that had been included were reviewed in full. After sorting, the following were investigated: (1) Whether VR treatment improved the musculoskeletal system as compared with other treatments; (2) whether there was any consistency in the musculoskeletal disorder of patients that received VR treatment. The selected articles were summarized and analyzed with descriptive statistics. The author, publication year, subject, intervention, outcome measures, and mean between-group differences (95% confidence interval) were extracted from the references by the two authors of this study. A consensus was reached through discussion when the authors had different opinions.

3. Result

A database search was made to exclude articles with a PEDro score of less than 5 and non-English publications. A total of 14 articles were included. These 14 articles were included in this scoping review (Figure 1).

3.1. Quality of the Included Studies

The quality of included studies was presented in Table 1. The mean PEDro score of the included articles was 6.14 (range, 5–7). All studies were randomized (100%). 8 studies carry out concealed allocation (57.14%), and all studies baseline comparability (100%). All studies were analyzed between-group comparison (100%) and 13 studies reported point estimates and variability (92.86%). All studies didn't carry out blind therapist. One study carried out blind subjects (7.14%) and 7 studies carried out blind assessors (50%). 10 studies have adequate outcome measurement (71.43%), and 5 studies have an intension-to-treat analysis (35.71%).

3.2. Description of Included Studies

Each article abstract (including author, musculoskeletal disorder, design, participants, intervention, comparison, and outcome measure) is organized in Table 2. In terms of age, a study about frozen shoulder investigated subjects older than 20 years of age [15]; a research about subacromial impingement syndrome (SAIS) studied subjects between 18–60 years old [22]; subjects of two articles discussing chronic cervical pain were older than 18 years old [17,18]; three studies that explored low back pain (LBP) had subjects between 18–50 years old [23], and those between 40–55 years old [24,25]; an investigation on pelvic floor muscle had subjects older than 50 years of age [26]; two researches discussed the treatment of acute burn wounds in adolescents aged 10–18 years [27,28]; three studies discussed the treatment for patients with TKR aged in the sixties [14,16,29]; an article discussing ankle sprains had subjects aged 18–64, belonging to the working-age group [30]. In terms of experimental intervention, most of the study regarding VR intervention lasted 15 to 30 min, 2 to 4 times per week for 2 to 6 weeks. One research conducted VR intervention for 3 weeks [16]; 3 articles discussed 4 weeks of VR intervention [15,17,24]; 2 studies described 5 weeks of VR intervention [18,26]; and another 2 articles discussed 6 weeks of VR intervention [22,30]. One study conducted VR treatment beginning the second day after TKA until 6 months [29]. There were 5 studies that compared VR intervention and no intervention at all [17,23,27,28,30]. The rest made comparisons between VR and other treatments.

3.3. Virtual Reality Resources Choosing

Virtual Reality was applied using several resources. In the 14 studies, one study used Kinect [15]; 5 studies used Wii [14,22,24,26,30]; 5 studies used VR glasses (one of the studies used headphones and joysticks) [17,18,25,27,28]; two studies used 3-D TV and 3-D shutter glasses [23,29]; and one study used enhanced reality with VR and mirror therapy [16].

3.4. Heterogeneity of Included RCT

The outcome could not be pooled into meta-analysis due to the following reasons. Clinical heterogeneity (Table 2) can be clearly observed from the participant, intervention, exercise mode, and outcome measures of the included studies. Diversity is seen in patient conditions, frequency and duration of VR intervention, whether or not the patient does home exercise, received patient health education, whether the experiment conducted was pure VR (only VR) or VR mixed with traditional physical therapy or with exercise therapy, whether the outcome measure contains follow-up, and whether different estimate measures were inconsistent at different times.

3.5. Effect of Virtual Reality versus Other Interventions

In the articles included, a total of twelve studies compared the effects of VR treatment and other intervention on orthopedic conditions (Table 3). The research on patients suffering from frozen shoulder for more than three months shows that four weeks of VR plus modalities (hot pack and ultrasound) produced a significant 8% increase in their shoulder range of motion (ROM) when compared to traditional exercise training, plus modalities [15]. Another research showed that after 6 months of short-term training and one-month of follow-up, the subacromial impingement syndrome (SAIS) patients without a rotator cuff problem on the VR group and home exercise group (scapular muscles training), were able to significantly reduce their disability and improve their quality of life. Furthermore, the VR group showed significant improvement of SAIS and scapular dyskinesis symptoms when compared with the home exercise group [22]. Another article showed that patients with chronic cervical pain who went through 5 weeks of VR and cervical kinematic training (KT) had a big difference in the global perceived change (variations in different areas of patient self-assessment, such as satisfaction, self-reported pain differences), which could last for three months when compared to those in the KT group [18]. A study also showed that after four weeks of training, the VR group of patients with chronic cervical pain displayed a significant difference in terms of pain, physical condition, fear of moving the neck, as well as in the mean and peak velocity from those in the laser beam projected group. However, there is no significant difference in cervical ROM during follow-up between the VR treatment group and the laser beam projected group [17]. Patients with chronic low back pain in another study were able to significantly improve pain, pressure algometry, disability, and the fear of low back pain after four weeks of VR training [24]. Another research proposed that VR with the supplementary traditional physical therapy can significantly reduce pain, fear, and increase functions for patients with subacute or chronic non-specific lower back pain [25]. Although a study comparing five weeks of pelvic floor muscle training via VR and traditional gym ball training, showed no significant difference in muscle strength, but a statistically significant difference in endurance was observed [26]. One study supported the idea that VR therapy during burn wound care can reduce adolescent pain [25]. Three included studies examined the effects of VR on patients with TKR [14,29]. The results of these two articles showed that VR treatment (physical therapy plus VR) did not produce a significant difference in terms of pain, ROM, walking speed, balance, and walking test for patients with total knee replacement (TKR), when compared with conventional therapy [14,16]. The other demonstrated that VAS scales were significantly lower in the experimental group than the control group during acute phase (at 3, 5, and 7 days after TKR) ($p < 0.05$) [29]. However, it did not reach the minimal clinically important difference (MCID) [31]. In the previously described study, VR intervention (one month, three months, six months after TKR) in the chronic phase can improve the functional recovery of the patients with TKR [29]. A study on the treatment of ankle sprains suggested that there is no significant difference in all parameters between VR treatment and traditional treatment [30].

3.6. Effect of Virtual Reality Versus No Intervention

In the included articles, four articles discussed the therapeutic effects of VR and no intervention on chronic cervical pain, burn wound, low back pain, and ankle sprains (Table 4). When applied to chronic cervical pain and burn wound, a statistically significant difference was present in some parameters, as described in the following section. Bohat et al. (2017) [17] studied patients with chronic cervical pain after four weeks of training and found that the VR group had significantly different results from the control group in disability, cervical angular velocity, time to peak velocity, and head follow-up task accuracy. However, in cervical ROM, physical health, and fear of moving the neck, no significant difference was observed [17]. Another study compared the results of a 3-day VR training of low-back pain patients with the results of the non-invasive group, and found no statistically significant difference in lumbar spine flexion ROM and pain improvement [23].

During the dressing application of patients with burn wounds, patients undergoing VR treatment received significantly lower doses of Entonox (analgesic) compared with those in the standard distraction group. However, there is no significant reduction in patient pain [28]. For patients with ankle sprains, no statistically significant difference was observed between the VR treatment and the control group [30].

Table 1. Physiotherapy Evidence Database (PEDro) Score for Included Studies ($n = 14$).

	Huang et al. 2014 [15]	Pekyavas et al. 2017 [22]	Bahat et al. 2015 [18]	Bahat et al. 2017 [17]	Kim et al. 2014 [24]	Thomas et al. 2016 [23]	Yilmaz Yelvar et al. 2017 [25]	Martinho et al. 2016 [26]	Kipping et al. 2012 [28]	Jeffs et al. 2014 [27]	Fung et al. 2012 [14]	Koo et al. 2018 [16]	Jin et al. 2018 [29]	Punt et al. 2016 [30]
	2014	2017	2015	2017	2014	2016	2017	2016	2012	2014	2012	2018	2018	2016
	Taiwan	Turkey	Australia	Australia	Korea	America	Turkey	Brazil	Australia	America	Canada	Korea	China	Switzerland
Eligibility criteria	Y	N	Y	N	N	Y	Y	Y	Y	Y	Y	Y	Y	Y
Random allocation	Y	Y	Y	Y	Y	Y	Y	Y	Y	Y	Y	Y	Y	Y
Concealed allocation	N	N	Y	Y	N	Y	N	Y	Y	Y	N	Y	N	Y
Baseline comparability	Y	Y	Y	Y	Y	Y	Y	Y	Y	Y	Y	Y	Y	Y
Blind subjects	N	N	N	N	N	N	N	N	N	Y	N	N	N	N
Blind therapists	N	N	N	N	N	N	N	N	N	N	N	N	N	N
Blind assessors	Y	Y	Y	Y	Y	Y	Y	N	Y	Y	Y	Y	Y	Y
Adequate follow-up	Y	Y	Y	N	Y	Y	Y	N	Y	N	Y	N	N	N
Intention-to-treat analysis	Y	N	N	Y	N	N	N	Y	Y	Y	N	N	Y	Y
Between-group comparisons	Y	Y	Y	Y	Y	Y	Y	Y	Y	Y	Y	Y	Y	Y
Point estimates and variability	Y	Y	Y	Y	Y	Y	Y	Y	Y	Y	N	Y	Y	Y
Total score (0–10)	7/10	5/10	7/10	7/10	5/10	6/10	6/10	6/10	7/10	7/10	5/10	6/10	5/10	7/10

Abbreviations: PEDro, Physiotherapy Evidence Database; Y: yes; N: no.

Table 2. Description of Included studies.

Title	Author	Part	Design	Participant (number) Age (years) = mean (SD)		Intervention	Exercise Mode (Frequency or Intensity)	Outcome Measures
Intelligent Frozen Shoulder Rehabilitation	Huang et al. 2014 [15]	Frozen shoulder	RCT	frozen shoulder syndrome > 3 months			20 min/time, 2 times/week (Total 4 weeks)	ROM, CMS assessment
				E	n = 20 Age (years) = 60.65 (11.84)	Hot pack + ultrasonic + VR		
				C	n = 20 Age (years) = 61.45 (12.84)	Hot pack + ultrasonic + traditional exercise training		
Comparison of virtual reality exergaming and home exercise programs in patients with subacromial impingement syndrome and scapular dyskinesis: Short term effect	Pekyavas et al. 2017 [22]	subacromial impingement syndrome(SAIS) & scapular dyskinesis	RCT	18–60 years old; Type II SAIS None rotator cuff problem				VAS(rest, activity, night), SPADI, Neer, Hawkins, SRT, SAT, LSST1-3
				E	n = 15 Age (years) = 40.33 (13.20)	VR + control period (after 6 weeks)	VR: 45 min/day, twice a week, for 6 weeks; Control: 1 month for home exercise	
				C	n = 15 Age (years) = 40.60 (11.77)	Exercise + control period (after 6 weeks)	Exercise: 45 min/day, twice a week, for 6 weeks; Control: 1 month for home exercise	
Cervical Kinematic Training with and without Interactive VR Training for Chronic Neck Pain—a Randomized Clinical Trial	Bahat et al. 2015 [18]	Chronic neck pain	RCT	Neck pain > 3 months, NDI > 10%			Total 30 min, at least 3 times a week, for 5 weeks	VAS, Neck Disability Index, TSK, ROM, Peak velocity, mean velocity, TIP%, Sway SD, Accuracy, Eyes closed balance, singer leg stance, step test
				E	n = 16 Age (years) = 40.63 (14.18)	VR + kinematic training		
				C	n = 16 Age (years) = 41.13 (12.59)	kinematic training (using laser point)		
Remote kinematic training for patients with chronic neck pain: a randomized controlled trial	Bahat et al. 2017 [17]	Chronic neck pain	RCT	Neck pain > 3 months, NDI > 12%			1 set 5 min, 20 min/day, 4 times/week, for 4 weeks	Neck Disability Index, Peak velocity, mean velocity, VAS, EQ5D, TSK, NVP, TTP%, Accuracy, ROM, GPE
				VR	n = 30 Age (years) = 48 (9.5)	VR		
				Laser	n = 30 Age (years) = 48 (12.5)	Laser point training		
				C	n = 30 Age (years) = 48 (13)	Not receive any treatment		
The Effects of VR-Based Wii Fit Yoga on Physical Function in Middle-Aged Female LBP Patients	Kim et al. 2014 [24]	LBP	RCT	LBP > 2 months				VAS, pressure algometer, ODI, RMDQ, FBQ
				E	n = 15 Age (years) = 44.33	VR	30 min/session, 3 session/week, for 4 weeks (1 session had 7 exercise program. 3 min of exercise and 1 min of rest)	
				C	n = 15 Age (years) = 50.46	Trunk stabilizing exercise + physical therapy	2 sets (30 min), 1set included 10 repetitions, physical therapy 30 min	
Feasibility and Safety of a Virtual Reality Dodgeball Intervention for Chronic Low Back Pain: A Randomized Clinical Trial	Thomas et al. 2016 [23]	LBP	RCT	18–50 years old with LBP > 3 months kinesiophobia ≥35			3 days (<48 h)	pain and harm, lumbar spine flexion ROM
				E	n = 26 Age (years) = 23.9 (6.8)	VR		
				C	n = 26 Age (years) = 26.7 (8.5)	Not receive any treatment		

Table 2. *Cont.*

Title	Author	Part	Design	Participant (number) Age (years) = mean (SD)		Intervention	Exercise Mode (Frequency or Intensity)	Outcome Measures
Is physiotherapy integrated virtual walking effective on pain, function, and kinesiophobia in patients with non-specific low-back pain? Randomised controlled trial	Yilmaz Yelvar et al. 2017 [25]	LBP	RCT	\multicolumn{2}{l}{non-specific LBP for longer than 2 months}				VAS, ODI, TKS, TUG, and 6MWT scores
				E	n = 23 Age (years) = 46.27 (10.93)	VR + Traditional physical therapy	5 times/week, for 2 weeks	
				C	n = 23 Age (years) = 52.81 (11.53)	Traditional physical therapy	5 times/week, for 2 weeks	
The effects of training by virtual reality or gym ball on pelvic floor muscle strength in postmenopausal women: a randomized controlled trial	Martinho et al. 2016 [26]	Pelvic floor muscle	RCT	\multicolumn{2}{l}{>50 years old women >1 year postmenopausal phase}				Maximum strength, average strength, endurance
				APT-VR	n = 30 Age (years) = 61.9 (8.6)	Abdominopelvic training by VR	1 session 5 min with 90 s resting, for 10 session. Twice a week, for 5 weeks	
				PFMT-GB	n = 30 Age (years) = 61 (8.5)	Pelvic floor muscle training using a gym ball	4 series of 10 fast & sustained (8 s maintain with 16 s resting), each exercise 5 times, twice a week, for 5 weeks	
Virtual reality for acute pain reduction in adolescents undergoing burn wound care: A prospective randomized controlled trial	Kipping et al. 2012 [28]	Burn wound	RCT	\multicolumn{2}{l}{11–18 years old burn wound Total Body Surface Area (TBSA) > 1%}				VAS, FLACC scale
				E	n = 20 Age (years) = 12.6 (1.3)	VR	Dressing period (3–58 min), only 1 time	
				C	n = 21 Age (years) = 13.5 (1.8)	Another distraction way or no distraction		
Effect of Virtual Reality on Adolescent Pain During Burn Wound Care	Jeffs et al. 2014 [27]	Burn wound	RCT	\multicolumn{2}{l}{10–17 years old}				Adolescent Pediatric Pain Tool, Spielberger State–Trait Anxiety InventoryFor Children, Pre-Procedure Questionnaire, Post-Procedure Questionnaire
				standard care	n = 10 Age (years) = 18.9 (2.8)	standard care	Dressing period only 1 time	
				passive distraction	n = 10 Age (years) = 12.6 (2.1)	passive distraction watching a movie		
				virtual reality	n = 8 Age (years) = 14.8 (2.0)	virtual reality		
Use of Nintendo Wii Fit™ in the Rehabilitation of Outpatients Following Total Knee Replacement: a Preliminary Randomized Controlled Trial	Fung et al. 2012 [14]	TKR	RCT	\multicolumn{2}{l}{requiring twice-weekly physiotherapy treatment for TKR rehabilitation Full lower extremity weight bearing}				active knee flexion/extension ROM, 2 min walk test, NPRS, ABCS, LEFS
				E	n = 27 Age (years) = 67.9 (9.5)	physiotherapy + VR	physiotherapy (45 min), 15 min VR until discharge	
				C	n = 23 Age (years) = 68.2 (12.8)	physiotherapy + lower extremity exercise	physiotherapy (45 min), 15 min lower extremity exercise until discharge	

Table 2. *Cont.*

Title	Author	Part	Design	Participant (number) Age (years) = mean (SD)		Intervention	Exercise Mode (Frequency or Intensity)	Outcome Measures
Enhanced Reality Showing Long-Lasting Analgesia after Total Knee Arthroplasty: Prospective, Randomized Clinical Trial	Koo et al. 2018 [16]	TKR	RCT	Full term	n = 20 Age (years) = 63.7 (5.09)	VR + physiotherapy for 2 weeks	VR + PT: 5 days/week, for 2 weeks	VAS, WOMAC, 6 min walk test, Timed-stands test
				Half term	n = 22 Age (years) = 65.0 (6.97)	VR + physiotherapy for 1 week before physiotherapy for 1 week	VR + PT for 1 week	
Virtual reality intervention in postoperative rehabilitation after total knee arthroplasty: a prospective and randomized controlled clinical trial	Jin et al. 2018 [29]	TKR	RCT	E	n = 33 Age (years) = 66.45 (3.49)	VR(begin 2nd days for TKA) + conventional rehabilitation	three sets of 30 repetitions	WOMAC, HSS, VAS, ROM.
				C	n = 33 Age (years) = 66.30 (4.41)	conventional rehabilitation	three sets of 30 repetitions	
Wii Fit™ Exercise Therapy for the Rehabilitation of Ankle Sprains: Its Effect Compared with Physical Therapy or No Functional Exercises at All	Punt et al. 2016 [30]	Ankle sprain	RCT	18–64 years old Grade I or II lateral ankle sprain requiring 4 weeks RICE and can pain free movement				FAAM-ADL, FAAM-sport, VAS-rest, VAS-walk
				VR	n = 30 Age (years) = 34.7 (10.7)	VR	30 min/time, 2 times/week, for 6 weeks	
				Physiotherapy	n = 30 Age (years) = 34.7 (11.3)	modalities, joint mobilization, muscle strengthening, proprioceptive exercise	30 min/time, 9 times/6 weeks	
				C	n = 30 Age (years) = 33.5 (9.5)	Not receive any treatment	-	

Abbreviations: *n* (number); E (experimental group); C (control group); VR (Virtual reality); min (minute); ROM (range of motion); CMS (Constant-Murley score); VAS (Visual Analog Scale); SPADI (Shoulder Pain and Disability Index); SRT (Scapular Retraction Test); SAT (Scapular Assistance Test); LSST (Lateral Scapular Slide Test); TSK (Tampa scale of kinesiophobia); TTP% (Time to peak velocity percentage); GPE (Global perceived effect); sway SD (standard deviation of the static head sway); EQ-5D(EQ-5D™, http://www.euroqol.org); NVP (Number of velocity peaks); ODI (Oswestry low-back pain disability index); RMDQ (Roland Morris disability questionnaire); FBQ (fear avoidance beliefs questionnaire); NPRS (Numeric Pain Rating Scale); LEFS (Lower Extremity Functional Scale); ABCS (Activity-specific Balance Confidence Scale); WOMAC (Western Ontario and McMaster Universities Osteoarthritis Index); FAAM (Foot and Ankle Ability Measure); ADL (activities of daily living); RICE (rest, ice, compression and elevation); FLACC (Faces, legs, activity, cry, consolability scale); Hospital for Special Surgery knee score (HSS); TKS (TAMPA Kinesiophobia Scale), TUG (timed-up and go test); 6MWT (6-Minute Walk Test); RCT (randomized controlled trial); LBP (low back pain); TKR (Total Knee Replacement).

Table 3. Effect of virtual reality (VR) versus another intervention.

Study		Outcome Measure	Mean Difference between VR Groups and Another Intervention	Significance of Difference between Groups
Huang et al. 2014 [15]		ROM	8%	Between groups $p < 0.05$
		CMS	NA	Between groups $p < 0.05$
	Neer	post-intervention/1 month follow-up	NA	$p = 0.02$
	SRT	post-intervention/1 month follow-up	NA	$p = 0.01$
	SAT	post-intervention/1 month follow-up	NA	$p = 0.047$
Pekyavas et al. 2017 [22]	VAS (rest, activity, night)	post-intervention/1 month follow-up	NA	-
	SPADI	post-intervention/1 month follow-up	NA	-
	Hawkins	post-intervention/1 month follow-up	NA	-
	LSST1-3	post-intervention/1 month follow-up	NA	-
	cervical flexion ROM	post-intervention	NA	Between groups $p < 0.05$
		3 months follow-up	NA	-
	Global Perceived change	post-intervention	NA	-
		3 months follow-up	NA	Between groups $p < 0.05$
	VAS	post-intervention/3 months follow-up	NA	-
Bahat et al. 2015 [18]	NDI	post-intervention/3 months follow-up	NA	-
	TSK	post-intervention/3 months follow-up	NA	-
	Velocity	post-intervention/3 months follow-up	NA	-
	TTP%	post-intervention/3 months follow-up	NA	-
	Accuracy	post-intervention/3 months follow-up	NA	-
	sway SD	post-intervention/3 months follow-up	NA	-
	Eyes closed balance	post-intervention/3 months follow-up	NA	-
	singer leg stance	post-intervention/3 months follow-up	NA	-
	V_{mean} (F,LR)	Post-pre intervention	NA	Between groups $p < 0.05$
	V_{peak} (LR)	Post-pre intervention	NA	Between groups $p < 0.05$
	V_{mean} (F,E,LR)	3 months follow up-pre intervention	NA	Between groups $p < 0.05$
	V_{peak} (E,LR)	3 months follow up-pre intervention	NA	Between groups $p < 0.05$
	VAS	Post-pre/3 months-pre	NA	Between groups $p < 0.05$
	EQ5D	Post-pre/3 months-pre	NA	Between groups $p < 0.05$
Bahat et al. 2017 [17]	Accuracy (F,RR,LR)	Post-pre intervention	NA	Between groups $p < 0.05$
	Accuracy (F)	3 months follow up-pre intervention	NA	Between groups $p < 0.05$
	TTP%	Post-pre/3 months-pre	NA	Between groups $p < 0.05$
	ROM	Post-pre/3 months-pre	NA	-
	NDI	Post-pre/3 months-pre	NA	-
	TSK	Post-pre/3 months-pre	NA	-
	NVP	Post-pre/3 months-pre	NA	-
	GPE	Post-pre/3 months-pre	NA	-

Table 3. *Cont.*

Study	Outcome Measure	Mean Difference between VR Groups and Another Intervention	Significance of Difference between Groups
Kim et al. 2014 [24]	VAS	NA	Between groups $p < 0.05$
	Pressure algometer	NA	
	ODI	NA	
	FBQ	NA	
	RMDQ	NA	-
	VAS	NA	
Yilmaz Yelvar et al. 2017 [25]	TKS	NA	Between groups $p < 0.05$
	TUG	NA	
	6 MWT scores	NA	
	Maximum strength	-0.08	$p = 0.1$
Martinho et al. 2016 [26]	average strength	0.01	$p = 0.6$
	Endurance	1.83	$p = 0.007$
Jeffs et al. 2014 [27]	Pain	23.7	$p = 0.029$
	Active knee flexion ROM	-0.33	-
	Active knee extension ROM	-0.6	-
Fung et al. 2012 [14]	2 min walk test	2.68	-
	NPPS	16.84	-
	ABCS	14.11	-
	LEFS	31.85	-
	VAS	NA	-
	WOMAC	NA	-
Koo et al. 2018 [16]	6 min walk test	NA	-
	Timed-stands test	NA	-
	VAS (at 3, 5, 7 days after TKR)	NA	$p < 0.05$
Jin et al. 2018 [29]	WOMAC (at 1, 3, 6 months after TKR)	NA	$p < 0.05$
	HSS (at 1, 3, 6 months after TKR)	NA	$p < 0.05$
	FAAM-ADL	NA	-
	FAAM-sport	NA	-
Punt et al. 2016 [30]	VAS-rest	NA	-
	VAS-walk	NA	-

Abbreviations: VR (Virtual reality); ROM (range of motion); CMS (Constant-Murley score); VAS (Visual Analog Scale); SPADI (Shoulder Pain and Disability Index); SRT (Scapular Retraction Test); SAT (Scapular Assistance Test); LSST (Lateral Scapular Slide Test); NDI (Neck Disability Index); TSK (Tampa scale of kinesiophobia); TIP% (Time to peak velocity percentage); GPE (Global perceived effect); sway SD (standard deviation of the static head sway); EQ-5D(EQ-5D™, http://www.euroqol.org); NVP (Number of velocity peaks); ODI (Oswestry low-back pain disability index); RMDQ (Roland Morris disability questionnaire); FBQ (fear avoidance beliefs questionnaire); NPRS (Numeric Pain Rating Scale); LEFS (Lower Extremity Functional Scale); ABCS (Activity-specific Balance Confidence Scale); WOMAC (Western Ontario and McMaster Universities Osteoarthritis Index); FAAM (Foot and Ankle Ability Measure); ADL (activities of daily living); v_{mean} (Mean velocity); Vpeak (Peak velocity); F (Flexion), E (Extension), LR (Left rotation), RR (Right rotation); the-marked mean $p >$ 0.05; NA (not available); Hospital for Special Surgery knee score (HSS); TKS (TAMPA Kinesiophobia Scale); TUG (timed-up and go test); 6 MWT (6-Minute Walk Test).

Table 4. Effect of VR versus no intervention.

Study	Outcome Measure	Mean Difference between VR Groups and Control Group	Significance of Difference between Groups
Bahat et al. 2017 [17]	NDI	NA	Between groups $p < 0.05$
	velocity	NA	
	TTP% (F,LR)	NA	
	Accuracy (F,RR)	NA	
	ROM	NA	-
	EQ5D	NA	-
	TSK	NA	-
	NVP	NA	-
Thomas et al. 2016 [23]	ROM	NA	-
	Pain	NA	-
Kipping et al. 2012 [28]	VAS	NA	-
	FLACC (dressing removal)	NA	Between groups $p < 0.05$
Punt et al. 2016 [30]	FAAM-ADL	NA	-
	FAAM-sport	NA	-
	VAS-rest	NA	-
	VAS-walk	NA	-

Abbreviations: VR (Virtual reality); NDI (Neck Disability Index); TIP% (Time to peak velocity percentage); ROM (range of motion); EQ-5D (EQ-5D™, http://www.euroqol.org); TSK (Tampa scale of kinesiophobia); NVP (Number of velocity peaks); VAS (Visual Analog Scale); FLACC (Faces, legs, activity, cry, consolability scale); FAAM (Foot and Ankle Ability Measure); ADL (activities of daily living); the-marked mean $p > 0.05$; NA (not available).

3.7. Effect of Virtual Reality on Acute and Chronic Musculoskeletal Pain

Although associated pain is not itself part of the root disorder, managing the pain of musculoskeletal disorders is a major part of general practice. Of the 14 musculoskeletal studies included, six were for acute pain, including the dressing of the burn wound [27,28], three were for TKR patients [14,16,29], one for patients with ankle sprain [30], and the rest of the eight articles were for chronic musculoskeletal pain patients, including patients with frozen shoulder, SAIS, Neck pain, LBP, and pelvic floor muscle training [15,17,18,22,24–26]. VR treatment seems to reduce the pain of burn patients, or it could reduce the use of analgesics [27,28]. No significant difference in all parameters was observed when TKR and ankle sprain patients received VR treatment as compared to conventional treatment [14,16,29,30]. And there is no MCID for VAS pain in its acute phase [29]. In the included articles, a significant difference in the main outcome was observed for all patients with chronic pain aside from the research conducted by Tomas et al. [23].

4. Discussion

Most virtual reality treatment research applications still focus on the VR treatment of central nervous system problems, such as stroke and cerebral palsy, while only a little research explores the therapeutic effect of VR treatment on patients with musculoskeletal disorders. At present, there is no research on the integration of virtual reality for patients with various musculoskeletal disorders and an analysis of its effects. Therefore, this scoping review searched and integrated multiple musculoskeletal disorders in VR applications. Analysis showed which patients with musculoskeletal disorders had better results after VR treatment.

In general, chronic pain usually lasts for more than 12 weeks, while acute pain usually lasts for 4 to 6 weeks [32]. Therefore, patients in the articles included in this study are those who experience chronic pain due to frozen shoulder (symptoms lasting more than 3 months), SAIS (symptoms lasting at least 2 months), neck pain (symptoms appear for more than 3 months), and LBP (symptoms persist for 2 or 3 months) [15,17,18,22–25]. The study on burn wound care included patients with acute pain due to burns. Fung et al. (2012) included TKR patients in their study under the condition of being able to apply a full load on the lower limbs after 2 weeks of physical therapy post-surgery. Another research made by Koo et al. studied TKR patients after 2 weeks of physical therapy post-surgery followed by VR treatment. In the preceding two TKR studies, patients belonged to the sub-acute and acute phase, and the pain that they felt was an acute pain [14,16]. As for another study, VR intervention was applied from one days to 6 months after TKR (longitudinal study). In the early postoperative period (3–7 days), VR intervention did not achieve any clinically better analgesic effect than traditional treatment [29]. The study on ankle sprains mentioned that patients with non-repetitive sprains can undergo emergency treatment for 4 weeks without pain followed by VR treatment; therefore, this does not belong to the category of chronic pain. From this systematic review, it was found that subjects that experienced more effective VR intervention tend to be patients with chronic orthopedic pain, or those with acute pain due to burn wounds. Patients with TKR and ankle sprains are not chronic pain patients, and results show that VR treatment is not more effective than other treatments.

Generally, patients suffering from chronic pain have lower levels of fitness than healthy people. This is because pain can affect the motor control strategies of people. Individuals tend to move in the least painful way; however, the least painful way is usually to refrain from moving. This causes a decrease in muscle size and strength; it repeatedly increases pain and stress, eventually producing to a vicious circle [33]. In the included research articles, the motions designed for patients with chronic orthopedic disorders are suitable for the joint movements of patients of this type. For example, in the virtual reality games for patients with frozen shoulder, the actions designed include shoulder elevation, shoulder IR/ER, and a shoulder abduction action, and suitable WII games are selected for shoulder impingement patients (such as the tennis game which involves shoulder capsule stretch, pectoral muscle stretch and shoulder elevation). For patients with other chronic orthopedic disorders, through somatosensory interactive games with larger movements, patients could try actions which they could not achieve. Furthermore, people usually focus on pain or impending pain; therefore, the use of VR is effective in distracting the attention of patients from pain. The distraction produced by VR reduces pain, induces movement, and promotes exercise. It also motivates patients to move. Most users describe that their experience of VR was pleasant, and it can relieve pain as well as reduce anxiety [20,34–36]. Nevertheless, VR treatment done under inadequate supervision may result in less than expected results [17,30]. VR intervention under supervision can increase the motivation or induce patients to receive movement training and boost their concentration. This systematic review found that VR treatment for patients with chronic pain, such as 4 weeks of VR plus modalities (hot pack and ultrasound) on patients with frozen shoulders produced a significant 8% increase in shoulder ROM when compared to traditional exercise training plus modalities [15]. Subacromial impingement syndrome (SAIS) patients underwent 6 weeks of VR training for 45 min/day, twice a week, and showed a significant improvement of SAIS and scapular dyskinesis symptoms than those in the home exercise group.

In addition, this result lasted for one month [22]. Another article that studied chronic cervical pain patients after 5 weeks of VR plus cervical kinematic training (KT) recounted a significant difference in global perceived change (patient self-reported changes in different areas, such as satisfaction, self-reported pain differences) when compared to the only KT group. The experienced outcome lasted for 3 months [18]. One research on low back pain showed that 4 weeks of VR training can alleviate pain, deep tissue pressure algometry, disability, and fear of low back pain. For the TKR patients, after one month to six months of VR intervention, the knee function is better than for those who received the traditional treatment [29]. One of the articles included in this study showed no significant difference in pain and lumbar spine flexion ROM after comparing 3 days of VR treatment for patients with lower back pain, and patients without VR treatment [23]. This scoping review shows that chronic patients may receive at least four weeks of VR treatment in order to experience a significant therapeutic effect. In addition, VR training seems to have a short-term effect for patients with chronic pain in the musculoskeletal system [17,18,22,25]. This is consistent with past research [36–38].

The results of this study show that VR treatment with a hand joystick significantly reduces the pain score of patients when removing dressings from patients with acute burns, or it will reduce the use of analgesics [27,28]. This is consistent with previous research [39–42]. Hoffman, et al. [40] showed that the use of VR for patients under severe pain can effectively reduce pain by 41%. It is speculated that VR can also be used to distract patients from severe acute pain during dressing change. Therefore, VR can be used to divert attention, thus reducing the use of analgesics.

In summary, VR treatment can reduce pain in acute burn wound care and chronic musculoskeletal disorders. It can effectively distract patients with chronic pain, and allow them to ignore the cumbersome rehabilitation training, consequently improving treatment motivation. In addition, VR treatment may be helpful in the psychological level and the establishment of confidence. For example, patients with burns or chronic disability may have a tendency to fall into depression because of the long course of the disorder. The use of VR can release psychological stress and reduce their fear of pain [19].

Virtual reality is also helpful in the control and perception of muscle movements. This systematic review includes the hard to control PFM, as well as waist and neck movements. The PFM training research included in this article [26] recommended the simple contraction of the lower abdominal muscles in the VR group. Previous studies pointed out that the lower abdominal muscles have a synergistic effect with PFM. Therefore, some scholars have suggested that if the patient does not know how to apply force during PFM contraction, training on abdominal transverse muscle contraction can be done to attain the same purpose [43]. Patients in the VR group interacted with the game screen and performed pelvic movements such as pelvic forward, backward, lateral tilt, and go around motions according to the easy-to-understand motion instructions provided by the Wii game screen. This made it possible for patients to understand how to control their pelvic motion, and at the same time, increased the control and perception of the PFM. The LBP patients included in this article used games that combined Wii and yoga for their training [24]. LBP patients usually have weak deep core muscles [44]. Yoga promotes the strengthening and relaxation of the waist muscles and ligaments. Through yoga, the body can be continuously aligned correctly. At the same time, the patients can clearly see their posture on the screen. The Wii board senses the weight and center of gravity of the body and trains LBP patients according to the steps in the game screen. For rehabilitation that needs repeated feedback and learning of exercises, VR can provide enthusiasm. Patients with neck pain can also use VR glasses to perform target tracking according to the instructions given by the game, and flex, stretch, and rotate the neck. Patients can adjust neck motion through the instant feedback given by the VR glasses [17,18]. The preceding discussions show that VR can be used to increase the control and training of PFM as well as the consciousness of waist and neck motion. Moreover, posture can be adjusted through VR instant feedback.

Depending on the different facilities which possess different visual perception methods, Virtual Reality can be divided into four types: (a) Desktop VR: Mouse, trackball, and joystick are the main computer transmission devices and a common PC screen was used as its output; (b) Simulator VR: In a specific environment, machines and equipment, added to an image screen, provided the Users simulation results; (c) Projection VR: With a large projection screen, several projectors, and stereo sound output devices, simulation scenes were projected around the user; (d) Immersion VR: Specific Input and output devices, such as helmet display, etc., were used in this type of simulation [1]. The result of the five included articles in the current study seemed to show some effectiveness of the immersion VR. VR glasses or VR TV output, 3D shuttle glasses or helmet display were used to allow the user to become fully immersed in the system, and computers were used to provide image or sound feedbacks (five out of five); Three of the five articles showed Wii (belong to the VR type (a) described as above) had achieved some effectiveness. Some patients may have nausea and dizziness due to the problems of the VR device, such as mismatched motion, motion parallax, viewing angle, limited reproduction of a real environment, and the imperfect simulation of human–world interactions. This condition occurring may affect its treatment effectiveness [45]. Facing the current economic development and the increase of the need of clinical care, we believe that it is necessary to explore the clinical effectiveness and applicability of the VR system. This highlights the importance of the ongoing discussions of the MCID on pain relief or on function increase in this article. The challenges in using the truly immersive

VR system include nausea or dizziness caused by immersing in the virtual world and investment costs (facilities, cost, personnel training) [35,45]. All of these also affect whether VR treatment is appropriate in clinical environment implementation.

Limitations

Because this system review includes first-rate RCT studies, fewer articles that compare the effects of VR therapy with other interventions on patients with musculoskeletal disorders are available. In some articles, the lack of raw numeric data makes it impossible to calculate the mean difference between the experimental and control groups. During the article retrieval process, language was also restricted; therefore, some language bias might exist. In addition, very few articles contain the minimal clinically important difference (MCID) on various parameters; hence, further discussion was not made.

5. Conclusions

VR treatment appears to have a significant effect upon pain relief, increased joint mobility, or the motor functions of patients with chronic painful musculoskeletal disorders. VR seems quite effective in relieving the pain of patients with acute burns as well. However, there is insufficient evidence in the current literature; hence, more research is needed to explore the therapeutic effects of VR treatment on musculoskeletal disorders. In the future, VR games maybe used for more patients with chronic musculoskeletal injuries. As to whether different types of VR would affect the effectiveness for rehabilitation results in musculoskeletal disorder patients, this should also be further investigated.

Acknowledgments: This study was partially funded by E-DA Hospital (EDAHT107029) and the Allied Advanced Intelligent Biomedical Research Center (A2IBRC) under the Higher Education Sprout Project of Ministry of Education.

References

1.   Burdea, G.C.; Coiffet, P. *Virtual Reality Technology*, 2nd ed.; Wiley-IEEE Press: Hoboken, NJ, USA, 2003.

2.   Wang, P.; Wu, P.; Wang, J.; Chi, H.-L.; Wang, X. A Critical Review of the Use of Virtual Reality in Construction Engineering Education and Training. *Int. J. Environ. Res. Public Health* **2018**, *15*, 1204. [CrossRef] [PubMed]

3.   Levac, D.; Glegg, S.; Colquhoun, H.; Miller, P.; Noubary, F. Virtual Reality and Active Videogame-Based Practice, Learning Needs, and Preferences: A Cross-Canada Survey of Physical Therapists and Occupational Therapists. *Games Health J.* **2017**, *6*, 217–228. [CrossRef] [PubMed]

4.   Levac, D.E.; Miller, P.E. Integrating virtual reality video games into practice: Clinicians' experiences. *Physiother. Theory Pract.* **2013**, *29*, 504–512. [CrossRef] [PubMed]

5.   Barton, G.J.; Hawken, M.B.; Foster, R.J.; Holmes, G.; Butler, P.B. The effects of virtual reality game training on trunk to pelvis coupling in a child with cerebral palsy. *J. Neuroeng. Rehabil.* **2013**, *10*, 15. [CrossRef] [PubMed]

6.   Broeren, J.; Rydmark, M.; Sunnerhagen, K.S. Virtual reality and haptics as a training device for movement rehabilitation after stroke: A single-case study. *Arch. Phys. Med. Rehabil.* **2004**, *85*, 1247–4250. [CrossRef] [PubMed]

7.   Chang, Y.J.; Chen, S.F.; Huang, J.D. A Kinect-based system for physical rehabilitation: A pilot study for young adults with motor disabilities. *Res. Dev. Disabil.* **2011**, *32*, 2566–2570. [CrossRef] [PubMed]

8.   Deutsch, J.E. Use of a low-cost, commercially available gaming console (Wii) for rehabilitation of an adolescent with cerebral palsy. *Phys. Ther.* **2008**, *88*, 1196. [CrossRef] [PubMed]

9.   Dos Santos Mendes, F.A.; Pompeu, J.E.; Modenesi Lobo, A.; Guedes da Silva, K.; Oliveira Tde, P.; Peterson Zomignani, A.; Pimentel Piemonte, M.E. Motor learning, retention and transfer after virtual-reality-based training in Parkinson's disease—Effect of motor and cognitive demands of games: A longitudinal, controlled clinical study. *Physiotherapy* **2012**, *98*, 217–223. [CrossRef]

10. Fischer, H.C.; Stubblefield, K.; Kline, T.; Luo, X.; Kenyon, R.V.; Kamper, D.G. Hand rehabilitation following stroke: A pilot study of assisted finger extension training in a virtual environment. *Top. Stroke Rehabil.* **2007**, *14*, 1–12. [CrossRef]

11. Sevick, M.; Eklund, E.; Mensch, A.; Foreman, M.; Standeven, J.; Engsberg, J. Using Free Internet Videogames in Upper Extremity Motor Training for Children with Cerebral Palsy. *Behav. Sci.* **2016**, *6*, 10. [CrossRef]

12. Bonnechere, B.; Jansen, B.; Omelina, L.; Van Sint Jan, S. The use of commercial video games in rehabilitation: A systematic review. *Int. J. Rehabil. Res.* **2016**, *39*, 277–290. [CrossRef]

13. The Definition of Musculoskeletal Disorders. 15 February 2018. Available online: https://www.who.int/news-room/fact-sheets/detail/musculoskeletal-conditions (accessed on 03 April 2019).

14. Fung, V.; Ho, A.; Shaffer, J.; Chung, E.; Gomez, M. Use of Nintendo Wii Fit in the rehabilitation of outpatients following total knee replacement: A preliminary randomised controlled trial. *Physiotherapy* **2012**, *98*, 183–188. [CrossRef] [PubMed]

15. Huang, M.C.; Lee, S.H.; Yeh, S.C.; Chan, R.C.; Rizzo, A.; Xu, W.; Wu, H.L.; Lin, S.H. Intelligent Frozen Shoulder Rehabilitation. *IEEE Intell. Syst.* **2014**, *29*, 22–28. [CrossRef]

16. Koo, K.-I.; Park, D.K.; Youm, Y.S.; Cho, S.D.; Hwang, C.H. Enhanced Reality Showing Long-Lasting Analgesia after Total Knee Arthroplasty: Prospective, Randomized Clinical Trial. *Sci. Rep.* **2018**, *8*, 2343. [CrossRef] [PubMed]

17. Sarig Bahat, H.; Croft, K.; Carter, C.; Hoddinott, A.; Sprecher, E.; Treleaven, J. Remote kinematic training for patients with chronic neck pain: A randomised controlled trial. *Eur. Spine J.* **2017**, *27*, 1309–1323. [CrossRef] [PubMed]

18. Sarig Bahat, H.; Takasaki, H.; Chen, X.; Bet-Or, Y.; Treleaven, J. Cervical kinematic training with and without interactive VR training for chronic neck pain—A randomized clinical trial. *Man. Ther.* **2015**, *20*, 68–78. [CrossRef] [PubMed]

19. Scapin, S.; Echevarria-Guanilo, M.E.; Boeira Fuculo Junior, P.R.; Goncalves, N.; Rocha, P.K.; Coimbra, R. Virtual Reality in the treatment of burn patients: A systematic review. *Burns* **2018**, *44*, 1403–1416. [CrossRef]

20. Hoffman, H.G.; Patterson, D.R.; Carrougher, G.J. Use of virtual reality for adjunctive treatment of adult burn pain during physical therapy: A controlled study. *Clin. J. Pain* **2000**, *16*, 244–250. [CrossRef]

21. Arlati, S.; Colombo, V.; Ferrigno, G.; Sacchetti, R.; Sacco, M. Virtual reality-based wheelchair simulators: A scoping review. *Assist. Technol.* **2019**, 1–12. [CrossRef]

22. Pekyavas, N.O.; Ergun, N. Comparison of virtual reality exergaming and home exercise programs in patients with subacromial impingement syndrome and scapular dyskinesis: Short term effect. *Acta Orthop. Traumatol. Turc.* **2017**, *51*, 238–242. [CrossRef]

23. Thomas, J.S.; France, C.R.; Applegate, M.E.; Leitkam, S.T.; Walkowski, S. Feasibility and Safety of a Virtual Reality Dodgeball Intervention for Chronic Low Back Pain: A Randomized Clinical Trial. *J. Pain* **2016**, *17*, 1302–1317. [CrossRef] [PubMed]

24. Kim, S.S.; Min, W.K.; Kim, J.H.; Lee, B.H. The Effects of VR-based Wii Fit Yoga on Physical Function in Middle-aged Female LBP Patients. *J. Phys. Ther. Sci.* **2014**, *26*, 549–552. [CrossRef] [PubMed]

25. Yilmaz Yelvar, G.; ırak1, Y.C.; Dalkılınc, M.; Demir, Y.P.; Guner, Z.; Boydak, A.E. Is physiotherapy integrated virtual walking effective on pain, function, and kinesiophobia in patients with non-specific low-back pain? Randomised controlled trial. *Eur. Spine J.* **2017**, *26*, 538–545. [CrossRef] [PubMed]

26. Martinho, N.M.; Silva, V.R.; Marques, J.; Carvalho, L.C.; Iunes, D.H.; Botelho, S. The effects of training by virtual reality or gym ball on pelvic floor muscle strength in postmenopausal women: A randomized controlled trial. *Braz. J. Phys. Ther.* **2016**, *20*, 248–257. [CrossRef] [PubMed]

27. Jeffs, D.; Dorman, D.; Brown, S.; Files, A.; Graves, T.; Kirk, E.; Meredith-Neve, S.; Sanders, J.; White, B.; Swearingen, C.J. Effect of virtual reality on adolescent pain during burn wound care. *J. Burn Care Res.* **2014**, *35*, 395–408. [CrossRef]

28. Kipping, B.; Rodger, S.; Miller, K.; Kimble, R.M. Virtual reality for acute pain reduction in adolescents undergoing burn wound care: A prospective randomized controlled trial. *Burns* **2012**, *38*, 650–657. [CrossRef]

29. Jin, C.; Feng, Y.; Ni, Y.; Shan, Z. Virtual reality intervention in postoperative rehabilitation after total knee arthroplasty: A prospective and randomized controlled clinical trial. *Int. J. Clin. Exp. Med.* **2018**, *11*, 6119–6124.

30. Punt, I.M.; Ziltener, J.L.; Monnin, D.; Allet, L. Wii Fit exercise therapy for the rehabilitation of ankle sprains: Its effect compared with physical therapy or no functional exercises at all. *Scand. J. Med. Sci. Sports* **2016**, *26*, 816–823. [CrossRef]

31. Tubach, F.; Ravaud, P.; Baron, G.; Falissard, B.; Logeart, I.; Bellamy, N.; Bombardier, C.; Felson, D.; Hochberg, M.; van der Heijde, D.; et al. Evaluation of clinically relevant changes in patient reported outcomes in knee and hip osteoarthritis: The minimal clinically important improvement. *Ann. Rheum. Dis.* **2005**, *64*, 29–33. [CrossRef]

32. Treede, R.D.; Rief, W.; Barke, A.; Aziz, Q.; Bennett, M.I.; Benoliel, R.; Cohen, M.; Evers, S.; Finnerup, N.B.; First, M.B.; et al. A classification of chronic pain for ICD-11. *Pain* **2015**, *156*, 1003–1007. [CrossRef]

33. Carpenter, D.M.; Nelson, B.W. Low back strengthening for the prevention and treatment of low back pain. *Med. Sci. Sports Exerc.* **1999**, *31*, 18–24. [CrossRef] [PubMed]

34. Sharar, S.R.; Alamdari, A.; Hoffer, C.; Hoffman, H.G.; Jensen, M.P.; Patterson, D.R. Circumplex Model of Affect: A Measure of Pleasure and Arousal During Virtual Reality Distraction Analgesia. *Games Health J.* **2016**, *5*, 197–202. [CrossRef] [PubMed]

35. Mosadeghi, S.; Reid, M.W.; Martinez, B.; Rosen, B.T.; Spiegel, B.M. Feasibility of an Immersive Virtual Reality Intervention for Hospitalized Patients: An Observational Cohort Study. *JMIR Ment. Health* **2016**, *3*, e28. [CrossRef] [PubMed]

36. Pourmand, A.; Davis, S.; Marchak, A.; Whiteside, T.; Sikka, N. Virtual Reality as a Clinical Tool for Pain Management. *Curr. Pain Headache Rep.* **2018**, *22*, 53. [CrossRef] [PubMed]

37. Garrett, B.; Taverner, T.; Masinde, W.; Gromala, D.; Shaw, C.; Negraeff, M. A rapid evidence assessment of immersive virtual reality as an adjunct therapy in acute pain management in clinical practice. *Clin. J. Pain* **2014**, *30*, 1089–1098. [CrossRef] [PubMed]

38. Jones, T.; Moore, T.; Choo, J. The Impact of Virtual Reality on Chronic Pain. *PLoS ONE* **2016**, *11*, e0167523. [CrossRef] [PubMed]

39. Chan, E.; Foster, S.; Sambell, R.; Leong, P. Clinical efficacy of virtual reality for acute procedural pain management: A systematic review and meta-analysis. *PLoS ONE* **2018**, *13*, e0200987. [CrossRef] [PubMed]

40. Hoffman, H.G.; Patterson, D.R.; Seibel, E.; Soltani, M.; Jewett-Leahy, L.; Sharar, S.R. Virtual reality pain control during burn wound debridement in the hydrotank. *Clin. J. Pain* **2008**, *24*, 299–304. [CrossRef]

41. Morris, L.D.; Louw, Q.A.; Crous, L.C. Feasibility and potential effect of a low-cost virtual reality system on reducing pain and anxiety in adult burn injury patients during physiotherapy in a developing country. *Burns* **2010**, *36*, 659–664. [CrossRef] [PubMed]

42. Maani, C.V.; Hoffman, H.G.; Morrow, M.; Maiers, A.; Gaylord, K.; McGhee, L.L.; DeSocio, P.A. Virtual reality pain control during burn wound debridement of combat-related burn injuries using robot-like arm mounted VR goggles. *J. Trauma* **2011**, *71*, S125–S130. [CrossRef]

43. Junginger, B.; Baessler, K.; Sapsford, R.; Hodges, P.W. Effect of abdominal and pelvic floor tasks on muscle activity, abdominal pressure and bladder neck. *Int. Urogynecol. J.* **2010**, *21*, 69–77. [CrossRef] [PubMed]

44. Hibbs, A.E.; Thompson, K.G.; French, D.; Wrigley, A.; Spears, I. Optimizing Performance by Improving Core Stability and Core Strength. *Sports Med.* **2008**, *38*, 995–1008. [CrossRef] [PubMed]

45. Park, M.; Im, H.; Kim, D.Y. Feasibility and user experience of virtual reality fashion stores. *Fash. Text.* **2018**, *5*, 1–17. [CrossRef]

Use of Secukinumab in a Cohort of Erythrodermic Psoriatic Patients

Giovanni Damiani [1,2,3,4,*,†], Alessia Pacifico [5,†], Filomena Russo [6],
Paolo Daniele Maria Pigatto [2,3], Nicola Luigi Bragazzi [7], Claudio Bonifati [5], Aldo Morrone [5],
Abdulla Watad [8,9,‡] and Mohammad Adawi [10,‡]

[1]   Department of Dermatology, Case Western Reserve University, Cleveland, OH 44124, USA
[2]   Clinical Dermatology, IRCCS Istituto Ortopedico Galeazzi, 20161 Milan, Italy; paolo.pigatto@unimi.it
[3]   Department of Biomedical, Surgical and Dental Sciences, University of Milan, 20122 Milan, Italy
[4]   Young Dermatologists Italian Network (YDIN), Centro Studi GISED, 24121 Bergamo, Italy
[5]   San Gallicano Dermatological Institute, IRCCS, 00144 Rome, Italy; alessia.pacifico@gmail.com (A.P.);
       claudio.bonifati@ifo.gov.it (C.B.); aldomorrone54@gmail.com (A.M.)
[6]   Dermatology Section, Department of Clinical Medicine and Immunological Science, University of Siena,
       53100 Siena, Italy; file.russo@libero.it
[7]   School of Public Health, Department of Health Sciences (DISSAL), University of Genoa, 16132 Genoa, Italy;
       robertobragazzi@gmail.com
[8]   NIHR Leeds Biomedical Research Centre, Leeds Teaching Hospitals NHS Trust, Leeds Institute of Rheumatic
       and Musculoskeletal Medicine, University of Leeds, Leeds LS7 4SA, UK; watad.abdulla@gmail.com
[9]   Department of Medicine 'B', Sheba Medical Center, Tel-Hashomer and Sackler Faculty of Medicine, Tel Aviv
       University, 5265601 Tel Aviv, Israel
[10]   Padeh and Ziv Hospitals, Azrieli Faculty of Medicine, Bar-Ilan University, 5290002 Ramat Gan, Israel;
       adawimo1802@gmail.com
*
†   These authors contributed equally to this work.

Abstract: Erythrodermic psoriasis (EP) is a dermatological emergency and its treatment with secukinumab is still controversial. Furthermore, no data exist regarding the prognostic value of drug abuse in such a condition. We performed a multi-center, international, retrospective study, enrolling a sample of EP patients (body surface area > 90%) who were treated with secukinumab (300 mg) during the study period from December 2015 to December 2018. Demographics and clinical data were collected. Drug abuses were screened and, specifically, smoking status (packages/year), cannabis use (application/week) and alcoholism—tested with the Alcohol Use Disorders Identification Test (AUDIT)—were assessed. All patients were followed for up to 52 weeks. We enrolled 13 EP patients, nine males, and four females, with a median age of 40 (28–52) years. Patients naïve to biologic therapy were 3/13. Regarding drug use, seven patients had a medium-high risk of alcohol addiction, three used cannabis weekly, and seven were smokers with a pack/year index of 295 (190–365). The response rate to secukinumab was 10/13 patients with a median time to clearance of three weeks (1.5–3). No recurrences were registered in the 52-week follow-up and a Psoriasis Area Severity Index (PASI) score of 90 was achieved. The entire cohort of non-responders (*n* = 3) consumed at least two drugs of abuse (alcohol, smoking or cannabis). Non-responders were switched to ustekinumab and obtained a PASI 100 in 24 weeks. However, given our observed number of patients using various drugs in combination with secukinumab in EP, further studies are needed to ascertain drug abuse prevalence in a larger EP cohort. Secukinumab remains a valid, effective and safe therapeutic option for EP.

Keywords: erythrodermic psoriasis; secukinumab; addiction; smoking; alcohol; cannabis

1. Introduction

Erythroderma is an uncommon and severe dermatological manifestation of a variety of diseases. The most common form of erythroderma is erythrodermic psoriasis (EP), which accounts for 1–2.25% of all psoriatic patients, with a male predominance as demonstrated by a male to female ratio of 3:1 [1]. EP clinically manifests with diffuse erythema (body surface area (BSA) > 75%) involving also skin folds with or without exfoliate dermatitis.

Several triggers have been described to elicit EP in predisposed subjects such as environmental factors (sunburn, alcoholism, and infections), drugs (lithium, anti-malarial drugs), and the rebound phenomenon following discontinuation of anti-psoriatic treatments (oral steroids or methotrexate) [1]. However, the pathogenesis of EP remains elusive, which can limit a physician's capability to deliver safe and effective therapy. In 2010, the National Psoriasis Foundation (NPF) published a guideline describing the current evidence regarding EP treatment, stating that cyclosporine and infliximab should be the first line treatment in acute and unstable patients, whilst methotrexate and acitretin are recommended in more stable patients [2].

Despite this clear advice, prominent limitations included that few high-quality studies assessing EP treatment were present in the literature [2]. In a clinical setting, EP treatment faces two other prominent challenges, namely the difficulty in differential diagnosis and in implementing a biological approach that rules out non-inflammatory conditions. Although histological confirmation is mandatory in suspected EP cases, it is sometimes challenging due to the potential lack of histological parameters resembling classical psoriasis, such as parakeratosis or acanthosis [1].

The exclusion of neoplastic causes (Sézary syndrome) is mandatory if biologics are the selected approach. In fact, in the last 5 years, neoplasia has been a relative contraindication [3]. The NPF guidelines did not include IL-17 inhibitors [2], such as secukinumab, and recently two case series studies described the use of secukinumab in EP patients [4,5]. Current evidence seems to support the use of secukinumab in EP patients, even though there is a dearth of data concerning potential predictors of responsiveness in these patients.

Remarkably, among psoriatic patients, alcohol use/abuse and smoking are described and linked to both psoriasis development and exacerbations but are not studied in EP [6–10]. Conversely, the prevalence of cannabis users among psoriatic patients and the effect of cannabis use on psoriasis are still missing. Furthermore, in vitro or murine studies explored keratinocyte changes only in response to a single cannabis compound [11]. Thus, due to the increasing prevalence of cannabis users in the general population and also its promoting role in medicine [11], reports focusing on the effect in psoriasis are needed.

The current study aimed to evaluate (i) first the efficacy and safety of secukinumab in psoriatic erythroderma and (ii) second to describe the prevalence of drug abuses, namely alcohol, tobacco, and cannabis smoking, in EP patients.

2. Experimental Section

This multi-center, international, retrospective, pilot study enrolled a sample of EP patients (BSA > 90%) treated with a loading dose of 300 mg subcutaneous secukinumab at weeks 0, 1, 2, 3 and 4, followed by 300 mg every 4 weeks, in the period from December 2015 to December 2018.

All erythrodermic patients were biopsied and malignancies were ruled out by complete blood count, blood smear, transaminases, lactate dehydrogenase (LDH), gamma-glutamyl transferase (GGT), anion gap, Sézary cell search, and total body computed tomography. Smoking history (pack/years), cannabis use (smoking episodes/week) and alcohol use (Alcohol Use Disorders Identification Test (AUDIT)) status were assessed.

AUDIT is a 10-question screening tool (0–40 points) developed by the World Health Organization (WHO) in order to evaluate alcohol consumption, drinking behavior, and alcohol-related complications. According to AUDIT, patients are stratified as follows: 0–7 points indicate a low risk, 8–15 points a medium risk, 16–19 points a high risk, and 20–40 points a probable addiction.

All EP patients underwent a 52-week follow-up to evaluate recurrent erythrodermic episodes.

Demographics and clinical charts were recorded, including: age; gender; previous Psoriasis Area Severity Index (PASI) score before erythroderma, if any; previous anti-psoriatic therapy; biologic therapy exposure; secukinumab response; side effects; drug use history; PASI and Dermatologic life quality index (DLQI) at weeks 8, 12, 16, 24, and 52. We stratified erythroderma clearance (BSA < 75%) based on PASI 75, PASI 90, PASI 100.

3. Results

3.1. Study Population

In the current study, 13 EP patients (female/male ratio equal to 9/4), with a median age of 40 (28–52), and body mass index of 24 (22–27) kg/m^2 were included. Family history of psoriasis was positive in 9/13 patients.

3.2. Drug History

In Table 1 we assessed drug history. Only 3/13 patients were naïve to biologic therapy. Among patients treated with biologics, eight had switched more than two biologics. Furthermore, 8/13 had a previous episode of erythroderma and six patients had more than two episodes. Drug history indicated that some of the EP patients had previously received therapeutic agents that could potentially trigger psoriasis, namely four underwent beta blockers, three received angiotensin II blockers (ARBs), two patients received angiotensin-converting enzyme (ACE) inhibitors, and one patient was previously treated with thiazide diuretics.

Table 1. Pharmacological history in our cohort.

Variables	EP ($n = 13$)
Last anti-psoriatic therapy (N (%))	
Methotrexate	1 (7.7)
Phototherapy	1 (7.7)
Adalimumab	4 (30.8)
Etanercept	2 (15.4)
Ustekinumab	2 (15.4)
Apremilast	1 (7.7)
Combination therapy (MTX + Etanercept)	3 (23.1)
Biologics naïve (N (%))	3 (23.1)
Biologics switching (N (%))	10 (76.9)
1	2 (20.0)
2	5 (50.0)
3	1 (10.0)
>3	2 (20.0)
Other drugs capable to aggravate psoriasis (N (%))	
Beta-blockers	4 (30.8)
ACE inhibitors	2 (15.4)
ARBs	3 (23.1)
Thiazides diuretics	1 (7.7)

ACE: Angiotensin-converting enzyme, ARBs: Angiotensin II receptor blockers, EP: erythrodermic psoriasis, MTX: Methotrexate.

3.3. Drug Abuses and Comorbidities

Drug abuse screening revealed that seven patients had a medium-high risk of alcohol abuse, three patients used cannabis on a weekly basis, and seven patients were smokers with a pack/year index of 295 (190–365). The comorbidities represented in our cohort included: dyslipidemia (five patients), hypertension (three patients), osteoporosis (two patients), atrial fibrillation (one patient) and pulmonary tuberculosis (one patient), respectively (Table 2).

Table 2. Prevalence of drug abuses in our cohort.

Addictions	EP (n = 13)
Smokers (N (%))	7 (53.8)
Pack/year (median (IQR))	295 (190–365)
AUDIT test (median ± SD)	9 (4–14)
Zone I (0–7 points) (N (%))	6 (46.2)
Zone II (8–15 points) (N (%))	6 (46.2)
Zone III (16–19 points) (N (%))	1 (7.7)
Zone IV (20–40 points) (N (%))	0 (0.0)
Cannabis use (N (%))	3 (23.1)

AUDIT: Alcohol Use Disorders Identification Test, EP: erythrodermic psoriasis, IQR: Interquartile range, SD: standard deviation.

3.4. Clinical Response to Secukinumab

Clinical and therapeutic data are summarized in Table 3. The median value of the last recorded PASI was 10 (7–15). Responders to secukinumab were 10/13 (Figure 1a,b) and the median clearing time was three (1.5–3) weeks.

Table 3. Clinical and therapeutic records in our cohort.

Variables	EP (n = 13)
Last control PASI (median (IQR))	10 (7–15)
Secukinumab responders (N (%))	10 (76.9)
Secukinumab non-responders (N (%))	3 (23.1)
Previous erythroderma episodes (N (%))	8 (61.5)
1	2 (25.0)
2	3 (37.5)
3	1 (12.5)
>3	2 (25.0)
Erythroderma clearing time (median (IQR), weeks)	3 (1–5.3)
PASI (median (IQR))	
Week 8	15 (13–17)
PASI 75 (N (%))	4 (30.8)
PASI 90 (N (%))	0 (0.0)
PASI 100 (N (%))	0 (0.0)
Week 12	4.5 (0–10)
PASI 75 (N (%))	5 (38.5)
PASI 90 (N (%))	3 (23.1)
PASI 100 (N (%))	4 (30.8)

Table 3. *Cont.*

Variables	EP (*n* = 13)
Week 16	2 (0–5)
PASI 75 (*N* (%))	1 (7.7)
PASI 90 (*N* (%))	5 (38.5)
PASI 100 (*N* (%))	4 (30.8)
Week 24	2 (0–2.75)
PASI 75 (*N* (%))	1 (7.7)
PASI 90 (*N* (%))	5 (38.5)
PASI 100 (*N* (%))	4 (30.8)
DLQI (median (IQR))	
Week 8	17 (13–22)
Week 12	12 (9–17)
Week 16	11 (7–16)
Week 24	8 (6–12)
Week 52	8 (5–12)
Side effects (*N* (%))	5 (38.5)
Recurrent oral candidiasis	1 (20.0)
Urticaria	1 (20.0)
Injection-site pain	3 (60.0)

DLQI: Dermatologic Life Quality Index, EP: erythrodermic psoriasis, IQR: Interquartile range, MTX: Methotrexate, PASI: Psoriasis Area Severity Index.

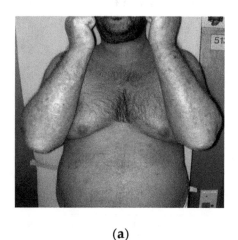 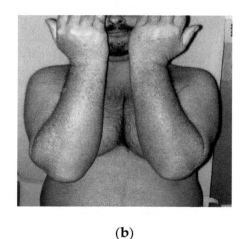

(a)   (b)

Figure 1. A 34-year-old patient with erythrodermic psoriasis that underwent secukinumab therapy. (**a**) Erythrodermic patient before treatment, (**b**) Patient after three weeks of secukinumab treatment.

Side effects were reported in 5/13 patients and remarkably were the only cause of treatment interruption, in contrast to other previously reported cases series [4,5]. All patients were on continuous secukinumab treatment and no recurrences were registered in the 52 weeks of follow up. After recovering from erythroderma at week eight, four patients achieved PASI 75, while none achieved PASI 90 or PASI 100. At week 52, five patients achieved PASI 90 and five achieved PASI 100. Interestingly, looking at the PASI trends of this cohort (Figure 2), all three non-responders used two out of three of the aforementioned drugs (alcohol, cannabis, and smoking) and no recorded comorbidities. Non-responders were switched to ustekinumab (90 mg) and obtained a PASI 100 in 24 weeks.

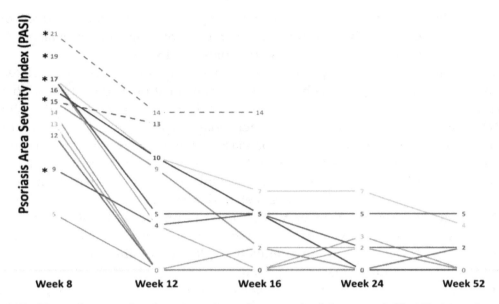

Figure 2. PASI trends in erythrodermic patients from week eight to week 52. * Patients that displayed more than one type of drug use (tobacco, cannabis, alcohol).

4. Discussion

Our study further supports that secukinumab is an effective therapy in EP and suggests that the use of recreational and accepted drugs (alcohol, cannabis, and tobacco) is prevalent in EP patients.

Furthermore, in the literature, EP patients treated with secukinumab had 16 [4] or 24 [5] months of follow up, lacking an assessment of long-term DLQI. Thus we assessed DLQI at 8, 12, 16, 24, and 52 weeks and found that secukinumab contributed to the improvement, not only in skin disease, but also in the long-term quality of life of EP patients. In our cohort, EP patients that responded to secukinumab did not exhibit recurrences and maintained long-term responsiveness to the drug. This study further supports the results described in a retrospective 52-week, observational, multicenter study, evaluated by Galluzzo et al., which suggested long-term efficacy of secukinumab in plaque psoriasis [12].

Focusing on EP patients, we assessed for the first time in detail the timing related to clearance of erythroderma, and after that, how secukinumab managed to clear the residual plaque psoriasis during the 52-week follow-up period. These two parameters together, are of pivotal importance in the clinical setting to guide therapeutic decisions made by dermatologists. In addition, the 52-week follow-up data highlighted that the EP responders to secukinumab achieved at least PASI 90 after clearing EP.

Among the three patients who did not respond to secukinumab therapy, one patient developed generalized urticaria at week three, the second patient experienced recurrent oral candidiasis and stopped the drug at week 12, and the third patient lost response at week 16. Remarkably, the second non-responder also smoked cannabis. Non-responders have not previously been treated with ustekinumab, and in accord with the recent real-life data on secukinumab non-responders, they were switched to ustekinumab and achieved a complete remission [13]. Ustekinumab is an IL-12/IL-23 blocker that targets the p40 subunit shared by these two cytokines. Furthermore, IL-12 plays a pivotal role in T helper cell type 1 (Th-1) polarization, as does IL-23 in Th-17 polarization [14]. We interpret the non-responsiveness of our patients as potentially due to the development of anti-secukinumab antibodies or up-regulation of Th-1-related pro-inflammatory cytokines, as previously demonstrated by Zaba et al. [15].

Evaluation of clinical characteristics in secukinumab non-responders indicated that all three had a familial history of EP and had used more than one drug, including smoking, alcohol, and cannabis. However, none of them were treated with any drug known to trigger psoriasis.

In the literature, the prevalence of drug abuse in the rare subset of EP is not reported, conversely, in plaque psoriasis patients several authors addressed the problem of drug abuse prevalence (alcohol and tobacco smoking) and its impact on anti-psoriatic therapies [7,8,16,17].

Alcohol intake and, consequently, also the abuse, may favor psoriasis-related systemic inflammation by promoting lipopolysaccharide (LPS) translocation from intestine to blood flow, increasing the pro-inflammatory activation of several immune cells, including lymphocytes (producing TNF-α and IFN-γ) and monocytes/macrophages (producing TNF-α), and directly by triggering keratinocytes pro-inflammatory activation via keratinocyte growth factor receptor (KGFR) [9]. These observations are further supported by Brenaut and colleagues, who conducted a meta-analysis on the epidemiological link between psoriasis and alcohol intake, and found that alcohol is a risk factor in developing psoriasis [17]. Furthermore, Qureshi et al. described a correlation between heavy beer intake and psoriasis severity during exacerbation [8]. This concept is translatable to EP patients, where erythroderma is an acute and very severe exacerbation of pre-existent psoriasis. Thus, alcohol abuse seems to increase TNF-α levels and may theoretically explain a possible lack or loss of response to IL-17 blockers, as with secukinumab in our EP patients.

Tobacco smoking and its link with psoriasis was assessed by Armstrong and colleagues in a large meta-analysis, involving 28 studies. They found an odds-ratio (OR) of 1.78 (95% confidence interval = 1.52–2.06) and a higher PASI in psoriatic smokers compared to non-smokers [16]. Remarkably, psoriasis severity gradually increases with the number of cigarettes smoked per day [17], but may benefit from a stop in smoking [18,19]. The nicotine contained in cigarettes activates nicotinic acetylcholine receptors (nAChRs) on the surface of dendritic cells, macrophages, endotheliocytes and keratinocytes, leading to an increased Th-1/Th-17 polarization of naïve T cells and to an increased production of pro-inflammatory cytokines, such as TNF-α, IL-12, IL-17, IL-23, IL-1β and IFN-γ [20]. These are all capable of decreasing the therapeutic effects of both TNF-α [7] and IL-17 blockers.

Conversely, fragmentary data exist regarding the effects of cannabis on the immune system and skin [21,22], but no data have been published about cannabis smoking in psoriatic patients or in murine models of psoriasis. However, some purified extracts derived from cannabis may inhibit in vitro keratinocyte proliferation [21] and Th-17 cell-related cytokine production in a dose-dependent manner [22]. Cannabinoids mainly interact with two receptors, cannabinoid-1 receptor (CB1R) and (CB2R), and both inhibit adenylate cyclase and activate mitogen-activated protein kinase (MAPK) [11]. This theoretically contrasts the anti-psoriatic function of apremilast, with regard to the intracellular cyclic adenosine monophosphate (AMPc) increase due to phosphodiesterase-4 inhibition. CB1R is prevalently present in keratinocytes, whilst CB2R is prevalent in immune cells, such as T cells and monocytes/macrophages [11]. Upon stimulation in the presence of purified cannabis extracts, namely cannabidiol (CBD) and tetrahydrocannabinol (THC), Th-17 cells massively decrease both transcription and release of IL-17A [22], which may theoretically act synergistically with IL-17 blockers. This aspect may be also confirmed by reports that list candidiasis as a side effect of both IL-17 blockers and chronic cannabis use [23]. Consequently, patients under IL-17 blockers that use cannabis may be exposed to a higher risk of candidiasis. Remarkably, Russo and colleagues pointed out that, in order to evaluate the global effect of cannabis, it is necessary to take into consideration the synergism existing among different cannabis compounds that altogether determine the final so-called entourage effect, capable of enhancing or even obscuring the properties of single compound [24]. Furthermore, no studies evaluated how smoking cannabis can modify these compounds and their biological effect. Thus, this is the first report to evaluate this relevant use of such drugs in a cohort of patients affected by EP, a chronic systemic inflammatory disease.

Moreover, both smoking and alcohol consumption were found to increase IL-17 and TNF-α production [9,12,16], corroborating our hypothesis that drug use may promote systemic inflammation, contributing to less favorable results from anti-psoriatic therapies.

The main limitation of the present study remains the small sample of enrolled patients, which was due to EP rarity and due to the fact secukinumab is still off-label in treating EP. Therefore, we cannot conclude that drug use in the non-responding patient group was causal. Other plausible reasons for the failed response in the small number of patients with addiction problems in the present cohort might well be insufficient compliance, even though all of our patients regularly attended dermatological appointments and reported to have auto-injected secukinumab.

5. Conclusions

Although not conclusive, our preliminary results in EP patients treated with secukinumab enlighten two presently unmet needs: (i) the need of therapy-specific biomarkers/prognostic factors and (ii) the prevalence of drug use in EP.

In conclusion, secukinumab may be a safe and effective treatment in EP, however, larger studies are needed to validate our results.

Author Contributions: Conceptualization, G.D. and A.W.; methodology, G.D., F.R. and N.L.B.; software, G.D. and N.L.B.; validation, G.D. and A.W.; formal analysis, G.D. and N.L.B.; investigation, G.D.; resources, M.A.; data curation, G.D. and N.L.B.; writing—original draft preparation, G.D. and C.B.; writing—review and editing, G.D., A.P., F.R., P.D.M.P., N.L.B., C.B., A.M., A.W. and M.A.; visualization, A.W. and M.A.; supervision, G.D., A.M. and M.A.; project administration, G.D., P.D.M.P., C.B. and A.M.; funding acquisition, M.A.

Acknowledgments: G.D. is supported by the P50 AR 070590 01A1 National Institute of Arthritis and Musculoskeletal and Skin Diseases.

References

1. Singh, R.K.; Lee, K.M.; Ucmak, D.; Brodsky, M.; Atanelov, Z.; Farahnik, B.; Abrouk, M.; Nakamura, M.; Zhu, T.H.; Liao, W. Erythrodermic psoriasis: Pathophysiology and current treatment perspectives. *Psoriasis (Auckl)* **2016**, *6*, 93–104.
2. Rosenbach, M.; Hsu, S.; Korman, N.J.; Lebwohl, M.G.; Young, M.; Bebo, B.F., Jr.; Van Voorhees, A.S.; National Psoriasis Foundation Medical Board. Treatment of erythrodermic psoriasis: From the medical board of the National Psoriasis Foundation. *J. Am. Acad. Dermatol.* **2010**, *62*, 655–662. [CrossRef] [PubMed]
3. Nast, A.; Gisondi, P.; Ormerod, A.D.; Saiag, P.; Smith, C.; Spuls, P.I.; Arenberger, P.; Bachelez, H.; Barker, J.; Dauden, E.; et al. European S3-Guidelines on the systemic treatment of psoriasis vulgaris–Update 2015–Short version–EDF in cooperation with EADV and IPC. *J. Eur. Acad. Dermatol. Venereol.* **2015**, *29*, 2277–2294. [CrossRef] [PubMed]
4. Mateu-Puchades, A.; Santos-Alarcón, S.; Martorell-Calatayud, A.; Pujol-Marco, C.; Sánchez-Carazo, J.L. Erythrodermic psoriasis and secukinumab: Our clinical experience. *Dermatol. Ther.* **2018**, *31*, e12607. [CrossRef] [PubMed]
5. Weng, H.J.; Wang, T.S.; Tsai, T.F. Clinical experience of secukinumab in the treatment of erythrodermic psoriasis: A case series. *Br. J. Dermatol.* **2018**, *178*, 1439–1440. [CrossRef] [PubMed]
6. Li, W.; Han, J.; Qureshi, A.A. Smoking and risk of incident psoriatic arthritis in US women. *Ann. Rheum. Dis.* **2012**, *71*, 804–808. [CrossRef]
7. Hojgaard, P.; Glintborg, B.; Hetland, M.L.; Hansen, T.H.; Lage-Hansen, P.R.; Petersen, M.H.; Holland-Fischer, M.; Nilsson, C.; Loft, A.G.; Andersen, B.N.; et al. Association between tobacco smoking and response to tumour necrosis factor alpha inhibitor treatment in psoriatic arthritis: Results from the DANBIO registry. *Ann. Rheum. Dis.* **2015**, *74*, 2130–2136. [CrossRef]
8. Qureshi, A.A.; Dominguez, P.L.; Choi, H.; Han, J.; Curhan, G. Alcohol intake and risk of incident psoriasis in US women: A prospective study. *Arch. Dermatol.* **2010**, *146*, 1364–1369. [CrossRef] [PubMed]
9. Farkas, A.; Kemeny, L. Alcohol, liver, systemic inflammation and skin: A focus on patients with psoriasis. *Skin Pharmacol. Physiol.* **2013**, *26*, 119–126. [CrossRef]
10. Poikolainen, K.; Reunala, T.; Karvonen, J.; Lauharanta, J.; Kärkkäinen, P. Alcohol intake: A risk factor for psoriasis in young and middle aged men? *BMJ* **1990**, *300*, 780–783. [CrossRef] [PubMed]

11. Katz-Talmor, D.; Katz, I.; Porat-Katz, B.S.; Shoenfeld, Y. Cannabinoids for the treatment of rheumatic diseases—Where do we stand? *Nat. Rev. Rheumatol.* **2018**, *14*, 488–498. [CrossRef]

12. Galluzzo, M.; Talamonti, M.; De Simone, C.; D'Adamio, S.; Moretta, G.; Tambone, S.; Caldarola, G.; Fargnoli, M.C.; Peris, K.; Bianchi, L. Secukinumab in moderate-to-severe plaque psoriasis: A multi-center, retrospective, real-life study up to 52 weeks observation. *Expert Opin. Biol. Ther.* **2018**, *18*, 727–735. [CrossRef]

13. Damiani, G.; Conic, R.R.Z.; de Vita, V.; Costanzo, A.; Regazzini, R.; Pigatto, P.D.M.; Bragazzi, N.L.; Pacifico, A.; Malagoli, P. When IL-17 inhibitors fail: Real-life evidence to switch from secukinumab to adalimumab or ustekinumab. *Dermatol. Ther.* **2018**, e12793. [CrossRef]

14. van Vugt, L.J.; van den Reek, J.M.P.A.; Hannink, G.; Coenen, M.J.H.; de Jong, E.M.G.J. Association of HLA-C*06:02 Status with Differential Response to Ustekinumab in Patients With Psoriasis: A Systematic Review and Meta-analysis. *JAMA Dermatol.* **2019**. [CrossRef]

15. Zaba, L.C.; Suárez-Fariñas, M.; Fuentes-Duculan, J.; Nograles, K.E.; Guttman-Yassky, E.; Cardinale, I.; Lowes, M.A.; Krueger, J.G. Effective treatment of psoriasis with etanercept is linked to suppression of IL-17 signaling, not immediate response TNF genes. *J. Allergy Clin. Immunol.* **2009**, *124*, 1022–1030.e395. [CrossRef] [PubMed]

16. Armstrong, E.J.; Harskamp, C.T.; Dhillon, J.S.; Armstrong, A.W. Psoriasis and smoking: A systematic review and meta-analysis. *Br. J. Dermatol.* **2014**, *170*, 304–314. [CrossRef] [PubMed]

17. Brenaut, E.; Horreau, C.; Pouplard, C.; Barnetche, T.; Paul, C.; Richard, M.A.; Joly, P.; Le Maître, M.; Aractingi, S.; Aubin, F.; et al. Alcohol consumption and psoriasis: A systematic literature review. *J. Eur. Acad. Dermatol. Venereol.* **2013**, *27*, 30–35. [CrossRef]

18. Fortes, C.; Mastroeni, S.; Leffondré, K.; Sampogna, F.; Melchi, F.; Mazzotti, E.; Pasquini, P.; Abeni, D. Relationship between smoking and the clinical severity of psoriasis. *Arch. Dermatol.* **2005**, *141*, 1580–1584. [CrossRef] [PubMed]

19. Richer, V.; Roubille, C.; Fleming, P.; Starnino, T.; McCourt, C.; McFarlane, A.; Siu, S.; Kraft, J.; Lynde, C.; Pope, J.E.; et al. Psoriasis and smoking: A systematic literature review and meta-analysis with qualitative analysis of effect of smoking on psoriasis severity. *J. Cutan. Med. Surg.* **2016**, *20*, 221–227. [CrossRef]

20. Armstrong, A.W.; Armstrong, E.J.; Fuller, E.N.; Sockolov, M.E.; Voyles, S.V. Smoking and pathogenesis of psoriasis: A review of oxidative, inflammatory and genetic mechanisms. *Br. J. Dermatol.* **2011**, *165*, 1162–1168. [CrossRef]

21. Wilkinson, J.D.; Williamson, E.M. Cannabinoids inhibit human keratinocyte proliferation through a non-CB1/CB2 mechanism and have a potential therapeutic value in the treatment of psoriasis. *J. Dermatol. Sci.* **2007**, *45*, 87–92. [CrossRef] [PubMed]

22. Kozela, E.; Juknat, A.; Kaushansky, N.; Rimmerman, N.; Ben-Nun, A.; Vogel, Z. Cannabinoids decrease the th17 inflammatory autoimmune phenotype. *J. Neuroimmune Pharmacol.* **2013**, *8*, 1265–1276. [CrossRef] [PubMed]

23. Dhadwal, G.; Kirchhof, M.G. The Risks and Benefits of Cannabis in the Dermatology Clinic. *J. Cutan. Med. Surg.* **2018**, *22*, 194–199. [CrossRef]

24. Russo, E.B. Taming THC: Potential cannabis synergy and phytocannabinoid-terpenoid entourage effects. *Br. J. Pharmacol.* **2011**, *163*, 1344–1364. [CrossRef] [PubMed]

16

The Efficacy and Safety of Doripenem in the Treatment of Acute Bacterial Infections

Chih-Cheng Lai [1], I-Ling Cheng [2], Yu-Hung Chen [2] and Hung-Jen Tang [3,*]

[1] Department of Intensive Care Medicine, Chi Mei Medical Center, Liouying 73657, Taiwan
[2] Department of Pharmacy, Chi Mei Medical Center, Liouying 73657, Taiwan
[3] Department of Medicine, Chi Mei Medical Center, Tainan 71004, Taiwan
* Correspondence: 8409d1@gmail.com

Abstract: This study aims to assess the efficacy and safety of doripenem on treating patients with acute bacterial infections. The Pubmed, Embase, and Cochrane databases were searched up to April 2019. Only randomized clinical trials comparing doripenem and other comparators for the treatment of acute bacterial infection were included. The primary outcome was the clinical success rate and the secondary outcomes were microbiological eradication rate and risk of adverse events. Eight randomized controlled trials (RCTs) were included. Overall, doripenem had a similar clinical success rate with comparators (odds ratio [OR], 1.15; 95% CI, 0.79–1.66, I2 = 58%). Similar clinical success rates were noted between doripenem and comparators for pneumonia (OR, 0.84; 95% CI, 0.46–1.53, I^2 = 72%) and for intra-abdominal infections (OR, 1.00; 95% CI, 0.57–1.72). For complicated urinary tract infection, doripenem was associated with higher success rate than comparators (OR, 1.89, 95% CI, 1.13–3.17, I^2 = 0%). The pool analysis comparing doripenem and other carbapenems showed no significant differences between each other (OR, 0.96, 95% CI, 0.59–1.58, I^2 = 63%). Doripenem also had a similar microbiological eradication rate with comparators (OR, 1.08; 95% CI, 0.86–1.36, I^2 = 0%). Finally, doripenem had a similar risk of treatment-emergent adverse events as comparators (OR, 0.98; 95% CI, 0.83–1.17, I^2 = 33%). In conclusion, the clinical efficacy of doripenem is as high as that of the comparator drugs in the treatment of acute bacterial infection; furthermore, this antibiotic is as well tolerated as the comparators.

Keywords: doripenem; acute bacterial infection; pneumonia; intra-abdominal infection; complicated urinary tract infection

1. Introduction

Carbapenems, including imipenem and meropenem, remain the mainstay of treatment for hospital-acquired infections, especially for the multidrug-resistant organism associated infections [1]. Doripenem is another important carbapenem, and has excellent bactericidal activity against most nosocomial pathogens according to several in vitro studies [2–5]. A global surveillance showed that doripenem was at least two-fold more potent in in vitro activities than imipenem and meropenem against *Pseudomonas aeruginosa*—an important nosocomial pathogen [3]. For another notorious pathogen—*Acinetobacter baumannii*, doripenem displayed comparable in vitro activities to imipenem and meropenem [4]. Clinically, doripenem is approved for the treatment of patients with complicated intra-abdominal infection (cIAI), complicated urinary tract infection (cUTI) and pyelonephritis, and healthcare-associated pneumonia (HAP) including ventilator-associated pneumonia (VAP) in Europe and in other countries, other than United States. Although Qu et al. [6] conducted a meta-analysis of doripenem for treating bacterial infections in 2015, only six clinical trials were enrolled and the number of patients was limited. Since then, two more studies investigating the efficacy of doripenem in comparison with other comparators were reported [7,8]. In Wagenlehner et al.'s study [7], 1033 randomized patients were enrolled, and they did the comparison between doripenem and ceftazidime-avibactam for the treatment of cUTI. In Oyake et al.'s study [8], they compared the empirical use of doripenem versus meropenem for febrile neutropenia in patients with acute leukemia. These two studies provided more patients and different types of infections compared to previse meta-analysis [6]. Therefore, we could conduct a comprehensive review and updated meta-analysis to assess the efficacy and safety of doripenem on treating patients with acute bacterial infections in comparison with other antibiotics, especially imipenem and meropenem.

2. Methods

2.1. Study Search and Selection

Studies were identified by a systematic review of the literature in the PubMed, Embase, and Cochrane databases until April 2019 using the following search terms—"doripenem," "infection," and "randomized" (Appendix A). Studies were considered eligible for inclusion if they directly compared the clinical effectiveness of doripenem with other antimicrobial agents in the treatment of adult patients with acute bacterial infections. Studies were excluded if they focused on in vitro activity, or pharmacokinetic-pharmacodynamic assessment. The articles of all languages of publication could be included. Two reviewers (I.-L.C. and Y.-H.C.) searched and examined publications independently. When they had disagreement, the third author (C.-C.L.) resolved the issue in time. The following data including year of publication, study design, type of infections, patients' demographic features, antimicrobial regimens, clinical and microbiological outcomes, and adverse events were extracted from every included study.

2.2. Definitions and Outcomes

The primary outcome was overall clinical success with resolution of clinical signs and symptoms of acute bacterial infection, or recovery to the pretreatment state at the end of treatment. Secondary outcomes included the microbiological eradication rate and adverse events. A microbiological eradication was defined as eradication (the baseline pathogen was absent) and presumed eradication (if an adequate source specimen was not available to culture, but the patient was assessed as clinically cured). Treatment-emergent adverse events were recorded, irrespective of causality. In addition, the risk of discontinuing due to adverse event and the incidence of serious adverse events, and some common events, including diarrhea, nausea, headache, constipation, and seizure were recorded.

2.3. Data Analysis

This study used the Cochrane risk of bias assessment tool to assess the quality of enrolled randomized controlled trials (RCTs) and the risk of bias [9]. The software Review Manager, version 5.3, was used to conduct the statistical analyses. The degree of heterogeneity was evaluated with the Q statistic generated from the χ^2 test. The proportion of statistical heterogeneity was assessed by the I^2 measure. Heterogeneity was considered significant when the p-value was less than 0.10 or the I^2 was more than 50%. The random-effects model was used when the data were significantly heterogeneous, and the fixed-effect model was used when the data were homogenous. Pooled odds ratios (OR) and 95% confidence intervals (CI) were calculated for outcome analyses. Sensitivity analysis was performed to ensure that the findings were not significantly affected by any individual study

3. Results

3.1. Study Selection and Characteristics

The search program yielded 499 references, including 263 from Pubmed, 170 from Embase, and 66 from Cochrane database. Then, 258 articles were screened after excluding 241 duplicated articles. Finally, a total of eight RCTs [7,8,10–15] fulfilling the inclusion criteria were included in this meta-analysis (Figure 1). All of studies were designed to compare the clinical efficacy and safety of doripenem with other antibiotics for patients with acute bacterial infection (Table 1) [7,8,10–15]. During the initial enrollment, doripenem and comparators were applied to 1736 and 1763 patients, respectively. Six studies [7,10–13,15] of them were multicenter studies. Three studies [10–12] focused on pneumonia, including two [12,16] on ventilator-associated pneumonia and one [10] on nosocomial pneumonia. Two studies focused on complicated urinary tract infections (cUTI) [7,13] and intra-abdominal infections (IAI) [14,15]. Only one study investigated febrile neutropenia [8]. Five studies [8,11,12,14,15] compared doripenem with other carbapenems including imipenem in three studies [11,12,14] and meropenem in two studies [8,15]. The regimen of doripenem was 1 g every eight hours in two studies [8,11] and 500 mg every eight hours in the other six studies [7,10,12–15]. For the two studies using double dose of doripenem (1 g every eight hour), the study drug (doripenem or meropenem) was used for at least five days in one study [8] and another one [11] compared seven-day doripenem versus 10-day imipenem-cilastatin. Figure 2 shows the analyses of risk of bias.

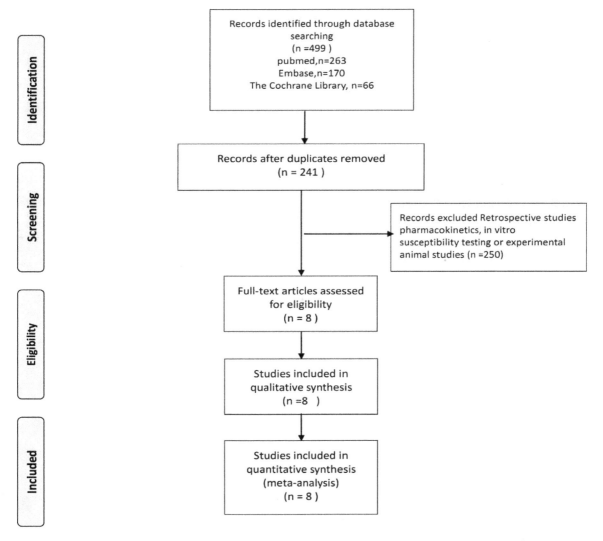

Figure 1. Flowchart of the study selection process.

Table 1. Characteristics of included studies.

Reference	RCT Study Design	Duration	Study Population	No. of Patients		Age of the Patients		Dose Regimen	
				Doripenem	Comparator	Doripenem	Comparator	Doripenem	Comparator
[10]	Randomized, open-label, multicenter trial	2004–2006	Nosocomial pneumonia	225	223	57.5	59.3	Doripenem 500 mg every 8 h	Piperacillin/tazobactam 4.5 g every 6 h
[15]	Prospective, multicenter, randomized, double-blind	2004–2006	Complicated intra-abdominal infection	237	239	46.9	46.4	Doripenem 500 mg every 8 h	Meropenem 1.0 g every 8 h
[12]	Prospective, multicenter, randomized, open-label trial	2004–2006	Ventilator-associated pneumonia	262	263	50.7	50.3	Doripenem 500 mg every 8 h	Imipenem/cilastatin 1 g every 8 h or 500 mg every 6 h
[13]	Prospective, multicenter, double-blind trial	2003–2006	Complicated UTI	377	376	51.2	51.1	Doripenem 500 mg every 8 h	Levofloxacin 250 mg everyday
[11]	Randomized, double-blind, multicenter trial	2008–2011	Ventilator-associated pneumonia	115	112	57.5	54.6	Doripenem 1 g every 8 h	Imipenem/cilastatin 1 g every 8 h
[14]	Randomized, open-label trial	2010–2013	Moderate or severe acute cholangitis or cholecystitis	62	65	74	73	Doripenem 500 mg every 8 h	Imipenem/cilastatin 500 mg every 8 h
[7]	Randomized, multicenter, double-blind, trials	2012–2014	Complicated UTI	393	417	53.3	51.4	Doripenem 500 mg every 8 h	Ceftazidime-avibactam 2000 mg/500 mg every 8 h
[8]	Randomized, open-label prospective trial	2011–2013	Febrile neutropenia in patients with acute leukemia or MDS-refractory anemia with excess blasts	65	68	57	56	Doripenem 1 g every 8 h	Meropenem 1.0 g every 8 h

MDS, myelodysplastic syndrome; UTI, urinary tract infection; RCT, randomized controlled trial.

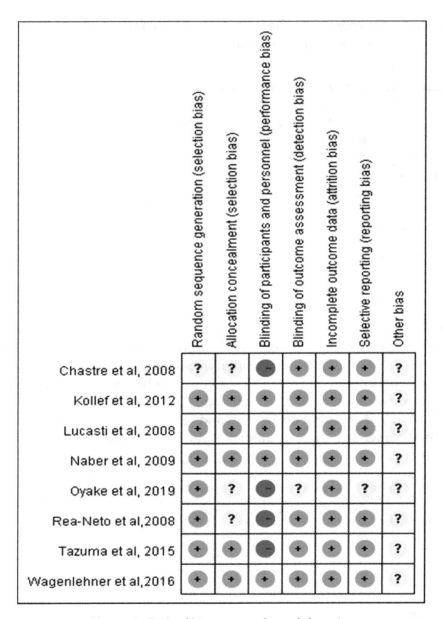

Figure 2. Risk of bias per study and domain.

3.2. Clinical Success

Overall, doripenem had a similar clinical success rate with comparators (OR, 1.15; 95% CI, 0.79–1.66, $I^2 = 58\%$, Figure 3). Sensitivity analysis after randomly deleting an individual study each time to reflect the influence of the single data set to the pooled OR showed similar findings in most occasions. There was only one exception, when we deleted Kollef et al.'s study [11], doripenem showed better clinical success rate than other comparators in the pool analysis of the remaining seven studies [7,8,10,12–15] (OR, 1.33; 95% CI, 1.03–1.72, $I^2 = 0\%$). In the different subgroup of patients with pneumonia, cUTI, and intra-abdominal infection, similar clinical success rates were noted between two different regimens for pneumonia (OR, 0.84; 95% CI, 0.46–1.53, $I^2 = 72\%$) and for IAI (OR, 1.00; 95% CI, 0.57–1.72). For cUTI, doripenem was associated with a higher success rate than comparators (OR, 1.89, 95% CI, 1.13–3.17, $I^2 = 0\%$). Three studies [11,12,14] compared the effect of doripenem and imipenem, and there was no difference in terms of clinical success rate between these two regimens (OR, 0.76; 95% CI, 0.38–1.55, $I^2 = 66\%$). Two studies [8,15] compared doripenem and meropenem, their clinical success rates were similar (OR, 1.31, 95% CI, 0.75–2.28, $I^2 = 34\%$). The pool analysis of these five studies comparing doripenem and other carbapenems showed no significant differences between each other (OR, 0.96, 95% CI, 0.59–1.58, $I^2 = 63\%$).

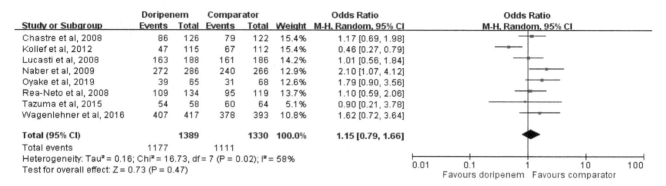

Figure 3. Overall clinical success rates of doripenem and comparators in the treatment of acute bacterial infections.

3.3. Microbiological Eradication

Only six studies [7,10,12–15] reported the data of microbiological eradication rate, and the pool analysis showed that doripenem had a similar microbiological eradication rate with comparators (OR, 1.08; 95% CI, 0.86–1.36, $I^2 = 0\%$, Figure 4). Sensitivity analysis showed similar results. In the different subgroup of patients with pneumonia and IAI, similar microbiological eradication rates were found for both regimens (for pneumonia, OR, 1.25; 95% CI, 0.79–1.97, $I^2 = 0\%$; for IAI, OR, 1.04; 95% CI, 0.49–2.17, $I^2 = 54\%$). While comparing doripenem and other carbapenems in the pool analysis of four studies [7,12,14,15], the microbiological eradication rates were similar between these two regimens (OR, 1.13; 95% CI, 0.85–1.51, $I^2 = 0\%$).

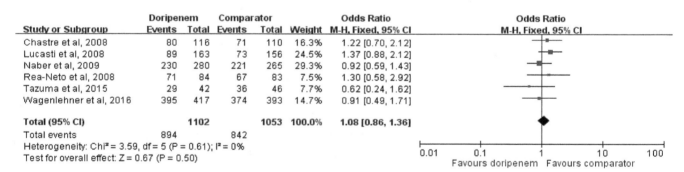

Figure 4. Overall microbiological eradication rates of doripenem and comparators in the treatment of acute bacterial infections.

3.4. Adverse Events

Six studies [7,8,11,13–15] reported the incidence of treatment-emergent adverse events, the doripenem had a similar risk with other antibiotics (OR, 0.98; 95% CI, 0.83–1.17, $I^2 = 33\%$, Figure 5). Serious adverse events were reported in six studies [7,10,12–15], the overall incidence was similar between doripenem and other antibiotics (OR, 1.06; 95% CI, 0.85–1.31, $I^2 = 43\%$). Six studies [7,10,12–15] reported the risk of discontinuing drug due to adverse event, the risk was similar between doripenem and comparators (OR, 0.75, 95% CI, 0.35–1.61, $I^2 = 61\%$). Regarding some common adverse events, doripenem was associated with the similar risk as comparators in terms of diarrhea (OR, 0.91, 95% CI, 0.64–1.28, $I^2 = 0\%$) in the pool analysis of eight studies [7,8,10–15], nausea (OR, 0.93, 95% CI, 0.45–1.93, $I^2 = 62\%$) among five studies [11–15], headache (OR, 1.10, 95% CI, 0.82–1.48, $I^2 = 0\%$) among three studies [13–15], and constipation (OR, 0.96, 95% CI, 0.61–1.52, $I^2 = 0\%$) among three studies [11,13,14]. In the pooled analysis of four studies [10,12,13,15] that reported the risk of seizure, doripenem was associated with a similar lower risk as comparators (OR, 0.37, 95% CI, 0.15–0.92, I^2 = 0%). Moreover, no seizure attack was reported to be related to doripenem in these four studies [10,12,13,15].

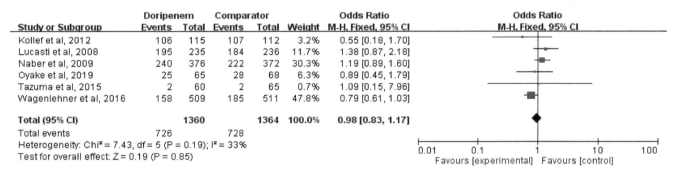

Figure 5. Risk of treatment-emergent adverse events of doripenem and comparators in the treatment of acute bacterial infections.

4. Discussion

This meta-analysis based on eight RCTs found that doripenem had a similar clinical success rate of treating acute bacterial infections with other comparators. The similar efficacy in terms of clinical response and microbiological eradication was found between doripenem and other carbapenems, including meropenem and imipenem. In addition, this result was not affected by the different types of infections—pneumonia, cUTI, or IAIs. Even for several specific types of infection—cholangitis, cholecystitis, appendicitis, lower urinary tract infection, and acute pyelonephritis—no statistical differences in terms of clinical efficacy was found between doripenem and comparators in the included studies [13–15]. In fact, in addition to Kollef et al.'s study [11], that showed doripenem was found to have non-significant higher rates of clinical failure and mortality compared to imipenem [7,10,12–15]. The difference between Kollef et al.'s study [11] and the other seven studies [7,10,12–15] may be explained by the fact that Kollef et al. compared a fixed seven-day course of doripenem with a fixed 10-day course of imipenem-cilastatin for treating VAP. Seven days of antibiotic treatment may have been too short for the patients with VAP, so the clinical outcome of VAP treated with a seven-day course of doripenem was worse than with a 10-day course of imipenem-cilastatin. In this meta-analysis, while we did sensitivity analysis after deleting this negative study [11] for doripenem, we found that the pooled analysis of the other seven studies [7,8,10,12–15] showed that doripenem was associated with better clinical outcome than comparators. Although this finding hints that the effect of doripenem may be better, or at least as good as, other antimicrobial agents in the treatment of acute bacterial infections, if doripenem can be used as long as the comparators, we still need further study to confirm this issue. Before that, the findings of this meta-analysis indicate that the clinical efficacy of doripenem is not inferior to other antimicrobial agents in the treatment of acute bacterial infections. Finally, several studies [16–18] demonstrated that doripenem was associated with lower medical resource utilization and hospital cost in the treatment of HAP and VAP versus comparators, including imipenem. Overall, doripenem could be both a life- and cost-saving antibiotic and could be recommended as the appropriate antibiotic in the treatment of acute bacterial infections, including pneumonia, cUTI, and cIAI.

In this meta-analysis, we also compared the microbiological response of doripenem with other antibiotics for acute bacterial infection. Overall, we found the microbiological eradication rates were similar between doripenem and comparators. Moreover, a similar trend was noted in the sensitivity analysis and subgroup analysis of pneumonia and IAIs. Finally, doripenem was comparable to other carbapenems, including imipenem and meropenem, in terms of microbiological eradication rate in the subgroup analysis. All these findings may be well explained by previous in vitro studies [3,4,19–21] that showed doripenem had a greater or similar in vitro activity against bacteria, including multi-drug resistant organisms. In this meta-analysis, we did not assess we did not evaluate the association between in vitro activity and the in vivo response of different organisms, especially for antibiotic-resistant pathogens, because the associated information was limited. However, this meta-analysis demonstrates that doripenem is comparable to other antimicrobial agents in both the clinical and microbiological responses of treating acute bacterial infections.

In addition to the assessment of clinical efficacy and microbiological eradication, the safety issue is another important concern in the treatment of acute bacterial infection by doripenem. In this analysis, the risks of overall treatment-emergent adverse effects, common adverse effects (diarrhea, nausea, headache and constipation), serious adverse effects, and the risk of discontinuing the drug due to adverse effects were similar between doripenem and comparators. Seizure is another important concern for patients using carbapenems. In this meta-analysis, four studies [10,12,13,15] reported the incidence of seizure, and the doripenem group had a lower risk of seizure than comparators. Moreover, although six seizure events were reported in this meta-analysis, all these events occurred in patients with underlying risk factors and were not clearly related to doripenem. Therefore, all these findings indicate that doripenem may be as safe as conventional regimens in the treatment of acute bacterial infections.

This meta-analysis has several limitations. First, we did not evaluate the effect of doripenem and comparators against specific organisms in each type of bacterial infection and the confounding effect of the antibiotic resistance of these pathogens. Besides, the immune status and the age effect were not assessed in this meta-analysis due to limited information. Second, the use of doripenem for treating pneumonia remains a serious concern due to the negative findings of Kolleff et al.'s study [11] that showed a shorter course (seven days) of doripenem was associated with a worse outcome than a longer course (10 days) of imipenem for patients with VAP. However, doripenem was commonly used for treating pneumonia in many countries [22], and several studies [10,12,23–25] showed the clinical outcomes of pneumonia treated by doripenem were favorable. In the subgroup analysis of this meta-analysis, we found the clinical and microbiological responses of doripenem for treating pneumonia were as good as comparators. But, as only three RCTs [10–12] focusing on pneumonia were enrolled in this meta-analysis, the number of studies is limited, thus further study is warranted to clarify this issue.

In conclusion, based on the analysis of eight RCTs, no differences in terms of clinical success and microbiological eradication rates were found between doripenem and comparators in the treatment of acute bacterial infections. Moreover, doripenem was well tolerated and had comparable safety profiles to other antimicrobial agents.

Author Contributions: Conceptualization, I.-L.C., Y.-H.C. and C.-C.L.; formal analysis, I.-L.C. and Y.-H.C.; writing—original draft, C.-C.L.; writing—review and editing, H.-J.T.

Conflicts of Interest: The authors declare no conflicts of interest.

Appendix A : List of Terms of the Search Strategy

Pubmed
1. "doripenem" [MeSH Terms]
2. "doripenem" [All Fields]
3. 1 OR 2
4. "infection" [MeSH Terms]
5. "infection" [All Fields]
6. 4 OR 5
7. "randomized" [All Fields]
8. "randomised" [All Fields]
9. 7 OR 8
10. 3 AND 6 AND 9
Embase

1. "doripenem"/exp
2. "doripenem"
3. 1 OR 2
4. "infection"
5. "randomized"
6. "randomised"
7. 5 OR 6
8. 3 AND 4 AND 7
Cochrane
1. doripenem
2. infection
3. #1 AND #2

References

1.   Kalil, A.C.; Metersky, M.L.; Klompas, M.; Muscedere, J.; Sweeney, D.A.; Palmer, L.B.; Napolitano, L.M.; O'Grady, N.P.; Bartlett, J.G.; Carratalà, J.; et al. Management of adults with hospital-acquired and ventilator-associated pneumonia: 2016 Clinical practice guidelines by the Infectious Diseases Society of America and the American Thoracic Society. *Clin. Infect. Dis.* **2016**, *63*, e61–e111. [CrossRef] [PubMed]

2.   Mazzei, T. The pharmacokinetics and pharmacodynamics of the carbapanemes: Focus on doripenem. *J. Chemother.* **2010**, *22*, 219–225. [CrossRef] [PubMed]

3.   Castanheira, M.; Jones, R.N.; Livermore, D.M. Antimicrobial activities of doripenem and other carbapenems against *Pseudomonas aeruginosa*, other nonfermentative bacilli, and *Aeromonas* spp. *Diagn. Microbiol. Infect. Dis.* **2009**, *63*, 426–433. [CrossRef] [PubMed]

4.   Douraghi, M.; Ghalavand, Z.; Nateghi Rostami, M.; Zeraati, H.; Aliramezani, A.; Rahbar, M.; Mohammadzadeh, M.; Ghourchian, S.; Boroumand, M.A.; Abdollahi, A. Comparative *in vitro* activity of carbapenems against clinical isolates of *Acinetobacter baumannii*. *J. Appl. Microbiol.* **2016**, *121*, 401–407. [CrossRef] [PubMed]

5.   Li, Y.; Lv, Y.; Xue, F.; Zheng, B.; Liu, J.; Zhang, J. Antimicrobial resistance surveillance of doripenem in China. *J. Antibiot. Tokyo* **2015**, *68*, 496–500. [CrossRef] [PubMed]

6.   Qu, X.Y.; Hu, T.T.; Zhou, W. A meta-analysis of efficacy and safety of doripenem for treating bacterial infections. *Braz. J. Infect. Dis.* **2015**, *19*, 156–162. [CrossRef] [PubMed]

7.   Wagenlehner, F.M.; Sobel, J.D.; Newell, P.; Armstrong, J.; Huang, X.; Stone, G.G.; Yates, K.; Gasink, L.B. Ceftazidime-avibactam versus doripenem for the treatment of complicated urinary tract infections, including acute pyelonephritis: RECAPTURE, a phase 3 randomized trial program. *Clin. Infect. Dis.* **2016**, *63*, 754–762. [CrossRef] [PubMed]

8.   Oyake, T.; Takemasa-Fujisawa, Y.; Sugawara, N.; Mine, T.; Tsukushi, Y.; Hanamura, I.; Fujishima, Y.; Aoki, Y.; Kowata, S.; Ito, S.; et al. Doripenem versus meropenem as first-line empiric therapy of febrile neutropenia in patients with acute leukemia: A prospective, randomized study. *Ann. Hematol.* **2019**, *98*, 1209–1216. [CrossRef] [PubMed]

9.   Higgins, J.P.; Altman, D.G.; Gotzsche, P.C.; Juni, P.; Moher, D.; Oxman, A.D.; Savovic, J.; Schulz, K.F.; Weeks, L.; Sterne, J.A.; et al. The Cochrane Collaboration's tool for assessing risk of bias in randomised trials. *BMJ* **2011**, *343*, d5928. [CrossRef]

10.   Rea-Neto, A.; Niederman, M.; Lobo, S.M.; Schroeder, E.; Lee, M.; Kaniga, K.; Ketter, N.; Prokocimer, P.; Friedland, I. Efficacy and safety of doripenem versus piperacillin/tazobactam in nosocomial pneumonia: A randomized, open-label, multicenter study. *Curr. Med. Res. Opin.* **2008**, *24*, 2113–2126. [CrossRef] [PubMed]

11.   Kollef, M.H.; Chastre, J.; Clavel, M.; Restrepo, M.I.; Michiels, B.; Kaniga, K.; Cirillo, I.; Kimko, H.; Redman, R. A randomized trial of 7-day doripenem versus 10-day imipenem-cilastatin for ventilator-associated pneumonia. *Crit. Care* **2012**, *16*, R218. [CrossRef] [PubMed]

12.   Chastre, J.; Wunderink, R.; Prokocimer, P.; Lee, M.; Kaniga, K.; Friedland, I. Efficacy and safety of intravenous infusion of doripenem versus imipenem in ventilator-associated pneumonia: A multicenter, randomized study. *Crit. Care Med.* **2008**, *36*, 1089–1096. [CrossRef] [PubMed]

13. Naber, K.G.; Llorens, L.; Kaniga, K.; Kotey, P.; Hedrich, D.; Redman, R. Intravenous doripenem at 500 milligrams versus levofloxacin at 250 milligrams, with an option to switch to oral therapy, for treatment of complicated lower urinary tract infection and pyelonephritis. *Antimicrob. Agents Chemother.* **2009**, *53*, 3782–3792. [CrossRef] [PubMed]

14. Tazuma, S.; Igarashi, Y.; Inui, K.; Ohara, H.; Tsuyuguchi, T.; Ryozawa, S. Clinical efficacy of intravenous doripenem in patients with acute biliary tract infection: A multicenter, randomized, controlled trial with imipenem/cilastatin as comparator. *J. Gastroenterol.* **2015**, *50*, 221–229. [CrossRef]

15. Lucasti, C.; Jasovich, A.; Umeh, O.; Jiang, J.; Kaniga, K.; Friedland, I. Efficacy and tolerability of IV doripenem versus meropenem in adults with complicated intra-abdominal infection: A phase III, prospective, multicenter, randomized, double-blind, noninferiority study. *Clin. Ther.* **2008**, *30*, 868–883. [CrossRef] [PubMed]

16. Kollef, M.H.; Nathwani, D.; Merchant, S.; Gast, C.; Quintana, A.; Ketter, N. Medical resource utilization among patients with ventilator-associated pneumonia: Pooled analysis of randomized studies of doripenem versus comparators. *Crit. Care* **2010**, *14*, R84. [CrossRef]

17. Kongnakorn, T.; Mwamburi, M.; Merchant, S.; Akhras, K.; Caro, J.J.; Nathwani, D. Economic evaluation of doripenem for the treatment of nosocomial pneumonia in the US: Discrete event simulation. *Curr. Med. Res. Opin.* **2010**, *26*, 17–24. [CrossRef] [PubMed]

18. Zilberberg, M.D.; Mody, S.H.; Chen, J.; Shorr, A.F. Cost-effectiveness model of empiric doripenem compared with imipenem-cilastatin in ventilator-associated pneumonia. *Surg. Infect. Larchmt* **2010**, *11*, 409–417. [CrossRef]

19. Drzewiecki, A.; Bulanda, M.; Talaga, K.; Sodo, A.; Adamski, P. Comparison of *in vitro* activity of doripenem, imipenem and meropenem against clinical isolates of *Enterobacteriaceae*, *Pseudomonas* and *Acinetobacter* in Southern Poland. *Pol. Przegl. Chir.* **2012**, *84*, 449–453.

20. Firsov, A.A.; Gilbert, D.; Greer, K.; Portnoy, Y.A.; Zinner, S.H. Comparative pharmacodynamics and antimutant potentials of doripenem and imipenem with ciprofloxacin-resistant *Pseudomonas aeruginosa* in an *in vitro* model. *Antimicrob. Agents Chemother.* **2012**, *56*, 1223–1228. [CrossRef]

21. Wali, N.; Mirza, I.A. Comparative In Vitro Efficacy of doripenem and imipenem against multi-drug resistant *Pseudomonas aeruginosa*. *J. Coll. Physicians Surg. Pak.* **2016**, *26*, 297–301. [PubMed]

22. Mustafa, M.; Chan, W.M.; Lee, C.; Harijanto, E.; Loo, C.M.; Van Kinh, N.; Anh, N.D.; Garcia, J. A PROspective study on the Usage patterns of Doripenem in the Asia-Pacific region (PROUD study). *Int. J. Antimicrob. Agents* **2014**, *43*, 353–360. [CrossRef] [PubMed]

23. Chao, C.M.; Chen, C.C.; Huang, H.L.; Chuang, Y.C.; Lai, C.C.; Tang, H.J. Clinical experience of patients receiving doripenem-containing regimens for the treatment of healthcare-associated infections. *PLoS ONE* **2016**, *11*, e0167522. [CrossRef] [PubMed]

24. Luyt, C.E.; Aubry, A.; Lu, Q.; Micaelo, M.; Brechot, N.; Brossier, F.; Brisson, H.; Rouby, J.J.; Trouillet, J.L.; Combes, A.; et al. Imipenem, meropenem, or doripenem to treat patients with *Pseudomonas aeruginosa* ventilator-associated pneumonia. *Antimicrob. Agents Chemother.* **2014**, *58*, 1372–1380. [CrossRef] [PubMed]

25. Muscedere, J.G.; Day, A.; Heyland, D.K. Mortality, attributable mortality, and clinical events as end points for clinical trials of ventilator-associated pneumonia and hospital-acquired pneumonia. *Clin. Infect. Dis.* **2010**, *51* (Suppl. 1), S120–S125. [CrossRef] [PubMed]

17

Prospective Evaluation of Intensity of Symptoms, Therapeutic Procedures and Treatment in Palliative Care Patients in Nursing Homes

Daniel Puente-Fernández [1], Concepción B. Roldán-López [2], Concepción P. Campos-Calderón [3,*], Cesar Hueso-Montoro [4], María P. García-Caro [4] and Rafael Montoya-Juarez [4]

[1]   Doctoral Program of Clinical Medicine and Public Health, University of Granada, 18071 Granada, Spain; danielpuentefdz@correo.ugr.es
[2]   Department of Statistics and Operational Research, Faculty of Medicine, University of Granada, 1016 Granada, Spain; iroldan@ugr.es
[3]   Alicante Biomedical Research Institute (ISABIAL), 03010 Alicante, Spain
[4]   Department of Nursing, Faculty of Health Sciences, Mind, Brain and Behaviour Research Institute, University of Granada, 18016 Granada, Spain; cesarhueso@ugr.es (C.H.-M.); mpazgc@ugr.es (M.P.G.-C.); rmontoya@ugr.es (R.M.-J.)

Abstract: The aim of the study is to evaluate the intensity of symptoms, and any treatment and therapeutic procedures received by advanced chronic patients in nursing homes. A multi-centre prospective study was conducted in six nursing homes for five months. A nurse trainer selected palliative care patients from whom the sample was randomly selected for inclusion. The Edmonton Symptoms Assessment Scale, therapeutic procedures, and treatment were evaluated. Parametric and non-parametric tests were used to evaluate month-to-month differences and differences between those who died and those who did not. A total of 107 residents were evaluated. At the end of the follow-up, 39 had (34.6%) died. All symptoms ($p < 0.050$) increased in intensity in the last week of life. Symptoms were more intense in those who had died at follow-up ($p < 0.05$). The use of aerosol sprays ($p = 0.008$), oxygen therapy ($p < 0.001$), opioids ($p < 0.001$), antibiotics ($p = 0.004$), and bronchodilators ($p = 0.003$) increased in the last week of life. Peripheral venous catheters ($p = 0.022$), corticoids ($p = 0.007$), antiemetics ($p < 0.001$), and antidepressants ($p < 0.05$) were used more in the patients who died. In conclusion, the use of therapeutic procedures (such as urinary catheters, peripheral venous catheter placement, and enteral feeding) and drugs (such as antibiotics, anxiolytics, and new antidepressant prescriptions) should be carefully considered in this clinical setting.

Keywords: palliative care; nursing homes; symptom assessment; drug therapy; therapeutics; longitudinal studies

1. Introduction

The World Health Organization (WHO) [1] and the European Association of Palliative Care (EAPC) [2] encourage an increase in the quality of dying in long-term care settings. In fact, several articles call for more research on end-of-life interventions in these centres, in order to improve care practice [3,4]. Meanwhile, nursing homes have become a plausible alternative in situations where the home is not the most suitable place for the end of life, due to clinical complexity or lack of resources [5].

Recent studies have indicated that there is a high prevalence of physical and psychological symptoms in nursing homes [3,6–8]. All of these symptoms increase in intensity and prevalence as the end of life approaches [4,9]. Most of the studies that have evaluated end-of-life symptoms in nursing homes are retrospective studies [3,6,9–11]. They may exhibit selection bias and problems caused by poorly recorded or unrecorded data. Prospective studies may be very helpful to properly assess the changes in symptom control when is death is about to occur.

Hospices in Spain are not widely developed, so end-of-life care must be provided by other institutions. In the case of elderly patients, this care is mostly provided by nursing homes. In these centres, most of the beds are privately funded (71%) [12], although some are partially government-funded. In Andalusia, only nursing homes with more than 60 beds are required to offer twenty-four hour nursing services and their own medical care [13].

Beyond this, little is known regarding routine therapeutic procedures and pharmacological treatments in palliative patients in nursing homes. In a recent retrospective study in Spanish hospitals, patients who were at the end stage of their lives received similar therapeutic and diagnosis procedures to acute care patients [14]. This is congruent with other papers published previously: procedures such as catheter insertion, the use of aspirators, and other actions that are common for patient care in a general hospital can make the difference between comfort and discomfort for end-of-life patients [8,15,16].

Regarding pharmacological treatments, a recent review highlighted that many patients continue to receive medications that are not prescribed as palliative treatments or for symptom control, despite being in the end stage of life [17]. A previous review [18] pointed out that few studies focus on pharmacological de-prescription in end-of-life and concluded that life expectancy is not often used as a criterion for medication discontinuation, even though unnecessary drugs might cause side effects that may increase suffering for patients.

In this context, the European Association of Palliative Care [19] emphasises that, in Spain, there are no specific documents on palliative care in long-term care facilities, nor publications regarding the provision of palliative care in this type of centres in Spain.

The purpose of this study is to prospectively explore perception of symptom control, pharmacological treatments, and therapeutic procedures received by palliative patients admitted to nursing homes in the last six months of life. This is one of the first studies to use a prospective approach, and the first one to show the end-of-life situation in Spanish nursing homes with this methodology. We hypothesize that, when death is near, intensity of symptoms and pharmacological treatments linked to symptom control will increase, whereas the frequency of routine therapeutic procedures will be the same as in previous months.

2. Experimental Section

2.1. Design

This is a multi-centre prospective study which has been conducted in nursing homes in Spain.

2.2. Sample

Six nursing homes were selected for convenience based on their institutional characteristics: Presence of a multidisciplinary team, the possible involvement of professionals, and the presence of both public and private beds. All centres included in the study have more than 50 beds. In each centre, one or two nurses with close knowledge of the patient who have been working at the nursing home for at least 6 months were responsible for data collection. All of the nurses that participated signed an informed consent form and received training prior to data collection. In order to control bias and to produce reliable data for the research, these professionals completed a training course designed to explain the study, to ensure that the same data collection methods were followed, and to avoid the dropout of patients at the follow-up stage. The research team was in contact with them via email, and they visited the centres regularly, i.e., at least once a month.

2.3. Recruitment

Each nursing home nurse recruited residents with chronic diseases that met the following criteria according to the Spanish Society of Palliative Care (SECPAL):

- Advanced, progressive, and incurable disease
- Little to no possibility of response to any specific treatment
- Presence of numerous problems or intense, multiple, multifactorial and changing symptoms
- Great emotional impact on patient, family, and staff
- Life expectancy limited to 6 months.

Within each nursing home, twenty patients were randomly selected among all the patients that met the aforementioned inclusion criteria. They were observed and the data of interest were recorded without interfering with the natural course of events. Data were collected between June 2016 and January 2017. All participants, patients, or representatives of patients (in the case of cognitively impaired patients) were fully informed and signed informed consent forms.

2.4. Data Collection Procedure

Nurses collected demographic and clinical information from the clinical records of the patients. A structured questionnaire was used to collect socio-demographic (age, gender, years in the centre, marital status, and number of children) and clinical (medical diagnosis, Charlson Comorbidity Index) data from patient records.

For the systematic symptom assessment, we used the Edmonton Symptom Assessment System (ESAS) [20]. The ESAS has been validated for both patient and care partner report in different settings, including those with older people with multiple morbidities [21]. ESAS was used regularly in all the nursing homes that participated in the study for symptom assessment. The patient version of the ESAS was self-administered by cognitively intact patients. For cognitively impaired residents, the professional version of the ESAS was completed by trained nurses. The relatives of the patients were not involved in data collection. Cognitive impairment was defined as the patient making three or more mistakes in the Pfeiffer test. The Pfeiffer test was used in all the nursing homes that participated in this study.

The prescription of therapeutic procedures such as urinary catheterisation, enteral feeding, peripheral venous catheter placement, use of aerosol sprays, oxygen therapy, and pharmacological treatments such as non-opioid analgesics, opioid analgesics, antibiotics, bronchodilators, corticosteroids, antiemetics, antihistamines, antidepressants, anxiolytics, hypnotics, and barbiturates was also evaluated.

Data were collected between June 2016 and January 2017. For this study, outcome data were collected from clinical records of the first month (T1) and of the following months (T2, T3, T4, and T5) if residents were still alive. For all the residents who died within these six months, the same data were collected from the clinical records of the last week before death (CT = closure test). All participants, residents, and the care partner were fully informed and signed informed consent forms.

2.5. Statistical Analysis

A descriptive analysis was carried out to describe the main characteristics of the study sample. Numerical variables were described with the mean and standard deviation (SD) and the median and interquartile range (P25-P75). Categorical variables were described using absolute frequencies and percentages. Quantitative data were assessed for normality using the Kolmogorov-Smirnov test, and all of the quantitative data collected were found to deviate significantly from the normal distribution ($p < 0.001$). Due to this, non-parametric inferential tests were used. Pearson's chi-squared test was used to evaluate between-group differences and McNemar's test was used to compare the prevalence rates. Wilcoxon's signed-rank test was used in order to compare month-by-month the symptoms reported using the ESAS for nursing home residents. Statistical analyses were conducted using IBM SPSS v.24. p-values of less than 0.05 were considered to be statistically significant.

2.6. Statement of Ethics

All participants (or when appropriate, a representative) signed a form to give their informed consent. The study received the approval of the Research Ethics Committee (PI-0619-2011). In compliance with Spanish Law (Article 16, Law 41/2002), patients' data were anonymised.

3. Results

Thirteen patients dropped out of the study. Two of them moved to another nursing home. Ten patients or representatives of patients refused to give their informed consent during follow-up. One of the residents died before the beginning of the follow-up. As a result, the final sample consisted of 107 residents. Most of them were women (63.6%) and they had a mean age of 84.6 (SD = 7.4) years. The characteristics can be seen in Table 1.

Table 1. Socio-demographic and clinical characteristics of the patients.

Socio-Demographic and Clinical Characteristics of the Patients.	Total Sample $n = 107$		Dying within 6 month $n = 39$		Alive $\geq$ 6 month $n = 68$		p
Age, md (P25-P75)	84	(81–89)	86	(83–95)	84	(78.5–89)	0.011^1
Female, n (%)	68	(63.6)	24	(64.8)	44	(62.9)	0.835^1
Years in the centre, md (P25-P75)	2	(1–4)	2	(0.6–5)	2	(1.3–4)	0.946^2
Marital status widower, n (%)	63	(60.8)	25	(67.6)	38	(54.3)	0.012^2
Number of children, md (P25-P75)	2	(0–3)	2	(0–2)	3	(2–5)	0.222^1
CCI, md (P25-P75)	3.5	(2–6)	4	(4–6)	3	(2–5)	0.007^1
Primary diagnosis							
Myocardial infarction, n (%)	6	(5.6)	2	(5.3)	4	(6.0)	1.000^2
Heart failure, n (%)	28	(26.2)	12	(31.6)	16	(23.3)	0.492^2
Peripheral vascular disease, n (%)	10	(9.3)	9	(23.7)	1	(1.5)	0.000^2
Thromboembolic disease, n (%)	7	(6.5)	6	(15.8)	1	(1.5)	0.009^2
Stroke or other cerebral lesions, n (%)	45	(42.1)	22	(57.9)	23	(34.3)	0.024^2
Hemiplegia, n (%)	14	(13.1)	7	(18.4)	7	(10.4)	0.370^2
Arterial hypertension, n (%)	63	(58.9)	15	(38.5)	41	(60.3)	0.044^2
Dementia	51	(47.7)	20	(52.6)	43	(64.2)	0.301^2
COPD, n (%)	25	(23.4)	12	(31.6)	13	(19.4)	0.233^2
Arrhythmia, n (%)	21	(19.6)	14	(36.8)	7	(10.4)	0.002^2
Renal disease, n (%)	19	(17.8)	6	(15.8)	13	(19.4)	0.794^2
Diabetes, n (%)	34	(31.8)	10	(27.8)	24	(38.1)	0.380^2
Tumour, n (%)	17	(15.9)	8	(20.5)	9	(13.2)	0.308^2
Solid tumour with metastasis, n (%)	10	(9.3)	4	(10.5)	6	(9.0)	1.000^2

Charlson Comorbidity Index, CCI; [1] Mann-Whitney U-test; [2] Pearson's chi-squared; COPD: chronic obstructive pulmonary disease.

Residents who died within the follow-up period (n = 39, 34.6%) were generally older and widowers, had a higher Charlson comorbidity index (CCI), and had more peripheral vascular and thromboembolic diseases, stroke or other cerebral lesions, arterial hypertension, and arrhythmia.

3.1. Perception of Symptom Intensity

In the comparison from T1 to T5, the perception of intensity of all symptoms was scored as moderate, except nausea and dyspnoea, which were scored as mild. No statistical differences were found in symptom intensity between T1 and T2 to T5 (Table 2). However, all differences were found to be statistically significant between T1 and symptoms in the last week of life (CT). In the comparison with CT, the median ratings for nausea ($p = 0.040$) and depression ($p = 0.033$) increased by up to 2 points; pain ($p = 0.026$), fatigue ($p = 0.003$), drowsiness ($p \leq 0.001$), dyspnoea ($p \leq 0.001$), and insomnia ($p = 0.032$) increased by up to 3 points; anxiety ($p = 0.001$), poor appetite ($p \leq 0.001$), and malaise ($p = 0.004$) increased in intensity by up to 4 points. In this case, all symptoms were scored as moderate except nausea, which was scored as mild, and fatigue and malaise, which were scored as severe.

Table 2. Month-by-month comparison of symptoms using Edmonton Symptom Assessment System (ESAS) for residents in nursing homes.

Symptoms	T1 vs. T2 (n = 102)		T1 vs. T3 (n = 95)		T1 vs. T4 (n = 84)		T1 vs. T5 (n = 82)		T1 vs. CT (n = 39)	
	md (P25-P75)	p^1	md (P25-P75)	p^1	md (P25-P75)	p^1	md (P25-P75)	p^1	md (P25-P75)	p^1
Pain										
T1	4 (2–6)	0.563	4 (2–6)	0.934	5 (2–7)	0.718	4 (2–6.5)	0.741	4 (2–7)	0.026
T(2-5) or CT	3.5 (2–6)		3.5 (2–6)		5 (2–7)		5 (2–7.5)		7 (2–9.5)	
Fatigue										
T1	5.5 (3–7)	0.225	5 (2–7)	0.485	5.5 (3–7)	0.443	4 (2.5–8)	0.559	5 (3–7)	0.003
T(2-5) or CT	5.5 (3–8)		5 (2–8)		5.5 (3–8)		5 (2.5–9)		8 (3.5–9)	
Nausea										
T1	0 (0–3)	0.721	0 (0–2)	0.728	0 (0–2.5)	0.228	0 (0–2)	0.836	0 (0–3)	0.040
T(2-5) or CT	0 (0–3)		0 (0–2)		0 (0–1)		1 (0–3)		2 (0–7)	
Depression										
T1	3 (0–6)	0.773	3 (0–6)	0.833	3 (0–6)	0.654	3 (0–6)	0.589	3 (0–7)	0.033
T(2-5) or CT	3 (0–5.5)		2 (0–7)		3.5 (1–6)		3.5 (1–7)		4.5 (1–9)	
Anxiety										
T1	3 (0–6)	0.298	3 (0–5.5)	0.470	3 (0–6)	0.889	3 (0–6)	0.553	3 (0–6)	0.001
T(2-5) or CT	2 (0–5)		2 (0–6)		3 (0–6)		4 (0–6)		7 (1–9)	
Drowsiness										
T1	2 (4–7)	0.357	4 (2–7)	0.777	3.5 (2–7)	0.985	3 (0.5–5)	0.850	4 (3–6)	<0.001
T(2-5) or CT	2 (1–7)		4 (1–6)		4 (1–7)		4 (1–5)		7 (6–10)	
Poor appetite										
T1	3 (0–6)	0.624	3 (0–6)	0.479	3 (0–7)	0.332	3 (0–6)	0.473	3 (1–7)	<0.001
T(2-5) or CT	4 (0–6)		2 (0–5.5)		2 (0–6.5)		2 (0–4)		7 (3–10)	
Malaise										
T1	5 (0–7)	0.114	5 (0–7)	0.284	5 (0–7)	0.210	4 (0–7)	0.357	5 (0–7)	0.004
T(2-5) or CT	4.5 (0–6)		4 (0–6)		5 (1–8)		4 (3–7)		9 (2–9.5)	
Dyspnoea										
T1	1 (0–6)	0.522	1 (0–6)	0.765	1 (0–6)	0.602	1 (0–6)	0.187	4 (0–6)	<0.001
T(2-5) or CT	1 (0–5)		1 (0–6)		0 (0–6.5)		0 (0–5.5)		7 (5–9)	
Insomnia										
T1	2.5 (0–6)	0.991	2 (0–6)	0.480	2.5 (0–7)	0.119	2 (0–6)	0.955	3 (0–7)	0.032
T(2-5) or CT	2 (0–6)		2 (0–5)		3 (0–6)		3 (0–6)		6 (1-9)	

Wilcoxon's signed-rank test[1]; T1: Initial follow-up time; T2, T3, T4, T5: Different follow-up times; CT: Closure Test. Week before death; P25: 25th percentile; P75: 75th percentile.

Residents who died during the follow-up period rated symptom intensity as higher for all symptoms, compared to those who were alive for the entire duration (Table 3).

Table 3. Comparison of symptoms using ESAS in residents of nursing homes who died with those who did not die.

Symptoms	Dying within 6 months n = 39 n(Range)	Alive ≥ 6 months n = 68 n(Range)	p^1
Pain, md (P25-P75)	7 (2–9)	4 (2–6)	0.012
Fatigue, md (P25-P75)	8 (3.5–9)	6 (3–8)	0.005
Nauseas, md (P25-P75)	1 (0–7)	0 (0–1)	0.003
Depression, md (P25-P75)	4 (1–9)	3 (0–6)	0.050
Anxiety, md (P25-P75)	4 (1–9)	3 (0–6)	0.002
Drowsiness, md (P25-P75)	7 (1–9)	4 (0–7)	< 0.001
Poor appetite, md (P25-P75)	7 (6–10)	4 (2–7)	< 0.001
Malaise, md (P25-P75)	9 (2–9.5)	5 (2–7)	< 0.001
Dyspnoea, md (P25-P75)	7 (5–9)	1 (0–6)	< 0.001
Insomnia, md (P25-P75)	6 (1–9)	2 (0–6)	0.011

[1]Mann-Whitney U-test.

3.2. Therapeutic Procedures and Pharmacological Treatments

No statistical differences were found in the comparison of therapeutic procedures between T1 and T2 to T5. Nevertheless, the analysis showed significant differences between T1 and CT (Table 4). The most repeated procedures (oxygen therapy ($p \leq 0.001$), use of aerosol sprays ($p = 0.008$), and peripheral venous catheter placement ($p = 0.039$)) had an increase of between 20 and 40 percentage points. Despite this, the percentage of procedures related to urinary catheters ($p = 1000$) and enteral feeding ($p = 0.221$) was not significantly different between T1 and CT.

Table 4. Comparison of therapeutic procedures and pharmacological treatments by months for patients in nursing homes.

Therapeutic Procedures/Pharmacological Treatments	T1 vs. T2 (n = 102)		T1 vs. T3 (n = 95)		T1 vs. T4 (n = 84)		T1 vs. T5 (n = 82)		T1 vs. CT (n = 37)		
	%	p^1	%	p^1	%	p^1	%	p^1	%	p^1	95% CI^2
					Therapeutic procedures						
Urinary catheter											
T1	14.7	1.000	14.7	1.000	11.9	0.752	14.6	0.267	21.1	1.000	
T(2-5) or CT	13.7		14.7		14.3		8.5		23.7		
Peripheral venous catheter placement											
T1	26.5	0.860	24.2	0.522	22.9	0.502	24.4	0.480	25.6	0.039	4.1–39.9
T(2-5) or CT	24.5		28.4		18.6		19.5		48.7		
Enteral feeding											
T1	11.8	1.000	14.0	1.000	15.5	1.000	14.6	0.789	5.3	0.221	
T(2-5) or CT	11.8		14.0		15.5		17.1		15.8		
Aerosol sprays											
T1	23.5	0.789	18.9	0.248	19.3	0.267	18.3	0.248	28.2	0.008	11.5–51.9
T(2-5) or CT	21.6		26.4		25.3		22.0		61.5		
Oxygen therapy											
T1	30.4	0.803	28.4	0.450	27.4	0.511	24.4	0.343	36.9	<0.001	17.6–65.3
T(2-5) or CT	32.4		31.9		33.3		29.3		79.5		
					Pharmacological treatments						
Non-opioid analgesics											
T1	58.8	0.263	54.7	0.345	54.8	0.404	51.2	0.170	71.8	0.628	
T(2-5) or CT	64.7		61.1		60.7		61.0		64.1		
Opioid analgesics											
T1	12.7	0.375	11.6	0.131	8.3	0.445	12.2	1.000	17.9	<0.001	25.6-57.3
T(2-5) or CT	15.7		16.8		11.9		11.0		61.5		
Antibiotics											
T1	21.6	0.185	20.0	0.109	21.4	0.136	17.1	0.211	30.8	0.004	14.9–53.4
T(2-5) or CT	29.4		29.5		31.0		25.6		66.7		
Bronchodilators											
T1	27.5	0.302	26.3	0.114	28.6	0.814	32.9	0.505	25.6	0.003	12.4–41.2
T(2-5) or CT	32.4		32.6		31.0		29.3		53.8		
Corticosteroids											
T1	20.6	1.000	18.9	1.000	15.5	0.453	17.1	1.000	28.2	0.267	
T(2-5) or CT	21.6		20.0		20.2		18.3		41.0		
Antiemetics											
T1	7.8	1.000	9.5	1.000	6.0	1.000	8.5	0.505	17.9	0.227	
T(2-5) or CT	7.8		9.5		7.1		12.2		30.8		
Antihistamines											
T1	7.8	1.000	6.3	0.500	6.0	1.000	3.7	1.000	10.3	0.248	
T(2-5) or CT	7.8		8.4		7.1		3.7		2.6		
Antidepressants											
T1	33.3	1.000	34.7	0.617	32.5	0.479	33.7	0.131	28.2	0.114	
T(2-5) or CT	33.3		32.6		30.1		27.7		12.8		
Anxiolytics											
T1	32.4	0.773	35.0	0.181	28.6	0.752	29.3	0.386	41.0	0.150	
T(2-5) or CT	30.4		28.4		25.7		34.1		25.6		
Hypnotics/barbiturates											
T1	49.0	0.267	46.3	1.000	41.7	0.383	50.0	0.424	51.3	1.000	
T(2-5) or CT	44.1		46.3		47.6		43.9		71.8		

^{1}McNemar's test; ^{2}Agresti Min 95% confidence interval for p2-p1.; T1: Initial follow-up time.; T2, T3, T4, T5: Different follow-up times.

Regarding pharmacological treatments, no significant differences were found between T1 and T2 to T5. However, some statistical differences were found between T1 and CT (Table 4). Opioid analgesics ($p \leq 0.001$), antibiotics ($p = 0.004$), bronchodilators ($p = 0.003$) had a significant increase in usage, that increase being of 45, 35, and 29 percentage points, respectively.

CT: Closure Test. Week before death. Statistical differences were found in the use of peripheral venous catheters ($p = 0.022$), aerosol sprays ($p = 0.001$), and oxygen therapy ($p = 0.001$) between the patients who died in the follow-up and those who survived (Table 5).

Table 5. Comparison of therapeutic procedures and pharmacological treatments in nursing home patients who died with those who did not die.

Therapeutic Procedures/Pharmacological Treatments	Dying within 6 months, $n = 39$	Alive ≥ 6 months, $n = 68$	$p*$	OR (95% CI)
Therapeutic procedures				
Urinary catheter, (%)	23.7	13.2	0.176	
Peripheral venous catheter placement, (%)	48.7	25.0	0.022	2.850 (1.238–6.562)
Enteral feeding, (%)	15.8	14.7	0.867	
Aerosol sprays, (%)	61.5	20.6	<0.001	6.171 (2.578–14.771)
Oxygen therapy, (%)	79.5	26.5	<0.001	10.764 (4.181–27.713)
Pharmacological treatments				
Non-opioid analgesics	65.8	54.4	0.350	
Opioid analgesics	63.2	10.3	<0.001	14.939 (5.372–41.546)
Antibiotics	65.8	16.2	<0.001	9.965 (3.930–25.268)
Bronchodilators	55.3	16.2	<0.001	6.401 (2.580–15.880)
Corticosteroids	42.1	16.2	0.007	3.769 (1.514–9.379)
Antiemetics	31.6	4.4	<0.001	10.000 (2.607–38.359)
Antihistamines	2.6	7.4	0.417	
Antidepressants	13.2	33.3	0.026	.278 (0.096–0.805)
Anxiolytics	26.3	29.4	0.909	
Hypnotics/barbiturates	52.6	48.5	0.839	

*Pearson's chi-squared; OR (95% CI), odds ratio (95% confidence interval of the odds ratio).

Finally, the comparison of pharmacological treatments showed differences for use of antibiotics ($p < 0.001$), bronchodilators ($p < 0.0001$), opioids ($p < 0.001$), corticosteroids ($p = 0.007$), antiemetics ($p < 0.001$), and antidepressants ($p = 0.026$) between those who died and the survivors (Table 5). The administration of these treatments was significantly greater in all deceased patients than in those who survived, except for antidepressants, whose usage was significantly lower.

4. Discussion

This is one of the first studies that prospectively describes the last months of life of nursing home residents, and the first that has been conducted in Spain. Our results suggest that there is a sudden increase in symptoms, therapeutic procedures, and pharmacological treatments in the last week of life, in comparison with previous follow-up times. In addition, an increasing number of invasive therapeutic procedures, which may result in decreased comfort for residents, was observed, such as urinary catheter placement, peripheral venous catheter placement, and enteral feeding. Similarly, increased drug use, such as antibiotics, anxiolytics, and new antidepressant prescriptions was also observed.

The perception of the intensity of symptoms remains stable between T1 and the following months, but increases substantially between T1 and the last week of life. This finding is consistent with the previous literature, which details a worsening of symptoms in the last days of life [6,9]. Nevertheless, it is necessary to point out that the consulted studies used prevalence, not intensity, to assess symptoms. Thompson et al. [10] conducted a prospective study in which they assessed pain in the last six months of life of residents in nursing homes, showing that the intensity of their pain remained stable during a short follow-up period, except in the last days of life, when it increased.

In the same way, in relation to therapeutic procedures, there are significant differences in the use of peripheral venous catheters, oxygen therapy, enteral feeding, and aerosol sprays in the last week of life compared to at T1. These differences are greater if we compare the therapeutic procedures between patients who died within the follow-up period and survivors. Regarding oxygen therapy and the use of aerosol sprays, Hendriks et al. [4] highlighted that, unlike what the results of the present study show, there was a decrease in the use of these procedures when death was near. Similarly, a retrospective study conducted in four Spanish hospitals [14] showed that oxygen therapy was a very frequently used intervention at the end of life. This study also reported that there is an increase in the use of peripheral venous catheters during the last days of life [14].

Enteral feeding is another intervention that might be considered to be futile [22], as this does not improve the wellbeing of patients in a significant way and may even be prolonging the dying process [22]. One of the factors that may influence the continuation of enteral feeding is that some professionals and relatives consider this intervention to be a measure of comfort that should not be removed [23].

With respect to urinary catheters, previous studies are not clear about the use of these interventions at the end of life. A literature review by Farrington et al. [24], which included clinical practice guidelines, pointed out that, even though some of the studies reviewed stated that urinary catheterisation could be used to provide comfort to patients, this procedure may cause or increase patient discomfort [24].

This could be interpreted as the performance of futile interventions in the last week of life in the nursing homes analysed.

As expected, the use of some medications linked to symptom control such as opioids, corticosteroids, and antiemetics increased in the last days of life. Opioids were one of the most used drugs in this study, which corresponds to what is described in the literature [4,9]. In relation to the use of non-opioid analgesics, Jansen et al., [25] unlike our study, reported an increase in the use of this group of drugs at the end of life.

On the other hand, there is a decrease in the use of antidepressants in the last week of life, although the consumption of other psychotropic drugs remains stable, compared to in previous months. The use of this kind of drug in end-of-life care is controversial: Some of them could be considered futile since they are not used to improve symptoms typical of the end of life [26]. The time delay before certain antidepressants have a noticeable effect is long (usually 4–6 weeks), so their usage may be considered futile for this reason. In fact, although psychotropic drugs may be indicated for the control of psycho-emotional symptoms, authors point out that they can cause undesirable side effects in the geriatric population and an increased risk of mortality [27].

Regarding the use of antibiotics at the end of life, our results indicate an increase in the last week of life. This may be due to the high percentage of patients with dementia in the sample, in whom infections are a common cause of death. Although, previous studies indicate that the use of antibiotics improves the prognosis of patients and the relief of symptoms [28–30], other studies provide evidence that not administering antibiotics improves comfort [31]. Furthermore, using antibiotics is not without risk in fragile patients with chronic diseases, due to drug reactions, drug-drug interactions, and infections [32]. Even so, there is no consensus as to whether or not they should be used at the end of life.

Furthermore, there has been no decrease in the prescription of drugs for any of the drugs evaluated. According to the consulted bibliography, one of those that would be expected to decrease according to current recommendations would be anxiolytics [33]. In our sample, the prescription of anxiolytics did not diminish at the end of life. According to Westbury [33], 'these psychotropic agents should be prescribed cautiously, at the lowest therapeutic doses for as short a time as possible, and be monitored regularly'. The literature consulted shows that identification of the terminal state increases the likelihood of a de-prescription occurring [34]. In the case of nursing homes, this identification is critical for facilitating patients' access to palliative care and, consequently, for improving the quality of care they receive, their satisfaction with it, and their symptoms [35]. Our results may be due to the lack of use of predictive survival tools that could be used in these centres. Therefore, in the absence of a prediction of the end of life, professionals do not question the utility of the interventions that can be carried out.

The present article tried to demonstrate part of the reality of the care provided by Spanish nursing homes, the study of which has had its importance emphasised by institutions, such as the EAPC. It would have been interesting to have assessed patient comfort, in order to clarify the suitability of controversial interventions, due to their possible futility in an end-of-life context. This work is a first approach to the end of life in Spanish nursing homes, being the stepping stone on which it can be developed into an intervention programme to improve end-of-life care in these centres. At the same time, it could well help to validate specific tools, in order to assess the quality of the dying process and to improve the detection of palliative care needs.

It should also be highlighted that some limitations of this study may affect the reliability of our results. It should be noted that the sample size is small in comparison with other published studies, so it has not been possible to complete further analyses. Furthermore, characteristics of this study's sample are similar to those in other studies conducted in nursing homes regarding age, sex, and diseases [4,6,9,36], so the results should be extrapolated carefully.

In this study, SECPAL criteria were used for case selection. Our results pointed out that only the 36.4% of patients of the sample have died, so a discussion on whether these criteria are the most appropriate is needed, particularly the limitation of a life expectancy of six months.

Several tools have been proposed to identify palliative care needs and prognosis [37]. For instance, White et al. [38] highlighted in a meta-analysis that the accuracy of the 'Surprise Question' referring to a one-year period was higher than 70% in trained professionals. For further studies, a year-long follow-up period could be considered.

5. Conclusions

In this prospective study, intensity of end-of-life symptoms increased in the last week of life. There is also an increase in therapeutic procedures and pharmacological treatments, but not all the procedures and drugs are linked to symptom management. Interventions (such as urinary catheters, peripheral venous catheter placement, and enteral feeding) and drugs (such as antibiotics, anxiolytics, and new antidepressant prescriptions) should be carefully considered in this clinical setting, in order to improve patient comfort and avoid futile treatments.

Primary care workers and stakeholders might support nursing home professionals in order to provide better symptom control and decide which interventions and drugs are to be recommended in the last days of life.

Author Contributions: Conceptualization, C.H.-M., M.P.G.-C. and R.M.-J.; data curation, D.P.-F. and C.P.C.-C.; formal analysis, C.B.R.-L.; investigation, D.P.-F. and C.B.R.-L.; methodology, C.H.-M., M.P.G.-C. and R.M.-J.; project administration, C.P.C.-C..; supervision, C.B.R.-L. and R.M.-J.; writing-original draft, D.P.-F., C.B.R.-L., C.P.C.-C., C.H.-M. and R.M.-J.; writing-review and editing, D.P.-F., C.B.R.-L., C.P.C.-C., C.H.-M. and R.M.-J. All authors have read and agreed to the published version of the manuscript.

Acknowledgments: We would like to thank all the patients, family members and professionals who have made this study possible. This manuscript is part of a PhD of Daniel Puente-Fernandez.

References

1. Hall, S.; Petkova, H.; Tsouros, A.D.; Costantini, M.; Higginson, I.J.; World Health Organization. *Palliative Care for Older People: Better Practices*; WHO Regional Office for Europe: Copenhagen, Denmark, 2011; p. 67.
2. Froggatt, K.A.; Reitinger, E.; Heimerl, K.; Hockley, J.; Brazil, K. Palliative Care in Long-Term Care Settings for Older People: EAPC Taskforce. *Eur. J. Palliat. Care* **2013**, *20*, 251–253.
3. Hendriks, S.A.; Smalbrugge, M.; Hertogh, C.M.P.M.; Van Der Steen, J.T. Dying with dementia: Symptoms, treatment, and quality of life in the last week of life. *J. Pain Symptom Manag.* **2014**, *47*, 710–720. [CrossRef] [PubMed]
4. Hendriks, S.A.; Smalbrugge, M.; Galindo-Garre, F.; Hertogh, C.M.P.M.; van der Steen, J.T. From Admission to Death: Prevalence and Course of Pain, Agitation, and Shortness of Breath, and Treatment of These Symptoms in Nursing Home Residents with Dementia. *J. Am. Med. Dir. Assoc.* **2015**, *16*, 475–481. [CrossRef]
5. Costa, V.; Earle, C.C.; Esplen, M.J.; Fowler, R.; Goldman, R.; Grossman, D.; Levin, L.; Manuel, D.G.; Sharkey, S.; Tanueputro, P.; et al. The determinants of home and nursing home death: A systematic review and meta-analysis. *BMC Palliat. Care* **2016**, *15*, 8. [CrossRef]

6.   Estabrooks, C.A.; Hoben, M.; Poss, J.W.; Chamberlain, S.A.; Thompson, G.N.; Silvius, J.L.; Norton, P.G. Dying in a Nursing Home: Treatable Symptom Burden and its Link to Modifiable Features of Work Context. *J. Am. Med. Dir. Assoc.* **2015**, *16*, 515–520. [CrossRef]

7.   Sandvik, R.K.; Selbaek, G.; Bergh, S.; Aarsland, D.; Husebo, B.S. Signs of Imminent Dying and Change in Symptom Intensity During Pharmacological Treatment in Dying Nursing Home Patients: A Prospective Trajectory Study. *J. Am. Med. Dir. Assoc.* **2016**, *17*, 821–827. [CrossRef] [PubMed]

8.   Hoben, M.; Chamberlain, S.A.; Knopp-Sihota, J.A.; Poss, J.W.; Thompson, G.N.; Estabrooks, C.A. Impact of Symptoms and Care Practices on Nursing Home Residents at the End of Life: A Rating by Front-line Care Providers. *J. Am. Med. Dir. Assoc.* **2016**, *17*, 155–161. [CrossRef] [PubMed]

9.   Koppitz, A.; Bosshard, G.; Schuster, D.H.; Hediger, H.; Imhof, L. Type and course of symptoms demonstrated in the terminal and dying phases by people with dementia in nursing homes. *Zeitschrift für Gerontol und Geriatr.* **2015**, *48*, 176–183. [CrossRef] [PubMed]

10.   Thompson, G.N.; Doupe, M.; Reid, R.C.; Baumbusch, J.; Estabrooks, C.A. Pain Trajectories of Nursing Home Residents Nearing Death. *J. Am. Med. Dir. Assoc.* **2017**, *18*, 700–706. [CrossRef] [PubMed]

11.   Smedbäck, J.; Öhlén, J.; Årestedt, K.; Alvariza, A.; Fürst, C.J.; Håkanson, C. Palliative care during the final week of life of older people in nursing homes: A register-based study. *Palliat. Support Care* **2017**, *15*, 417–424. [CrossRef]

12.   Campos-Calderón, C.; Montoya-Juárez, R.; Hueso-Montoro, C.; Hernández-López, E.; Ojeda-Virto, F.; García-Caro, M.P. Interventions and decision-making at the end of life: The effect of establishing the terminal illness situation. *BMC Palliat. Care* **2016**, *15*, 91. [CrossRef] [PubMed]

13.   Centro de Investigaciones Sociológicas. Informe Envejecimiento en Red. Centro de Investigaciones Sociológicas. Madrid. 2018. Available online: http://envejecimiento.csic.es/documentos/documentos/enred-estadisticasresidencias2017.pdf (accessed on 10 March 2020).

14.   *Decreto 168/2007 de 12 de Junio, por el que se Regula el Procedimiento para el Reconocimiento de la Situación de Dependencia y del Derecho a las Prestaciones del Sistema para la Autonomía y Atención a la Dependencia, así como los órganos Competentes para su Valoración.* Boletín Oficial de la Junta de Andalucía. núm. 119. 2007, pp. 38–42. Available online: https://www.juntadeandalucia.es/boja/2007/119/3 (accessed on 10 March 2020).

15.   Verhofstede, R.; Smets, T.; Cohen, J.; Eecloo, K.; Costantini, M.; Van Den Noortgate, N.; Deliens, L. End-of-Life Care and Quality of Dying in 23 Acute Geriatric Hospital Wards in Flanders, Belgium. *J. Pain Symptom Manag.* **2017**, *53*, 693–702. [CrossRef] [PubMed]

16.   Li, Q.; Zheng, N.T.; Temkin-Greener, H. Quality of end-of-life care of long-term nursing home residents with and without dementia. *J. Am. Geriatr. Soc.* **2013**, *61*, 1066–1073. [CrossRef] [PubMed]

17.   Poudel, A.; Yates, P.; Rowett, D.; Nissen, L.M. Use of Preventive Medication in Patients with Limited Life Expectancy: A Systematic Review. *J. Pain Symptom Manag.* **2017**, *53*, 1097–1110. [CrossRef]

18.   Tjia, J.; Velten, S.J.; Parsons, C.; Valluri, S.; Briesacher, B.A. Studies to Reduce Unnecessary Medication Use in Frail Older Adults: A Systematic Review. *Drugs Aging* **2013**, *30*, 285–307. Available online: http://link.springer.com/10.1007/s40266-013-0064-1 (accessed on 10 March 2020). [CrossRef]

19.   Arias-Casais, N.; Garralda, E.; Rhee, J.; Lima, L.; Pons-Izquierdo, J.; Clark, D.; Hasselaar, J.; Ling, J.; Mosoiu, D.; Centeno-Cortes, C. *EAPC Atlas of Palliative Care in Europe*; EAPC Press: Vilvoorde, Belgium, 2019.

20.   Carvajal, A.; Centeno, C.; Watson, R.; Bruera, E. A comprehensive study of psychometric properties of the Edmonton Symptom Assessment System (ESAS) in Spanish advanced cancer patients. *Eur. J. Cancer* **2011**, *47*, 1863–1872. [CrossRef]

21.   Nekolaichuk, C.; Watanabe, S.; Beaumont, C. The Edmonton Symptom Assessment System: A 15-year retrospective review of validation studies (1991–2006). *Palliat. Med.* **2008**, *22*, 111–122. [CrossRef]

22.   Krishna, L. Nasogastric feeding at the end of life: A virtue ethics approach. *Nurs. Ethics.* **2011**, *18*, 485–494. [CrossRef]

23.   Van der Riet, P.; Good, P.; Higgins, I.; Sneesby, L. Palliative care professionals' perceptions of nutrition and hydration at the end of life. *Int. J. Palliat. Nurs.* **2008**, *14*, 145–151. [CrossRef]

24.   Farrington, N.; Fader, M.; Richardson, A. Managing urinary incontinence at the end of life: An examination of the evidence that informs practice. *Int. J. Palliat. Nurs.* **2019**, *9*, 449–456. [CrossRef]

25.   Jansen, K.; Schaufel, M.A.; Ruths, S. Drug treatment at the end of life: An epidemiologic study in nursing homes. *Scand. J. Prim. Health Care* **2014**, *32*, 187–192. [CrossRef] [PubMed]

26. McNeil, M.J.; Kamal, A.H.; Kutner, J.S.; Ritchie, C.S.; Abernethy, A.P. The Burden of Polypharmacy in Patients near the End of Life. *J. Pain Symptom Manag.* **2016**, *51*, 178–183. [CrossRef] [PubMed]

27. Park, Y.; Franklin, J.M.; Schneeweiss, S.; Levin, R.; Crystal, S.; Gerhard, T.; Huybrechts, K.F. Antipsychotics and mortality: Adjusting for mortality risk scores to address confounding by terminal Illness. *J. Am. Geriatr. Soc.* **2015**, *63*, 516–523. [CrossRef] [PubMed]

28. Rosenberg, J.H.; Albrecht, J.S.; Fromme, E.K.; Noble, B.N.; McGregor, J.C.; Comer, A.C.; Furuno, J.P. Antimicrobial use for symptom management in patients receiving hospice and palliative care: A systematic review. *J. Palliat. Med.* **2013**, *16*, 1568–1574. [CrossRef]

29. Lam, P.T.; Chan, K.S.; Tse, C.Y.; Leung, M.W. Retrospective analysis of antibiotic use and survival in advanced cancer patients with infections. *J. Pain Symptom Manag.* **2005**, *30*, 536–543. [CrossRef]

30. Oh, D.Y.; Kim, J.H.; Kim, D.W.; Im, S.A.; Kim, T.Y.; Heo, D.S.; Kim, N.K. Antibiotic use during the last days of life in cancer patients. *Eur. J. Cancer Care (Engl.)* **2006**, *15*, 74–79. [CrossRef]

31. Givens, J.L.; Jones, R.N.; Shaffer, M.L.; Kiely, D.K.; Mitchell, S.L. Survival and comfort after treatment of pneumonia in advanced dementia. *Arch. Intern Med.* **2010**, *170*, 1102–1107. [CrossRef]

32. Juthani-Mehta, M.; Malani, P.N.; Mitchell, S.L. Antimicrobials at the End of Life: An Opportunity to Improve Palliative Care and Infection Management. *JAMA* **2015**, *314*, 2017–2018. [CrossRef]

33. Westbury, J.L.; Gee, P.; Ling, T.; Brown, D.T.; Franks, K.H.; Bindoff, I.; Peterson, G.M. RedUSe: Reducing antipsychotic and benzodiazepine prescribing in residential aged care facilities. *Med. J. Aust.* **2018**, *208*, 398–403. [CrossRef]

34. Van Den Noortgate, N.J.; Verhofstede, R.; Cohen, J.; Piers, R.D.; Deliens, L.; Smets, T. Prescription and Deprescription of Medication during the Last 48 Hours of Life: Multicenter Study in 23 Acute Geriatric Wards in Flanders, Belgium. *J. Pain Symptom Manag.* **2016**, *51*, 1020–1026. [CrossRef]

35. Stephens, C.E.; Hunt, L.J.; Bui, N.; Halifax, E.; Ritchie, C.S.; Lee, S.J. Palliative Care Eligibility, Symptom Burden, and Quality-of-Life Ratings in Nursing Home Residents. *JAMA Intern Med.* **2018**, *178*, 141–142. [CrossRef] [PubMed]

36. Brandt, H.E.; Ooms, M.E.; Deliens, L.; van der Wal, G.; Ribbe, M.W. The last two days of life of nursing home patients-a nationwide study on causes of death and burdensome symptoms in the Netherlands. *Palliat. Med.* **2006**, *20*, 533–540. [CrossRef] [PubMed]

37. Simmons, C.P.L.; McMillan, D.C.; McWilliams, K.; Sande, T.A.; Fearon, K.C.; Tuck, S.; Fallon, M.T.; Laird, B.J. Prognostic Tools in Patients with Advanced Cancer: A Systematic Review. *J. Pain Symptom Manag.* **2017**, *53*, 962–970. [CrossRef] [PubMed]

38. White, N.; Kupeli, N.; Vickerstaff, V.; Stone, P. How accurate is the 'Surprise Question' at identifying patients at the end of life? A systematic review and meta-analysis. *BMC Med.* **2017**, *15*, 139. [CrossRef]

Multidiscipline Stroke Post-Acute Care Transfer System: Propensity-Score-Based Comparison of Functional Status

Chung-Yuan Wang [1], Hong-Hsi Hsien [2], Kuo-Wei Hung [3], Hsiu-Fen Lin [4], Hung-Yi Chiou [5,6], Shu-Chuan Jennifer Yeh [7,8], Yu-Jo Yeh [7] and Hon-Yi Shi [7,8,9,10,*]

[1]   Department of Physical Medicine and Rehabilitation, Pingtung Christian Hospital, Pingtung 90059, Taiwan
[2]   Department of Internal Medicine, St. Joseph Hospital, Kaohsiung 80760, Taiwan
[3]   Division of Neurology, Department of internal medicine, Yuan's General Hospital, Kaohsiung 80249, Taiwan
[4]   Department of Neurology, Kaohsiung Medical University Hospital, Kaohsiung 80756, Taiwan
[5]   School of Public Health, Taipei Medical University, Taipei 11031, Taiwan
[6]   Center for Neurotrauma and Neuroregeneration, Taipei Medical University, Taipei 11031, Taiwan
[7]   Department of Healthcare Administration and Medical Informatics, Kaohsiung Medical University, Kaohsiung 80708, Taiwan
[8]   Department of Business Management, National Sun Yat-sen University, Kaohsiung 80424, Taiwan
[9]   Department of Medical Research, Kaohsiung Medical University Hospital, Kaohsiung 80756, Taiwan
[10] Department of Medical Research, China Medical University Hospital, China Medical University, Taichung 40447, Taiwan
*   Correspondence: hshi@kmu.edu.tw

Abstract: Few studies have investigated the characteristics of stroke inpatients after post-acute care (PAC) rehabilitation, and few studies have applied propensity score matching (PSM) in a natural experimental design to examine the longitudinal impacts of a medical referral system on functional status. This study coupled a natural experimental design with PSM to assess the impact of a medical referral system in stroke patients and to examine the longitudinal effects of the system on functional status. The intervention was a hospital-based, function oriented, 12-week to 1-year rehabilitative PAC intervention for patients with cerebrovascular diseases. The average duration of PAC in the intra-hospital transfer group (31.52 days) was significantly shorter than that in the inter-hospital transfer group (37.1 days) ($p < 0.001$). The intra-hospital transfer group also had better functional outcomes. The training effect was larger in patients with moderate disability (Modified Rankin Scale, MRS = 3) and moderately severe disability (MRS = 4) compared to patients with slight disability (MRS = 2). Intensive post-stroke rehabilitative care delivered by per-diem payment is effective in terms of improving functional status. To construct a vertically integrated medical system, strengthening the qualified local hospitals with PAC wards, accelerating the inter-hospital transfer, and offering sufficient intensive rehabilitative PAC days are the most essential requirements.

Keywords: stroke; post-acute care; medical referral system; propensity score matching

1. Introduction

Acute stroke is a major cause of mortality and disability [1,2]. Stroke patients can incur considerable costs for medical care, including nursing, rehabilitative, and long term care. Therefore, many countries are attempting to establish comprehensive and integrated healthcare systems for stroke patients [3,4]. Post-acute care (PAC), which refers to medical care services that support the individual patient in recovery from illness or management of chronic disability, is aimed at enhancing the functional status of patients discharged from acute hospitalization [2–5]. Discharges to PAC facilities have increased nearly 50% during the past 15 years, and PAC is a major contributor to hospitalization costs in the United States [5]. To control medical expenses, reform the medical referral system, and improve continuity of care, the Taiwan National Health Insurance Administration (NHIA) focused on stroke for its first national PAC project in 2014—post-acute care for cerebrovascular disease (PAC-CVD).

In Taiwan, beneficiaries are free to visit their preferred physicians and are not required to follow strict referral rules [6]. An efficient PAC system for stroke patients is needed to reduce unnecessary utilization of hospital resources and to ensure seamless care for these patients [7]. Stroke patients and their families expect that local hospitals can deliver PAC at a lower cost and with greater efficiency, effectiveness, and convenience. Our review of studies published in international journals, however, shows that most studies of PAC have analyzed a limited number of patients in a single hospital [8,9]. Additionally, few studies have used longitudinal data exceeding 1 year, and few studies have applied propensity score matching (PSM) in a natural experimental design to examine the longitudinal impacts of a medical referral system on functional status. Therefore, this study coupled a natural experimental design with PSM to assess the impact of the medical referral system in stroke patients and to examine the longitudinal effects of the medical referral system on functional status.

2. Materials and Methods

2.1. The PAC Program

In Taiwan, the multidisciplinary PAC stroke team consisted of neurologists, physiatrists, physical therapists, occupational therapists, speech therapists, and nurses. The PAC rehabilitation program was prescribed by the physiatrist, and it consisted of a complex program of universal activities that were performed at least three times per day. One hour of physical therapy, occupational therapy, or speech and swallowing therapy was carried out at each time. Notably, the fiscal incentive for a medical center to transfer a patient to a regional or a district hospital is mitigated by several factors, including the PAC-CVD transfer policy, the willingness of the stroke patient (or family) to accept further post-acute care in local hospitals, and whether the physician agrees to the transfer. These factors should cause health providers to reconsider the manner in which patient stays are controlled and to be mindful that the shortest lengths of stay (LOS) may not obtain the best outcome for the patient [10,11].

2.2. Study Design and Sample

The study population included all stroke patients admitted to PAC wards in four Taiwan hospitals between March 2014 and March 2018 (defined as ICD-9-CM codes 433.x, 434.x, and 436.x for ischemic stroke, and codes 430 and 431 for hemorrhagic stroke). The inclusion criteria were acute stroke and admission to PAC ward within 40 days after day of stroke onset. Another inclusion criterion was Modified Rankin Scale (MRS) level 2 to 4. Instead of focusing on patients who had received intensive in-patient rehabilitation, this national PAC project focused on the prevention of complications (e.g., pressure sores) in stroke patients who were bed-ridden (MRS 5). Patients who did not have major disability (MRS 0–1) were assumed to have undergone out-patient rehabilitation or were assumed to have resumed their pre-morbidity activities of daily living.

In observational studies, non-comparability between the intervention group and the comparison group can distort the estimation of the treatment effect [12,13]. The propensity score is a balancing score that can be used to compare groups that do not systematically differ. This study used PSM at the patient level to compare the baseline characteristics of the two groups, which increased the robustness of the analysis. A generalized estimating equation (GEE) model was used to cluster stroke patients treated by the same physician and to generate propensity scores for predicting the probability of the medical referral system. The covariates included patient demographics (age and gender), clinical attributes (stroke type, hypertension, hyperlipidemia, diabetes mellitus, atrial fibrillation, and previous stroke), quality of medical care (acute care LOS and PAC LOS), and pre-rehabilitation functional status. The caliper matching method ("greedy algorithm") was used for 1:1 PSM between the inter-hospital transfer group and the intra-hospital transfer group. Thus, 483 patients in the inter-hospital transfer group were compared with an "all participants matched set" of 483 patients in the intra-hospital transfer group (Figure 1). These PAC stroke patients completed the pre-rehabilitation and the 12th week and first year post-rehabilitation assessments.

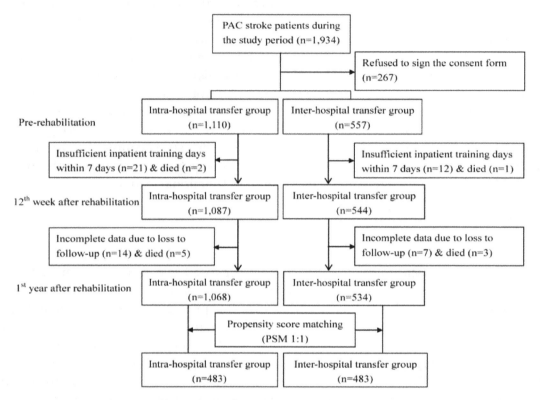

Figure 1. Flow chart of recruitment and study procedure.

2.3. Functional Status Instruments

The MRS scores of 0, 1, 2, 3, 4, and 5 are interpreted as no symptoms, no significant disability, slight disability, moderate disability, moderately severe disability, and severe disability, respectively [14]. The Barthel Index (BI) score was used to measure functional disability in daily life activities (e.g., eating, grooming, bathing, dressing, walking, transferring, staring, and controlling bladder and bowel) [15]. The score is for the 10-item BI ranges from 0 (totally dependent) to 100 (independent). The Functional Oral Intake Scale (FOIS) was used to assess functional oral intake in stroke patients with dysphagia [16]. The FOIS classifies swallowing function from level 1 (nothing by mouth) to level 7 (total oral diet with no restrictions). The Lawton-Brody Instrumental Activities of Daily Living Scale (IADL) is used to evaluate performance in daily life activities, including making telephone calls, shopping, preparing food, housekeeping, laundering, taking medicine, using transportation, and performing financial activities [17]. In the conventional use of the scale, women are scored in all eight domains, while men are not scored in the domains of preparing food, housekeeping, and laundering. The rationale for excluding these three domains in males is that performance of these tasks is subject to cultural differences in gender roles, which could compromise comparisons of the incidence of disability between men and women [18]. The EuroQoL five-dimensional (EQ-5D) measure is a self-assessment of mobility, self-care, usual activities, pain or discomfort, and anxiety or depression as part of a total health state [19]. The subject is required to score each item from 1 to 3 (no problem, some problem, or extreme problem, respectively). The Berg Balance Scale (BBS) is a scale of functional balance, including static and dynamic balance [20]. Each item on this 14-item scale is rated from 0 (poor balance) to 4 (good balance). The maximum score is 56. The Mini-Mental State Examination (MMSE) is the best-known short screening tool for cognitive impairment [21]. The MMSE tests orientation, attention, memory, language, and visual–spatial skills. The maximum score is 30 points. An MMSE score below an education-adjusted cut-off score indicates cognitive impairment. The Taiwan version of these measures has been validated as a reliable and valid tool for measuring functional status in both clinical practice and research [22].

2.4. Statistical Analysis

The unit of analysis in this study was the individual stroke patient. Descriptive statistics were tabulated to depict the stroke patient demographics. For clarification, the values predicted by the regression models were used to illustrate the results, starting from before initiation of PAC until completion of 12 weeks to 1 year of follow up in the two matched study groups. Thus, the GEE models were used to estimate difference-in-differences models used to examine the effectiveness of the medical referral system. For the predicted values, standard errors in differences and standard errors in difference-in-differences were estimated using a bootstrap technique involving 1000 replications, with sample sizes equivalent to that of the original sample [23].

Hierarchical linear regression models were used to examine the roles of the MRS after accounting for demographic characteristics, clinical attributes, quality of care, and pre-rehabilitative function status. Five-step hierarchical linear regression models were used to analyze differences between explanatory factors. In Model 1, explanatory factors included age, gender, stroke type, hypertension, hyperlipidemia, diabetes mellitus, atrial fibrillation, previous stroke, length of stay in acute care, length of stay in post-acute care, and pre-rehabilitation functional status. Model 2 included Model 1 and MRS = 2; Model 3 included Model 1 and MRS = 3; Model 4 included Model 1 and MRS = 4; Model 5 included Model 1, MRS, and medical referral system. In each model, the adjusted R-square was estimated while adjusting for covariates. For each model, the variance inflation factor (VIF) was used to assess multicollinearity. No models showed multicollinearity.

Statistical analyses were performed using Stata Statistical Package, version 13.0 (Stata Corp, College Station, TX, USA). All tests were two-sided, and p values less than 0.05 were considered statistically significant.

3. Results

Table 1 compares the inter-hospital transfer group and the intra-hospital transfer group before and after PSM. Before PSM, all assessed characteristics significantly differed between the two groups ($p < 0.05$). After PSM, no variables significantly differed between the two groups.

All PAC stroke patients had significantly improved scores for functional measures at the 1-year follow-up survey ($p < 0.001$) (Table 2). When the 12th week post-rehabilitation scores were used as the baseline, functional status showed significant improvements at the first year post-rehabilitation ($p < 0.001$). All subscale scores continued to improve throughout the follow-up period. Additionally, in both groups, functional status scores at the first year post-rehabilitation were significantly higher than the functional status scores at the 12th week post-rehabilitation and the functional status scores at pre-rehabilitation ($p < 0.001$). Throughout the follow-up period, the intra-hospital transfer group also had significantly higher scores for functional status measures compared to the inter-hospital transfer group ($p < 0.001$).

Table 3 shows that Model 1 revealed a significant association between patient demographics and scores for functional status measures at the first year post-rehabilitation during the study period ($p < 0.05$). In Models 2–4, patients with MRS = 2 showed very little functional status improvement after adjustment for patient demographics; however, patients with MRS = 3 and MRS = 4 showed improvements. That is, rehabilitative PAC improved quality of life in patients with moderate disability (MRS = 3) or moderately severe disability (MRS = 4) but not in patients with slight disability (MRS = 2). After adjustment for all relevant influential factors, the intra-hospital transfer group had greater improvements in functional status scores compared to the inter-hospital transfer group.

Table 1. Stroke patient characteristics *.

Variables		Before Propensity Score Matching			After Propensity Score Matching		
		Intra-Hospital Transfer Group (n = 1068)	Inter-Hospital Transfer Group (n = 534)	p Value	Intra-Hospital Transfer Group (n = 483)	Inter-Hospital Transfer Group (n = 483)	p Value
Demographics							
Age, years *		65.67 ± 12.38	63.96 ± 13.50	0.024	63.61 ± 13.10	63.96 ± 13.24	0.834
Gender	Female	450(42.1%)	186(34.8%)	0.014	171(35.4%)	169(35.0%)	0.784
	Male	618(57.9%)	348(65.2%)		312(64.6%)	314(65.0%)	
Clinical Attributes							
Stroke type	Ischemic	942(88.2%)	396(74.2%)	<0.001	363(75.0%)	360(74.5%)	0.880
	Hemorrhagic	126(11.8%)	138(25.8%)		120(25.0%)	123(25.5%)	
Hypertension	Yes	698(65.4%)	405(75.8%)	<0.001	372(77.0%)	367(76.0%)	0.221
Hyperlipidemia	Yes	332(31.1%)	227(42.5%)	<0.001	202(41.8%)	206(42.6%)	0.507
Diabetes mellitus	Yes	419(39.2)	200(37.5%)	0.570	182(37.7%)	181(37.5%)	0.990
Atrial fibrillation	Yes	67(6.3%)	55(10.3%)	0.013	47(9.7%)	49(10.1%)	0.887
Previous stroke	Yes	173(16.2%)	98(18.4%)	0.803	87(18.0%)	89(18.4%)	0.879
Quality of Medical Care							
Acute care LOS, days *		13.01 ± 27.83	24.45 ± 34.61	<0.001	23.75 ± 11.84	24.50 ± 11.56	0.356
PAC LOS, days *		31.52 ± 17.75	37.1 ± 12.59	<0.001	35.75 ± 12.34	36.50 ± 11.88	0.506
Pre-rehabilitation functional status							
BI *		41.91 ± 23.10	34.67 ± 23.48	<0.001	35.75 ± 20.11	34.00 ± 18.21	0.269
FOIS *		5.95 ± 3.04	5.38 ± 2.25	<0.001	5.53 ± 2.75	5.14 ± 2.84	0.927
EQ5D *		10.67 ± 1.86	10.40 ± 1.78	0.015	10.80 ± 1.82	10.93 ± 2.05	0.261
IADL *		1.41 ± 1.20	1.15 ± 1.12	<0.001	1.32 ± 1.14	1.27 ± 1.05	0.694
BBS *		15.30 ± 14.99	16.91 ± 17.27	0.097	14.00 ± 17.26	15.50 ± 17.71	0.972
MMSE *		20.15 ± 7.90	18.50 ± 9.66	0.001	20.75 ± 11.15	19.75 ± 10.47	0.908

Note: LOS, length of stay; PAC, post-acute care; QOL, quality of life; BI, Barthel Index; FOIS, Functional Oral Intake Scale; EQ5D, EuroQoL five-dimensional; IADL, Instrumental Activities of Daily Living Scale; BBS, Berg Balance Scale; MMSE, Mini-Mental State Examination. * Values are expressed as mean ± standard deviation or n (%).

Table 2. Comparison of functional status between intra-hospital transfer group and inter-hospital transfer group, before and after rehabilitation ($n = 1195$).

Functional Status Measure	Group	Before Rehabilitation (T1) Mean ± SD	12th Week After Rehabilitation (T2) Mean ± SD	Difference †	p Value	First Year After Rehabilitation (T3) Mean ± SD	Difference †	p Value
BI	Intra-hospital transfer	41.91 ± 23.10	51.50 ± 24.10	9.59	<0.001	68.84 ± 26.49	17.34	<0.001
	Inter-hospital transfer	34.67 ± 23.48	42.28 ± 25.96	7.61	<0.001	54.29 ± 27.20	12.01	0.002
	Difference ‡	7.24	9.22	1.98	<0.001	14.55	5.33	<0.001
FOIS	Intra-hospital transfer	5.95 ± 3.04	5.98 ± 1.82	0.03	0.037	6.41 ± 1.32	0.43	0.006
	Inter-hospital transfer	5.38 ± 2.25	5.68 ± 1.89	0.30	0.002	6.26 ± 1.47	0.58	0.044
	Difference ‡	0.57	0.30	−0.27	<0.001	0.15	−0.15	<0.001
EQ5D	Intra-hospital transfer	10.67 ± 1.86	9.81 ± 1.65	−0.86	<0.001	8.15 ± 2.23	−1.66	<0.001
	Inter-hospital transfer	10.40 ± 1.79	10.02 ± 1.70	−0.38	0.004	9.19 ± 1.88	−0.83	0.001
	Difference ‡	0.27	−0.21	−0.48	<0.001	−1.04	−0.83	<0.001
IADL	Intra-hospital transfer	1.41 ± 1.20	1.84 ± 1.32	0.43	<0.001	2.87 ± 1.75	1.03	<0.001
	Inter-hospital group	1.15 ± 1.13	1.36 ± 1.31	0.21	0.054	1.86 ± 1.57	0.5	0.023
	Difference ‡	0.26	0.48	0.22	<0.001	1.01	0.53	<0.001
BBS	Intra-hospital transfer	15.30 ± 14.99	26.32 ± 17.56	11.02	<0.001	34.58 ± 17.79	8.26	<0.001
	Inter-hospital transfer	16.91 ± 17.27	24.40 ± 19.25	7.49	<0.001	29.91 ± 19.35	5.51	0.022
	Difference ‡	−1.61	1.92	3.53	<0.001	4.67	2.75	<0.001
MMSE	Intra-hospital transfer	20.15 ± 7.90	21.62 ± 7.79	1.47	0.020	22.73 ± 7.39	1.11	0.078
	Inter-hospital transfer	18.50 ± 9.66	19.64 ± 10.80	1.14	0.090	21.25 ± 9.41	1.61	0.260
	Difference ‡	1.65	1.98	0.33	<0.001	1.48	−0.5	<0.001

Note: BI, Barthel Index; FOIS, Functional Oral Intake Scale; EQ5D, EuroQoL five-dimensional; IADL, Instrumental Activities of Daily Living Scale; BBS, Berg Balance Scale; MMSE, Mini-mental State Examination. † Difference indicates mean score for functional status at the 12th week after rehabilitation, mean score for functional status before rehabilitation, or mean score for functional status at the first year after rehabilitation. ‡ Difference indicates mean score for functional status in intra-hospital transfer group, or mean score for functional status in inter-hospital transfer group at each time point.

Table 3. Change in coefficient of multiple correlations associated with addition of subsequent variables to the model *.

Model	BI		FOIS		EQ5D		IADL		BBS		MMSE	
	R^2	R^2 Change	R^2	R^2 Change	R^2	R^2 Change	R^2	R^2 Change	R^2	R^2 Change	R^2	R^2 Change
1st level	0.64	-	0.28	-	0.38	-	0.51	-	0.48	-	0.79	-
2nd level	0.64	0.00	0.28	0.00	0.39	0.01	0.52	0.01	0.48	0.00	0.79	0.00
3rd level	0.64	0.00	0.29	0.01	0.44	0.06	0.55	0.04	0.51	0.03	0.79	0.00
4th level	0.64	0.00	0.29	0.01	0.44	0.06	0.55	0.04	0.51	0.03	0.79	0.00
5th level	0.67	0.03	0.29	0.01	0.49	0.11	0.58	0.07	0.53	0.05	0.79	0.00

Note: BI, Barthel Index; FOIS, Functional Oral Intake Scale; EQ5D, EuroQoL five-dimensional; IADL, Instrumental Activities of Daily Living Scale; BBS, Berg Balance Scale; MMSE, Mini-mental State Examination. * Model 1 included age, gender, stroke type, hypertension, hyperlipidemia, diabetes mellitus, atrial fibrillation, previous stroke, length of stay in acute care, length of stay in post-acute care, and pre-rehabilitation functional status; Model 2 included Model 1 and Modified Rankin Scale (MRS) = 2; Model 3 included Model 1 and MRS = 3; Model 4 included Model 1 and MRS = 4; Model 5 included Model 1, MRS, and medical referral system.

4. Discussion

Our data for the percentage of stroke patients with vascular risk factors were consistent with previous reports. After PSM, the percentages of stroke patients with hypertension, hyperlipidemia, diabetes mellitus, atrial fibrillation in our study were 77%, 42%, 37%, and 10%, respectively. Previous studies of stroke patients have reported hypertension in 63–80%, hyperlipidemia in 40–49%, diabetes mellitus in 34–42%, and atrial fibrillation in 7.3–11% [24,25]. A review of studies performed in Asia found that Taiwan has a higher prevalence of hypertension, diabetes mellitus, and hyperlipidemia compared to Japan, Korea and Singapore [26]. A previous Taiwan study of stroke incidence and recurrence during 2000–2011 also reported that, although the prevalence of diabetes mellitus, hyperlipidemia and atrial fibrillation increased during this period, the rates of primary ischemic stroke and 1-year recurrence of stroke decreased by 9% and 18% respectively [27]. Factors that can have important effects on stroke incidence and recurrence include medication control, early detection of diseases, diet control, body weight control, life style adjustment and exercise.

To achieve a vertically integrated medical system, post-stroke care should be patient-centered, and inter-hospital transfer of stroke patients must be seamless. In Australia, stroke patients treated at hospitals with stroke coordinators had lower LOS and higher quality of evidence-based care compared to those treated at hospitals without stroke coordinators [28]. In the Taiwan national PAC project reported here, the case manager assigned to each stroke patient ensured efficient transfer of the patient to a local hospital. Therefore, the mean LOS for patients in acute stage was much lower in the intra-hospital transfer group compared to the inter-hospital transfer group (13.01 and 24.45 days, respectively). Since minimizing the time from admission to inter-hospital transfer decreases total LOS and total cost, implementation of a case manager and an efficient inter-hospital transfer system are essential for an integrated medical system. Other possible reasons in the inter-hospital transfer group include geographical variations in the distribution of physicians and medical resources, and differences in care quality and expertise among hospitals and individual providers. For stroke patients in acute stage, those treated at teaching hospitals and certified primary stroke centers have a lower mortality rate, greater availability of rehabilitative care, and lower ADL dependence status [29]. A possible reason for the superior outcomes obtained by teaching hospitals and certified primary care centers for stroke is that they tend to have a high volume of stroke patients, and clinicians who treat a high volume of patients tend to achieve high skill levels.

Before PSM, compared to the intra-hospital transfer group, the inter-hospital transfer group in this study had a lower functional status before PAC and more comorbidity (hypertension, hyperlipidemia, atrial fibrillation). Most of the patients in inter-hospital transfer group had been treated at a medical center. Compared to stroke patients treated at medical centers tend to have a higher severity of disability, are more likely to require intubation (e.g., tracheostomy tube, nasogastric tube, and urinary catheter tube), and tend to require more time to stabilize. These differences might explain why the inter-hospital transfer group in our study had a longer mean LOS in acute stage compared to the intra-hospital transfer group. However, further studies are needed to compare the service path and treatment costs in patients with varying severity of stroke and in stroke patients treated at different hospital levels.

After the acute stage, local low-volume rehabilitation facilities can usually provide adequate care [30]. Several studies have reported that, compared to skilled nursing facilities, intensive inpatient rehabilitation facilities achieve higher functional outcomes in PAC for stroke [30,31]. Additionally, duration of hospital stay and in-hospital mortality are related to socioeconomic status [32]. Therefore, increasing socioeconomic inequality over time has markedly increased inequality in stroke survival. Direct non-healthcare costs (including informal care costs, paid care costs and transportation costs) and rehabilitation costs are the largest post-stroke care costs [33,34]. Stroke patients who receive PAC and rehabilitation at local hospitals can reduce the physical, mental and economic burdens on their families. Our study analyzed data obtained from four local southern Taiwan hospitals that had the largest volumes of stroke inpatients in PAC. Therefore, the data obtained in this work are highly representative of hospitals throughout Taiwan and have immediate applications.

In Japan, the rehabilitation is 3 hours, and the average LOS in rehabilitation facilities after discharge from tertiary hospitals is approximately 74.7 days [35]. The Taiwan PAC-CVD program provides the maximum of 12 weeks of services. Reimbursements are similar regardless of the hospital accreditation level (regional or district) and the equipment costs of the hospital. The PAC-CVD project enables stroke patients to access rehabilitation programs that are more intensive (in terms of frequency and duration of treatment) compared to those available under current NHIA provisions. The PAC-CVD project was expected to offer a continuous care model to restore function and reduce disability in stroke patients [8,9]. Most PAC-CVD studies published thus far have been studies of a limited case number in a single hospital [8,9]. In the post-acute stage, the mean LOS in the intra-hospital transfer group and the inter-hospital transfer group was 31.52 and 37.1 days, respectively. Another study of a large population of stroke patients reported a mean PAC stay of only 15.1 days [36]. Notably, the LOS of stroke patients in different countries is related to differences in post-stroke policy. For example, the average LOS for inpatient rehabilitation after stroke is approximately 1 month in Ireland, Switzerland, and Thailand [37]. In contrast, the average LOS inpatient rehabilitation after stroke is only 15.8 days in the United States, which is much shorter than that in western countries (e.g., 32.7 days in Germany, 35.3 days in Canada) [38–40]. The main reasons for the short LOS in the United States are the high economic burden of inpatient care for stroke patients and the availability of various well-established PAC rehabilitation facilities (e.g., inpatient rehabilitation hospitals, skilled nursing facilities, home health agency services, long term care hospitals) [4]. According to our multi-center data, the LOS for stroke patients who undergo PAC in Taiwan is similar to that in other countries. Notably, our data indicated that the effectiveness of rehabilitation training during the 12th week to the first year is better than in the first 12 weeks. These data confirm that a continuous rehabilitative PAC program is essential.

A study by Dewilde concluded that MRS level is a major determinant of medical resource use [41]. For this national PAC-CVD project, the MRS level was the main criterion for participation. Initially, only patients with MRS levels of 2 to 4 were eligible for transfer to hospitals with PAC wards. However, some people have proposed excluding patients in MRS level 2 or including patients in MRS level 5. In 2019, the Taiwan NHIA excluded MRS level 2 patients from this national PAC-CVD project. This study found that after adjusting for all relevant influential factors, the quality of life improvement was smaller in patients at MRS level 2 compared to patients at other MRS levels. Therefore, these data support the decision made by the Taiwan NHIA. In terms of maximizing efficiency in the use of limited healthcare resources, the decision to limit inpatient rehabilitation to patients with MRS 3 to 4 was not only justifiable, but necessary.

Although all research questions were adequately and satisfactorily addressed, two limitations are noted. This study only collected data for acute stroke patients for 40 days after stroke onset. Furthermore, this study only analyzed patients treated at four hospitals in south Taiwan. However, the numbers of patients treated in the PAC-programs at these hospitals were among the four highest of all district hospitals in south Taiwan. Further studies are needed to compare a PAC group and a control group in other regions of Taiwan and under current NHI regulations. Additionally, the two groups in this study were matched for demographic characteristics, clinical attributes, quality of care, and pre-rehabilitative functional status. Future studies could consider the use of inverse probability weighting rather than PSM.

5. Conclusions

In conclusion, this study showed that rehabilitative PAC improved outcomes of stroke rehabilitation. To achieve a vertically integrated medical system for stroke rehabilitation, the key requirements are improving the PAC ward qualifications of local hospitals, accelerating inter-hospital transfer, and ensuring a sufficient duration of intensive rehabilitative PAC. Early rehabilitation is important for successful restoration of health, confidence, and self-care ability in these patients.

Author Contributions: Study concept and design, C.-Y.W. and H.-Y.S.; acquisition of data, H.-H.H., K.-W.H., H.-F.L., H.-Y.C., S.-C.J.Y., and Y.-J.Y.; analysis and interpretation of data, C.-Y.W. and H.-Y.S.; drafting of the manuscript, C.-Y.W. and H.-Y.S.; revision of the manuscript, H.-H.H., K.-W.H., H.-F.L., H.-Y.C., S.-C.J.Y., and Y.-J.Y.; approval of the manuscript, all authors.

Acknowledgments: We thank all the individuals who participated in this study, without which this study would not have been possible.

References

1. Prabhakaran, S.; Ruff, I.; Bernstein, R.A. Acute stroke intervention: A systematic review. *JAMA* **2015**, *313*, 1451–1462. [CrossRef] [PubMed]

2. Sturm, J.W.; Dewey, H.M.; Donnan, G.A.; Macdonell, R.A.; McNeil, J.J. Handicap after stroke: How does it relate to disability, perception of recovery, and stroke subtype? The north North East Melbourne Stroke Incidence Study (NEMESIS). *Stroke* **2002**, *33*, 762–768. [CrossRef] [PubMed]

3. Burke, R.E.; Juarez-Colunga, E.; Levy, C.; Prochazka, A.V.; Coleman, E.A.; Ginde, A.A. Rise of post-acute care facilities as a discharge destination of US hospitalizations. *JAMA Intern. Med.* **2015**, *175*, 295–296. [CrossRef] [PubMed]

4. Huckfeldt, P.J.; Mehrotra, A.; Hussey, P.S. The Relative Importance of Post-Acute Care and Readmissions for Post-Discharge Spending. *Health Serv. Res.* **2016**, *51*, 1919–1938. [CrossRef] [PubMed]

5. Redberg, R.F. The role of post-acute care in variation in the Medicare program. *JAMA Intern. Med.* **2015**, *175*, 1058. [CrossRef] [PubMed]

6. Chen, C.C.; Cheng, S.H. Does pay-for-performance benefit patients with multiple chronic conditions? Evidence from a universal coverage health care system. *Health Policy Plan.* **2016**, *31*, 83–90. [CrossRef] [PubMed]

7. Lee, H.C.; Chang, K.C.; Lan, C.F. Factors associated with prolonged hospital stay for acute stroke in Taiwan. *Acta Neurol. Taiwan* **2008**, *17*, 17–25. [PubMed]

8. Wang, C.Y.; Chen, Y.R.; Hong, J.P.; Chan, C.C.; Chang, L.C.; Shi, H.Y. Rehabilitative post-acute care for stroke patients delivered by per-diem payment system in different hospitalization paths: A Taiwan pilot study. *Int. J. Qual. Health Care* **2017**, *29*, 779–784. [CrossRef] [PubMed]

9. Lai, C.L.; Tsai, M.M.; Luo, J.Y.; Liao, W.C.; Hsu, P.S.; Chen, H.Y. Post-acute care for stroke—A retrospective cohort study in Taiwan. *Patient Prefer. Adherence* **2017**, *11*, 1309–1315. [CrossRef]

10. Huang, S.T.; Yu, T.M.; Ke, T.Y.; Wu, M.J.; Chuang, Y.W.; Li, C.Y.; Chiu, C.W.; Lin, C.L.; Liang, W.M.; Chou, T.C.; et al. Intensive Periodontal Treatment Reduces Risks of Hospitalization for Cardiovascular Disease and All-Cause Mortality in the Hemodialysis Population. *J. Clin. Med.* **2018**, *7*, 344. [CrossRef]

11. Cheng, C.Y.; Hsu, C.Y.; Wang, T.C.; Jeng, Y.C.; Yang, W.H. Evaluation of Cardiac Complications Following Hemorrhagic Stroke Using 5-Year Centers for Disease Control and Prevention (CDC) Database. *J. Clin. Med.* **2018**, *7*, 519. [CrossRef] [PubMed]

12. Rosenbaum, P.R.; Rubin, D.B. The central role of the propensity score in observational studies for causal effects. *Biometrika* **1983**, *70*, 41–55. [CrossRef]

13. D'Agostino, R.B. Tutorial in biostatistics. Propensity score methods for bias reduction in the comparison of a treatment to a non-randomized control group. *Stat Med.* **1998**, *17*, 2265–2281. [CrossRef]

14. Banks, J.L.; Marotta, C.A. Outcomes validity and reliability of the modified Rankin scale: Implications for stroke clinical trials: A literature review and synthesis. *Stroke* **2007**, *38*, 1091–1096. [CrossRef] [PubMed]

15. Wolfe, C.D.; Taub, N.A.; Woodrow, E.J.; Burney, P.G. Assessment of scales of disability and handicap for stroke patients. *Stroke* **1991**, *22*, 1242–1244. [CrossRef] [PubMed]

16. Crary, M.A.; Mann, G.D.; Groher, M.E. Initial psychometric assessment of a functional oral intake scale for dysphagia in stroke patients. *Arch. Phys. Med. Rehabil.* **2005**, *86*, 1516–1520. [CrossRef] [PubMed]

17. Lawton, M.P.; Brody, E.M. Assessment of older people: Self-maintaining and instrumental activities of daily living. *Gerontologist* **1969**, *9*, 179–186. [CrossRef]

18. Alexandre, T.S.; Corona, L.P.; Nunes, D.P.; Santos, J.L.; Duarte, Y.A.; Lebrão, M.L. Disability in instrumental activities of daily living among older adults: Gender differences. *Rev. Saude Publica* **2014**, *48*, 379–389. [CrossRef]

19. Rabin, R.; de Charro, F. EQ-5D: A measure of health status from the EuroQol group. *Ann. Med.* **2001**, *33*, 337–343. [CrossRef]

20. Chou, C.Y.; Chien, C.W.; Hsueh, I.P.; Sheu, C.F.; Wang, C.H.; Hsieh, C.L. Developing a short form of the Berg Balance Scale for people with stroke. *Phys. Ther.* **2006**, *86*, 195–204.

21. Folstein, M.F.; Folstein, S.E.; McHugh, P.R. "Mini-mental state". A practical method for grading the cognitive state of patients for the clinician. *J. Psychiatr. Res.* **1995**, *12*, 189–198. [CrossRef]

22. Guo, N.W.; Lui, H.C.; Wong, P.F.; Liao, K.K.; Yan, S.H.; Lin, K.P. Chinese version and norms of the Mini-Mental State Examination. *J. Rehabil. Med. Assoc. Taiwan* **1988**, *16*, 52–59.

23. Efron, B.; Tibshirani, R. *An Introduction to the Bootstrap*; Chapman & Hall: New York, NY, USA, 1993.

24. Hsieh, C.Y.; Wu, D.P.; Sung, S.F. Trends in vascular risk factors, stroke performance measures, and outcomes in patients with first-ever ischemic stroke in Taiwan between 2000 and 2012. *J. Neurol. Sci.* **2017**, *378*, 80–84. [CrossRef] [PubMed]

25. Cheng, J.H.; Zhang, Z.; Ye, Q.; Ye, Z.S.; Xia, N.G. Characteristics of the ischemic stroke patients whose seizures occur at stroke presentation at a single institution in Eastern China. *J. Neurol. Sci.* **2018**, *387*, 46–50. [CrossRef] [PubMed]

26. Hsieh, F.I.; Chiou, H.Y. Stroke: Morbidity, Risk Factors, and Care in Taiwan. *J. Stroke* **2014**, *16*, 59–64. [CrossRef] [PubMed]

27. Lee, M.; Wu, Y.L.; Ovbiagele, B. Trends in Incident and Recurrent Rates of First-Ever Ischemic Stroke in Taiwan between 2000 and 2011. *J. Stroke* **2016**, *18*, 60–65. [CrossRef] [PubMed]

28. Purvis, T.; Kilkenny, M.F.; Middleton, S.; Cadilhac, D.A. Influence of stroke coordinators on delivery of acute stroke care and hospital outcomes: An observational study. *Int. J. Stroke* **2018**, *13*, 585–591. [CrossRef]

29. Bettger, J.P.; Thomas, L.; Liang, L.; Xian, Y.; Bushnell, C.D.; Saver, J.L.; Fonarow, G.C.; Peterson, E.D. Hospital Variation in Functional Recovery After Stroke. *Circ. Cardiovasc. Qual. Outcomes* **2017**, *10*, e002391. [CrossRef]

30. Graham, J.E.; Deutsch, A.; O'Connell, A.A.; Karmarkar, A.M.; Granger, C.V.; Ottenbacher, K.J. Inpatient rehabilitation volume and functional outcomes in stroke, lower extremity fracture, and lower extremity joint replacement. *Med. Care* **2013**, *51*, 404–412. [CrossRef]

31. Alcusky, M.; Ulbricht, C.M.; Lapane, K.L. Postacute Care Setting, Facility Characteristics, and Poststroke Outcomes: A Systematic Review. *Arch. Phys. Med. Rehabil.* **2018**, *99*, 1124–1140. [CrossRef]

32. Blattner, M.; Price, J.; Holtkamp, M.D. Socioeconomic class and universal healthcare: Analysis of stroke cost and outcomes in US military healthcare. *J. Neurol. Sci.* **2018**, *386*, 64–68. [CrossRef] [PubMed]

33. Fattore, G.; Torbica, A.; Susi, A.; Giovanni, A.; Benelli, G.; Gozzo, M.; Toso, V. The social and economic burden of stroke survivors in Italy: A prospective, incidence-based, multi-centre cost of illness study. *BMC Neurol.* **2012**, *12*, 137. [CrossRef] [PubMed]

34. Rajsic, S.; Gothe, H.; Borba, H.H.; Sroczynski, G.; Vujicic, J.; Toell, T.; Siebert, U. Economic burden of stroke: A systematic review on post-stroke care. *Eur. J. Health Econ.* **2019**, *20*, 107–134. [CrossRef] [PubMed]

35. Miyai, I.; Sonoda, S.; Nagai, S.; Takayama, Y.; Inoue, Y.; Kakehi, A.; Kurihara, M.; Ishikawa, M. Results of new policies for inpatient rehabilitation coverage in Japan. *Neurorehabil. Neural. Repair.* **2011**, *25*, 540–547. [CrossRef] [PubMed]

36. Peng, L.N.; Lu, W.H.; Liang, C.K.; Chou, M.Y.; Chung, C.P.; Tsai, S.L.; Chen, Z.J.; Hsiao, F.Y.; Chen, L.K. Functional Outcomes, Subsequent Healthcare Utilization, and Mortality of Stroke Postacute Care Patients in Taiwan: A Nationwide Propensity Score-matched Study. *J. Am. Med. Dir. Assoc.* **2017**, *18*, 990.e7–990.e12. [CrossRef] [PubMed]

37. Kuptniratsaikul, V.; Kovindha, A.; Massakulpan, P.; Permsirivanich, W.; Kuptniratsaikul, P.S. Inpatient rehabilitation services for patients after stroke in Thailand: A multi-centre study. *J. Rehabil. Med.* **2009**, *41*, 684–686. [CrossRef] [PubMed]

38. Lewis, Z.H.; Hay, C.C.; Graham, J.E.; Lin, Y.L.; Karmarkar, A.M.; Ottenbacher, K.J. Social Support and Actual Versus Expected Length of Stay in Inpatient Rehabilitation Facilities. *Arch. Phys. Med. Rehabil.* **2016**, *97*, 2068–2075. [CrossRef] [PubMed]

39. Meyer, M.; Britt, E.; McHale, H.A.; Teasell, R. Length of stay benchmarks for inpatient rehabilitation after stroke. *Disabil. Rehabil.* **2012**, *34*, 1077–1081. [CrossRef] [PubMed]

40. Verpillat, P.; Dorey, J.; Guilhaume-Goulant, C.; Dabbous, F.; Brunet, J.; Aballéa, S. A chart review of management of ischemic stroke patients in Germany. *J. Mark. Access Health Policy* **2015**, *3*. [CrossRef]

41. Dewilde, S.; Annemans, L.; Peeters, A.; Hemelsoet, D.; Vandermeeren, Y.; Desfontaines, P.; Brouns, R.; Vanhooren, G.; Cras, P.; Michielsens, B.; et al. Modified Rankin scale as a determinant of direct medical costs after stroke. *Int. J. Stroke* **2017**, *12*, 392–400. [CrossRef]

Permissions

List of Contributors

Tino Prell
Department of Neurology, Jena University Hospital, 07740 Jena, Germany
Center for Healthy Ageing, Jena University Hospital, 07740 Jena, Germany

Frank Siebecker
Praxis Neurologie, 48291 Telgte, Germany

Michael Lorrain
Neuroärzte Gerresheim-Pempelfort, 40625 Düsseldorf, Germany

Lars Tönges
Department of Neurology, St. Josef-Hospital, Ruhr-University Bochum, 44801 Bochum, Germany

Tobias Warnecke
Department of Neurology, University of Muenster, 48149 Münster, Germany

Jochen Klucken
Department of Molecular Neurology, Universitätsklinikum Erlangen, Schwabachanlage 6, 91054 Erlangen Neurology, Ev. Amalie Sieveking Hospital, 22359 Hamburg, Germany
AG Digital Health Pathways, Fraunhofer Institute for Integrated Circuits, Am Wolfsmantel 33, 91058 Erlangen, Germany
Münster Medical Center Hamburg-Eppendorf, 20246 Hamburg, Germany

Ingmar Wellach
Department of Neurology, Ev. Amalie Sieveking Hospital, 22359 Hamburg, Germany
Office for Neurology and Psychiatry Hamburg Walddörfer, 22359 Hamburg, Germany

Carsten Buhmann
Department of Neurology, University Medical Center Hamburg-Eppendorf, 20246 Hamburg, Germany

Martin Wolz
Department of Neurology, Elblandklinikum Meißen, 01662 Meißen, Germany

Stefan Lorenzl
Professorship for Palliative Care, Paracelsus Medical University, 5020 Salzburg, Austria
Department of Palliative Medicine, Ludwig-Maximilians-University Munich, 81377 Munich, Germany

Department of Neurology, Klinikum Agatharied, 83734 Hausham, Germany

Heinz Herbst
Neurozentrum Sophienstrasse, 70178 Stuttgart, Germany

Carsten Eggers
Department of Neurology, University Hospital Marburg, 35037 Marburg, Germany

Tobias Mai
Department of Nursing, University Hospital Frankfurt, Goethe University, 60590 Frankfurt, Germany

Oscar Corli
Department of Oncology, Laboratory of Methodology for Clinical Research, Unit of Pain and Palliative Care Research, Istituto di Ricerche Farmacologiche Mario Negri IRCCS, 20156 Milan, Italy

Luca Porcu
Department of Oncology, Laboratory of Methodology for Clinical Research, Unit of Methodological Research, Istituto di Ricerche Farmacologiche Mario Negri IRCCS, 20156 Milan, Italy

Claudia Santucci and Cristina Bosetti
Department of Oncology, Laboratory of Methodology for Clinical Research, Unit of Cancer Epidemiology, Istituto di Ricerche Farmacologiche Mario Negri IRCCS, 20156 Milan, Italy

Shao-Huan Lan
School of Pharmaceutical Sciences and Medical Technology, Putian University, Putian 351100, Fujian, China

Shen-Peng Chang
Department of Pharmacy, Chi Mei Medical Center, Liouying 73657, Taiwan

Chih-Cheng Lai and Chien-Ming Chao
Department of Intensive Care Medicine, Chi Mei Medical Center, Liouying 73657, Taiwan

Li-Chin Lu
School of Management, Putian University, Putian 351100, Fujian, China

José Ramon Calvo
Healthcare Department, Praxair Spain, 28020 Madrid, Spain

Cátia Caneiras
Institute of Environmental Health (ISAMB), Faculty of Medicine, Universidade de Lisboa, 1649-028 Lisboa, Portugal
Healthcare Department, Praxair Portugal Gases, 2601-906 Lisboa, Portugal

Cristina Jácome
CINTESIS-Center for Health Technologies and Information Systems Research, Faculty of Medicine, University of Porto, 4200-450 Porto, Portugal
Respiratory Research and Rehabilitation Laboratory (Lab3R), School of Health Sciences (ESSUA), University of Aveiro, 3810-193 Aveiro, Portugal

Sagrario Mayoralas-Alises
Service of Pneumology, Hospital Universitario Moncloa, 28008 Madrid, Spain
Healthcare Department, Praxair Spain, 28020 Madrid, Spain

João Almeida Fonseca
CINTESIS-Center for Health Technologies and Information Systems Research, Faculty of Medicine, University of Porto, 4200-450 Porto, Portugal
MEDCIDS-Department of Community Medicine, Health Information and Decision, Faculty of Medicine, University of Porto, 4200-450 Porto, Portugal
Allergy Unit, Instituto and Hospital CUF, 4460-188 Porto, Portugal

Joan Escarrabill
Hospital Clínic de Barcelona, 08036 Barcelona, Spain
Master Plan for Respiratory Diseases (Ministry of Health) & Observatory of Home Respiratory Therapies (FORES), 08028 Barcelona, Spain
REDISSEC Health Services Research on Chronic Patients Network, Instituto de Salud Carlos III, 28029 Madrid, Spain

João Carlos Winck
Faculty of Medicine, University of Porto, 4200-319 Porto, Portugal

Chong-Chi Chiu
Department of General Surgery, Chi Mei Medical Center, Liouying 73657, Taiwan
Department of General Surgery, Chi Mei Medical Center, Tainan 71004, Taiwan
Department of Electrical Engineering, Southern Taiwan University of Science and Technology, Tainan 71005, Taiwan

Wen-Li Lin
Department of Cancer Center, Chi Mei Medical Center, Liouying 73657, Taiwan

Dong-il Chun, Jahyung Kim and Sung Hun Won
Department of Orthopaedic Surgery, Soonchunhyang University Hospital Seoul, 59, Daesagwan-ro, Yongsan-gu, Seoul 04401, Korea

Chien-Cheng Huang
Department of Emergency Medicine, Chi-Mei Medical Center, Tainan 71004, Taiwan
Department of Senior Services, Southern Taiwan University of Science and Technology, Tainan 71005, Taiwan

Jyh-Jou Chen
Department of Gastroenterology and Hepatology, Chi Mei Medical Center, Liouying 73657, Taiwan

Shih-Bin Su
Department of Occupational Medicine, Chi Mei Medical Center, Liouying 73657, Taiwan
Department of Occupational Medicine, Chi Mei Medical Center, Tainan 71004, Taiwan
Department of Leisure, Recreation and Tourism Management, Southern Taiwan University of Science and Technology, Tainan 71005, Taiwan

Chao-Jung Tsao
Department of Oncology, Chi Mei Medical Center, Liouying 73657, Taiwan

Shang-Hung Chen
National Institute of Cancer Research, National Health Research Institutes, Tainan 70403, Taiwan

Jhi-Joung Wang
Department of Medical Research, Chi Mei Medical Center, Tainan 71004, Taiwan
AI Biomed Center, Southern Taiwan University of Science and Technology, Tainan 71005, Taiwan

Munjae Lee and Sewon Park
Research Institute for Future Medicine, Samsung Medical Center, Seoul 06351, Korea
Department of Medical Device Management and Research, SAIHST, Sungkyunkwan University, Seoul 06355, Korea

Kyu-Sung Lee
Department of Medical Device Management and Research, SAIHST, Sungkyunkwan University, Seoul 06355, Korea
Department of Urology, Samsung Medical Center, Sungkyunkwan University School of Medicine, Seoul 06351, Korea

María Rosa García-Merino
Health District of Córdoba Sur, 14940 Córdoba, Spain

Encarnación Blanco-Reina and Inmaculada Bellido-Estévez
Pharmacology and Therapeutics Department, School of Medicine, Instituto de Investigación Biomédica de Málaga-IBIMA, University of Málaga, 29016 Málaga, Spain

Jenifer Valdellós
Health District of Málaga-Guadalhorce, 29009 Málaga, Spain

Ricardo Ocaña-Riola
Escuela Andaluza de Salud Pública, 18011 Granada, Spain
Instituto de Investigación Biosanitaria ibs.GRANADA, 18012 Granada, Spain

Lorena Aguilar-Cano
Physical Medicine and Rehabilitation Department, Hospital Regional Universitario, 29010 Málaga, Spain

Gabriel Ariza-Zafra
Geriatrics Department, Complejo Hospitalario Universitario, 02006 Albacete, Spain

Sangyoung Kim
SCH Biomedical Informatics Research Unit, Soonchunhyang University Seoul Hospital, Seoul 04401, Korea

Hyeon-Jong Yang
Department of Pediatrics, Soonchunhyang University Hospital Seoul, 59, Daesagwan-ro, Yongsan-gu, Seoul 04401, Korea

Jae Heon Kim
Department of Urology, Soonchunhyang University Hospital Seoul, 59, Daesagwan-ro, Yongsan-gu, Seoul 04401, Korea

Jae-ho Cho
Department of Orthopaedic Surgery, Chuncheon Sacred Heart Hospital, Hallym University, 77, Sakju-ro, Chuncheon-si 24253, Korea

Young Yi
Department of Orthopaedic Surgery, Seoul Foot and Ankle Center, Inje University, 85, 2-ga, Jeo-dong, Jung-gu, Seoul 04551, Korea

Woo Jong Kim
Department of Orthopaedic Surgery, Soonchunhyang University Hospital Cheonan, 31, Soonchunhyang 6-gil, Dongnam-gu, Cheonan 31151, Korea

Masanari Kuwabara
Intensive Care Unit and Department of Cardiology, Toranomon Hospital, Tokyo 105-8470, Japan
Cardiovascular Center, St. Luke's International Hospital, Tokyo 104-8560, Japan

Koichiro Niwa
Cardiovascular Center, St. Luke's International Hospital, Tokyo 104-8560, Japan

Ichiro Hisatome
Division of Regenerative Medicine and Therapeutics, Tottori University Graduate School of Medical Sciences, Tottori 683-8503, Japan

Carlos A. Roncal-Jimenez, Ana Andres-Hernando Richard J. Johnson and Miguel A. Lanaspa
Division of Renal Diseases and Hypertension, School of Medicine, University of Colorado Denver, Aurora, CO 80045, USA

Petter Bjornstad
Division of Renal Diseases and Hypertension, School of Medicine, University of Colorado Denver, Aurora, CO 80045, USA
Children's Hospital Colorado and Barbara Davis Center for Childhood Diabetes, Aurora, CO 80045, USA

Mehmet Kanbay
Division of Nephrology, Department of Medicine, Koc University School of Medicine, Istanbul 34450, Turkey

Chang-Hua Chen
Division of Infectious Disease, Department of Internal Medicine, Changhua Christian Hospital, Changhua 500, Taiwan
Center for Infection Prevention and Control, Changhua Christian Hospital, Changhua 500, Taiwan
Program in Translational Medicine, National Chung Hsing University, Taichung County 402, Taiwan
Rong Hsing Research Center for Translational Medicine, National Chung Hsing University, Taichung County 402, Taiwan

Li-Jhen Lin
Center for Infection Prevention and Control, Changhua Christian Hospital, Changhua 500, Taiwan

Yu-Min Chen
Department of Pharmacy, Changhua Christian Hospital, Changhua 500, Taiwan

Yu Yang
Division of Nephrology, Department of Internal Medicine, Changhua Christian Hospital, Changhua 500, Taiwan

Yu-Jun Chang
Epidemiology and Biostatistics Center, Changhua Christian Hospital, Changhua 500, Taiwan

Hua-Cheng Yen
Department of Neurosurgery, Changhua Christian Hospital, Changhua 500, Taiwan

Min Ho Jo
Department of Internal Medicine, Institute of Gastroenterology, Yonsei University College of Medicine, Seoul 03722, Korea

Tae Seop Lim, Mi Young Jeon and Hye Won Lee
Department of Internal Medicine, Institute of Gastroenterology, Yonsei University College of Medicine, Seoul 03722, Korea
Yonsei Liver Center, Severance Hospital, Seoul 03722, Korea

Beom Kyung Kim, Jun Yong Park, Do Young Kim, Sang Hoon Ahn, Kwang-Hyub Han and Seung Up Kim
Department of Internal Medicine, Institute of Gastroenterology, Yonsei University College of Medicine, Seoul 03722, Korea
Yonsei Liver Center, Severance Hospital, Seoul 03722, Korea
Institute of Gastroenterology, Severance Hospital Yonsei University College of Medicine, Seoul 03722, Korea

Ki-Sun Lee
Department of Biomedical Engineering, College of Medicine, Seoul National University, Seoul 03080, Korea
Department of Clinical Dentistry, College of Medicine, Korea University, Seoul 02841, Korea
Department of Prosthodontics, Korea University An-san Hospital, Gyung-gi do 15355, Korea

Seok-Ki Jung
Department of Orthodontics, Korea University Ansan Hospital, Gyung-gi do 15355, Korea

Jae-Jun Ryu
Department of Prosthodontics, Korea University Anam Hospital, Seoul 02841, Korea

Sang-Wan Shin
Department of Advanced Prosthodontics, Graduate School of Clinical Dentistry, Korea University, Seoul 02841, Korea
Institute of Clinical Dental Research, Korea University, Seoul 02841, Korea

Jinwook Choi
Department of Biomedical Engineering, College of Medicine, Seoul National University, Seoul 03080, Korea

Institute of Medical & Biological Engineering, Medical Research Center, Seoul 03080, Korea

Hui-Ting Lin and Yen-I Li
Department of Physical Therapy, I-Shou University No. 8, Yida Road, Yan-chao District, Kaohsiung 82445, Taiwan

Wen-Pin Hu
Department of Bioinformatics and Medical Engineering, Asia University. 500, Lioufeng Road,Wufeng, Taichung 41354, Taiwan

Chun-Cheng Huang
Department of Rehabilitation, E-DA Hospital, No.1, Yida Road, Yan-chao District, Kaohsiung 82445, Taiwan

Yi-Chun Du
Department of Electrical Engineering, Southern Taiwan University of Science and Technology, No. 1, Nan-Tai Street, Yungkang District, Tainan 71005, Taiwan

Giovanni Damiani
Department of Dermatology, Case Western Reserve University, Cleveland, OH 44124, USA
Clinical Dermatology, IRCCS Istituto Ortopedico Galeazzi, 20161 Milan, Italy
Department of Biomedical, Surgical and Dental Sciences, University of Milan, 20122 Milan, Italy
Young Dermatologists Italian Network (YDIN), Centro Studi GISED, 24121 Bergamo, Italy

Nicola Luigi Bragazzi
Clinical Dermatology, IRCCS Istituto Ortopedico Galeazzi, 20161 Milan, Italy
Department of Biomedical, Surgical and Dental Sciences, University of Milan, 20122 Milan, Italy

Alessia Pacifico, Claudio Bonifati and Aldo Morrone
San Gallicano Dermatological Institute, IRCCS, 00144 Rome, Italy

Filomena Russo
Dermatology Section, Department of Clinical Medicine and Immunological Science, University of Siena, 53100 Siena, Italy

Paolo Daniele Maria Pigatto
School of Public Health, Department of Health Sciences (DISSAL), University of Genoa, 16132 Genoa, Italy

Cesar Hueso-Montoro, María P. García-Caro and Rafael Montoya-Juarez
Department of Nursing, Faculty of Health Sciences, Mind, Brain and Behaviour Research Institute, University of Granada, 18016 Granada, Spain

Abdulla Watad
NIHR Leeds Biomedical Research Centre, Leeds Teaching Hospitals NHS Trust, Leeds Institute of Rheumatic and Musculoskeletal Medicine, University of Leeds, Leeds LS7 4SA, UK
Department of Medicine 'B', Sheba Medical Center, Tel-Hashomer and Sackler Faculty of Medicine, Tel Aviv University, 5265601 Tel Aviv, Israel

Mohammad Adawi
Padeh and Ziv Hospitals, Azrieli Faculty of Medicine, Bar-Ilan University, 5290002 Ramat Gan, Israel

Chih-Cheng Lai
Department of Intensive Care Medicine, Chi Mei Medical Center, Liouying 73657, Taiwan

I-Ling Cheng and Yu-Hung Chen
Department of Pharmacy, Chi Mei Medical Center, Liouying 73657, Taiwan

Hung-Jen Tang
Department of Medicine, Chi Mei Medical Center, Tainan 71004, Taiwan

Daniel Puente-Fernández
Doctoral Program of Clinical Medicine and Public Health, University of Granada, 18071 Granada, Spain

Concepción B. Roldán-López
Department of Statistics and Operational Research, Faculty of Medicine, University of Granada, 1016 Granada, Spain

Concepción P. Campos-Calderón
Alicante Biomedical Research Institute (ISABIAL), 03010 Alicante, Spain

Chung-Yuan Wang
Department of Physical Medicine and Rehabilitation, Pingtung Christian Hospital, Pingtung 90059, Taiwan

Hong-Hsi Hsien
Department of Internal Medicine, St. Joseph Hospital, Kaohsiung 80760, Taiwan

Kuo-Wei Hung
Division of Neurology, Department of internal medicine, Yuan's General Hospital, Kaohsiung 80249, Taiwan

Hsiu-Fen Lin
Department of Neurology, Kaohsiung Medical University Hospital, Kaohsiung 80756, Taiwan

Hung-Yi Chiou
School of Public Health, Taipei Medical University, Taipei 11031, Taiwan
Center for Neurotrauma and Neuroregeneration, Taipei Medical University, Taipei 11031, Taiwan

Yu-Jo Yeh
Department of Healthcare Administration and Medical Informatics, Kaohsiung Medical University, Kaohsiung 80708, Taiwan

Shu-Chuan Jennifer Yeh
Department of Healthcare Administration and Medical Informatics, Kaohsiung Medical University, Kaohsiung 80708, Taiwan
Department of Business Management, National Sun Yat-sen University, Kaohsiung 80424, Taiwan

Hon-Yi Shi
Department of Healthcare Administration and Medical Informatics, Kaohsiung Medical University, Kaohsiung 80708, Taiwan
Department of Business Management, National Sun Yat-sen University, Kaohsiung 80424, Taiwan
Department of Medical Research, Kaohsiung Medical University Hospital, Kaohsiung 80756, Taiwan
Department of Medical Research, China Medical University Hospital, China Medical University, Taichung 40447, Taiwan

Index

A

Adverse Events, 13-14, 17, 20-21, 23-24, 28, 30, 140, 144-145, 201-202, 206-207

Analgesia, 13-14, 19-20, 190-191

Analgesic Response, 13, 15-16

Anastomotic Leakage, 61, 69

Antibiotic Resistance, 23, 32, 208

Antibiotics, 15, 23-24, 27, 30-31, 125, 140, 202-203, 206-207, 211, 213, 216-219

Antimicrobial Agents, 24, 140, 202, 207-208

Atherosclerosis, 99, 109, 119-120

Average Pain Intensity, 14, 16, 20

B

Bacterial Infection, 23, 31, 201-203, 207-208

Bioimpedance Analysis, 148-150, 152-156, 159

Bloodstream, 68, 121, 125, 130, 132-133

Body Mass Index, 78, 83, 86-87, 89-91, 108, 110, 114-116, 148, 150, 152-156, 173, 194

C

Cancer Pain, 13-14, 20-21

Cardiometabolic Diseases, 107-110, 113, 117-119

Cardiovascular Disease, 78, 85-86, 99-100, 107-108, 117, 119-120, 231

Catheter, 121-125, 127-138, 211-213, 215-217, 219, 229

Ceftaroline, 23-25, 27-33, 145

Ceftriaxone, 23-25, 27-33

Chemotherapy, 61, 71

Chronic Diseases, 47, 76-86, 100, 104, 158, 212, 218

Chronic Kidney Disease, 85-86, 107-116, 119-120

Chronic Respiratory Failure, 34-35, 55

Clinical Efficacy, 23-24, 27, 30-32, 139-141, 143-145, 191, 201, 203, 207-208, 210

Clinical Research, 3-4, 13, 34, 55, 88, 90, 158

Cognitive Impairment, 3, 97, 213, 224-225

Colonoscopy, 60-61, 68, 71

Colorectal Cancer, 58-59, 61, 65-75, 160

Comorbidities, 14, 31, 88, 91-93, 108, 119, 195-196

Computed Tomography, 60, 148-150, 152-156, 160, 193

D

Dementia, 3, 218-221

Dental Panoramic Radiographs, 162-163, 173-174

Diabetes, 8, 51, 76, 78, 91-94, 98-100, 103-117, 119-120, 150, 152-154, 156-158, 160, 223, 225-226, 228-229

Diabetic Foot Ulcer, 99-104

Dose Escalation, 13, 15-16, 19

Dyslipidemia, 78, 107-119, 195

E

Enterobacteriaceae, 23, 140, 145, 147, 210

Epidemiology, 10, 12-13, 35, 85, 99-100, 104-105, 107, 121, 135, 158, 160, 173

Eravacycline, 139-147

Escherichia Coli, 28, 140

F

Functional Impairment, 2, 88

H

Healthcare Professionals, 3, 53

Hemodialysis, 104, 106, 121-124, 133-138, 231

Heparin, 121-124, 134-138

Home Mechanical Ventilation, 34-35, 55-57

Home Respiratory Therapy, 34-35

Hyperalgesia, 14, 19-21

Hypercholesterolemia, 76, 78-83

Hypertension, 76, 78, 90-94, 98, 107-120, 150, 152-154, 156-158, 195, 223, 225-226, 228-229

Hyperuricemia, 107-108, 112, 117-119

Hypouricemia, 107, 109-110, 112-113, 116-117, 120

Hypouricemic Subjects, 107, 109-111, 113, 117-118

I

Inpatient Treatment, 2, 12

Intensive Care Unit, 24, 71, 107

Intra-abdominal Infection, 139, 146, 201, 205, 210

L

Laparoscopic Resection, 59, 62-63, 71-73

Laparoscopic Surgery, 58-59, 68, 71, 73-74

Long-term Oxygen Therapy, 34, 56-57

Lymph Nodes, 58, 61, 63, 65, 67, 70, 73

M

Magnetic Resonance Imaging, 60, 149

Medication, 2-4, 6, 8-11, 51, 87-91, 94, 96, 109, 111, 117-118, 212, 220-221, 229

Morbidity, 23, 35, 66, 76-78, 80, 82, 122, 223, 232

Morphine, 13-14, 20-21

Mortality, 23-24, 28, 31, 35, 58, 66, 68, 70, 76, 85-88, 96, 100, 119-123, 125, 129-130, 132-135, 139, 144-145, 148, 158-160, 162, 172, 207, 210, 218, 221-222, 229, 231-232

N
Neurologists, 1-2, 6, 9, 223
Neuromuscular Diseases, 34, 37, 42

O
Obesity, 37-38, 40, 42, 45, 59, 72, 76, 78-83, 85-86, 90, 98, 119-120, 159-161
Obstructive Sleep Apnea, 34, 42-43, 57
Oncologic Outcome, 59, 67-68
Open Surgery, 58-59, 71-74
Opioids, 13-14, 19-22, 211, 217-218
Osteoarthritis, 90, 94, 185, 191
Osteoporosis, 162-164, 167-174, 195
Outpatient Clinics, 6-9

P
Palliative Care, 1, 3-4, 9, 12-14, 21, 211-212, 218-221
Parkinson's Disease, 1-3, 10-12, 176, 189
Pathogens, 23-24, 27-29, 31-33, 137, 140, 145, 147, 201, 208
Peripheral Arterial Disease, 99-101, 105
Pneumonia, 23-25, 27-33, 58, 61, 63, 65, 71, 201, 203, 205-210, 221

Polymedication, 88-91, 94, 97
Pseudomonas Aeruginosa, 23, 201, 209-210

R
Randomized Controlled Trials, 23-24, 72, 135-136, 139, 175, 201-202
Renal Disease, 121, 136

S
Sarcopenia, 148, 150-151, 154-161
Serum Uric Acid, 107, 110, 114-116, 119-120
Skeletal Muscle, 148, 150-156, 158-161
Surgical Complication, 59, 67

U
Urate, 107-118, 120

W
Wound Infection, 58, 61, 63, 65, 71

X
X-ray Absorptiometry, 149, 159-161, 163